Hypnosis in Sex Therapy

A Guide for Clinical Hypnotherapists and Medical Hypnotists

Hypnosis in Sex Therapy

A Guide for Clinical Hypnotherapists and Medical Hypnotists

Tracie O'Keefe

About Dr Tracie O'Keefe, DCH, BHSc, ND

Tracie is a sex researcher, teacher and therapist, clinical psychotherapist, clinical hypnotherapist, counsellor, clinical supervisor, naturopath, medical nutritionist, medical herbalist, and Director of the Australian Health and Education Centre (AHEC) in Sydney, Australia.

Tracie has worked in the sex, gender and sexuality community since being at college in 1970. She has been in private practice since 1994 at the London Medical Centre in the UK before becoming the full-time director of AHEC in 2001. In clinical practice she has seen thousands of patients dealing with sexual health issues.

Tracie holds a degree in complementary medicine, a degree in clinical hypnotherapy, a post-graduate advanced diploma in psychotherapy and hypnosis, and a doctorate in clinical hypnotherapy (DCH). She is a registered mental health professional and member of the College of Psychotherapy of the Psychotherapy and Counselling Federation of Australia (PACFA), a member of the Australian Hypnotherapists Association (AHA), Australian Society of Clinical Hypnotherapists (ASCH) and a member of the Australian Naturopathic Practitioners Association (ANPA).

She has presented her work at many conferences and universities across the globe and continues to teach and pass on her skills, whilst continuing in clinical practice.

Dedication

I dedicate this book to all those people I have worked
with for you to have a higher level of sexual
and loving pleasure.

I honour you and your journey,
and I am humbled by your trust.

Disclaimer:
This book is designed to provide general information only for health professionals who treat or plan to treat clients with sexual health issues. This information is provided and sold with the knowledge that the publisher and author do not offer any medical, legal, financial or other professional advice. In the case of a need for any such expertise, consult with the appropriate professional. This book does not contain all information available on the subject.

This book has not been created to be specific to any individuals' or organisations' situation or needs. Every effort has been made to make this book as accurate as possible. However, there may be typographical and/or content errors. Therefore, this book should serve only as a general guide and not as the ultimate source of subject information.

The examples stated in the book are not intended to represent or guarantee that anyone will achieve the same or similar results. Each individual's success depends on their background, dedication, desire and motivation.

Any and all information contained in this book or any related materials are not intended to take the place of medical advice from a healthcare professional. Any action taken based on the contents found in this book or related materials is to be used at the sole discretion and sole liability of the reader.

Under no circumstances, including, but not limited to, negligence, shall the author or O'Keefe & Fox Industries Pty Ltd be liable for any special or consequential damages that result from the use of, or the inability to use, the book and related materials in this book, even if O'Keefe & Fox Industries Pty Ltd or an O'Keefe & Fox Industries Pty Ltd authorised representative has been advised of the possibility of such damages.

This book contains information that might be dated and is intended only to educate and entertain. The author and publisher shall have no liability or responsibility to any person or entity regarding any loss or damage incurred, or alleged to have incurred, directly or indirectly, by the information contained in this book.

FIRST EDITION, 2025

Published by Australian Health & Education Centre, an imprint of O'Keefe & Fox Industries Pty Ltd, Suite 2, Level 5: Wellshare, 428 George St, The Dymocks Building Sydney, NSW 2000, Australia

Website: www.tracieokeefe.com
International wholesale enquiries through Ingram.

Copyediting: Katrina Fox
Cover design: Aleksandar Novovic
Text layout: Marites Bautista
Cover image: Adobe Stock

ISBN: 978-0-9875109-7-6

"Sex and love are of the highest forms of connection that each human being is entitled to in their own way in harmony with the world. The are the honey of the bee, cooling of the breeze, warmth of the sun and passions of a life well lived."

— Tracie O'Keefe

Table of Contents

Acknowledgements

I want to acknowledge the Gadigal people of the Eora Nation whose land I rest upon while carrying out this research and project. I respect your elders past, present and emerging.

Thank you once again to my beautiful wife Katrina Fox for guidance on the editing. You never fail to be objective, smart and kind.

To my assistant Rosalie Vinluan who continually backs me up in my practice on a daily basis.

To the hosts of all the sex parties I attended, the sex workers who shared their knowledge, and the academics and researchers who educated me with their knowledge and research.

To my lovely hypnosis and psychotherapy colleagues who trained me and provided endless hours of clinical supervision during my career. There are so many of you, you know who you are, and I treasured every moment under your tutelage.

The librarians who I sort of borrowed books on sex from as a teenager. Just to let you know, I did return them all, although you never noticed they were gone. I am sorry but nowhere else had that material in those days and I did put the knowledge to good use so perhaps you might pardon my audacity.

Most of all, those brave clients who trusted me with their innermost, delicate, sexual issues and were willing to be guided and helped by me. You are my heroes who dared to travel a journey to a better sex life. I learnt the most about sex and therapy from every one of you.

Introduction

According to research, more than half the human race experiences sexual dysfunction at some point in their lives. However, very few seek help or even know where to access appropriate healthcare professionals.

Currently psychosexual therapy with hypnosis is beginning to get academic traction and clinical recognition. Research is amassing in modern-day medicine and therapy literature. But the danger is that as clinicians we begin to treat sex solely as a science and need to remember that sex is as much an art as well, and everyone is the artist of their own experience.

Sex therapy was offered as far back as in ancient Sumerian brothels more than 2,500 years ago, and due to human nature, probably a long time before. It's reasonable to assume that hypnotic techniques were also used. We have evidence that hypnosis was used as far back as ancient Egyptian healing temples.

From a clinical perspective my work as a sexologist, researcher, educator and therapist is grounded and informed by science and research, both quantitative and qualitative. Then it is profoundly influenced by biological, psychological and sociological considerations, plus my own sexual history. That formulates a broader picture of how I help my clients, guided by clinical experience.

People with psychosexual dysfunction are constrained by the traumas and barriers that have been built up inside their minds, by themselves, others and experience. This also alters their physiology, sexual experiences and the sexual response cycle.

Sex is such a wonderful, life-enriching experience and, with the right guidance, it becomes satisfying and memorable. But many people never get that guidance, so they drown in a sea of sexual dysfunction.

Hypnosis is one of the strongest and fastest sciences and arts used to rearrange the personal psyche, thinking, values, beliefs, behaviours, knowledge, experiences, and constraints, and can rapidly promote psychosexual health. It's not the only way but I have found it can accelerate the process exponentially, above standard psychosexual therapy.

So, for me as a psychosexual therapist talking about and helping clients with sex and hypnosis every week at work, it is just a perfectly normal day at the office. And it is also a special day because everyone who is helped is another happy, sexual human being.

I help people with their sexual issues with hypnotherapy every week in my clinic. Fifty-five years later, after I started a sexuality self-help group at college in 1970, I'm still talking with people about sex. All kinds of sexual issues that people have never spoken to anyone else about before. Issues they would sometimes never disclose to their partners, friend or doctor.

As therapists we are often their last hope for resolution, restoration of sexual function and a good sex life. I believe it's important that we learn as many hypnotic and sex skills and techniques as we can to help the client in their sex lives.

The use of hypnotherapy and psychosexual therapy I find not only makes the process of therapy go much faster but also can give a more permanent change. For those of us who work in hypnosis we already know how quick behavioural and experiential transformations can happen and you can learn to apply that to sex therapy.

This work is not for all therapists as it requires you to find a way to be comfortable working daily with sexual issues. This is so you are not only comfortable with sex, but the client's unconscious and conscious mind knows that you glory in its wholesomeness and beauty.

I remember sneaking into the reference library on my hands and knees as a teenager, where books on sex were kept, to take out medical texts on sex. You were supposed to be 18 or in some libraries at least 21 in those days, but of course I wasn't. I smuggled them back when I had read them, just in case their absence would sound an alarm.

It was a long time before the internet. Women's liberation, gay, sex and gender diverse rights, and social attitudes were very different. To speak openly about sex could have been considered poor taste, foul-mouthed or you were avant-garde and risqué.

Being born with a form of intersex and needing surgery, I didn't have intercourse until I was 22, but by that time I had amassed a considerable amount of knowledge on the subject.

Between the ages of 22 and 37 I embarked upon a quest to have sex for England, although I did not restrict myself to one culture or country. It was every kind of sex with endless amounts of lovers. Being naturally omnisexual I imposed no restrictions on age, sex, class, colour, ability or sexual persuasion on who those lovers were, just as long as they were adults.

In my clinic over the years I have been able to help thousands of clients have much better sex lives. Each generation reinvents their concepts of what good sex is but running through that can be thousands of years of knowledge and techniques that can help everyone.

This book shows some practices of hypnosis in sex therapy I have used in my clinics over the decades with clients who sought help. Here I also give a background in sex therapy that you will need to know and 40 case studies using hypnotic and psychosexual techniques.

It is a window into my clinical practice of sex therapy and hypnosis so that those of you who are hypnosis practitioners can work in sex therapy, affording you more guidance and insights to help your clients.

The work can afford you multiple learnings in a systemic, progressive way and help you build your professional confidence in the field of hypnosis with psychosexual matters.

Immerse yourself and enjoy the journey.

HOW TO USE THIS BOOK

This book is different from my previous works because I am showing you more aspects of what I do in my clinic. The methodology is different because I must change my methods according to how the client presents and the field in which I am working.

There are no rote methods here to cure all. Everyone who presents in sex therapy needs help specially designed for them, as an individual. I may treat several people presenting with the same complaint several different ways.

There are common themes and techniques, however, that you as a hypnotherapist can put together to aid your clients, but you can never treat all clients the same. Neither sex therapy nor hypnotherapy successfully works that way.

These techniques are both simple and highly technical. We make it simple for the client but behind that we need to work in a targeted, technically-informed way, because that is the expertise we are being paid for.

Each chapter is self-contained around one aspect of sex therapy or a particular sexual problem we are treating. Some themes are visited many times as you learn to build your skills and gain your clinical knowledge.

Since the book is for beginners, students and seasoned professionals, the breadth of information is vast and amassed over half a century. Don't cherry pick what you read because in treating sexual health issues with hypnosis you need to understand biology, psychology, sociology and hypnotherapy theory and practice.

This is the global lenses through which I help people and through which you need to look to see the whole patient/ client. I am a deeply technical clinician and what may seem sexual magic to the client is achieved by hundreds of clinical observations and hypnotic interventions.

As I say, the client is more than their individual parts.

TECHNICAL BACKGROUND MATERIAL

You arrive at this text with many different levels of skills and training in your career which is always a continual learning process. The first five chapters teach you the background you need to know to be effective in using hypnotherapy with sexual issues.

You may already have that background or you may not, but I encourage you to focus on that material to begin or advance your studies. I operate from a psychosocial, biological perspective because I was trained in both the hard and soft sciences.

I am science-informed, not evidence-based, because every client is different, and I need to negotiate and explore the paradigms of individual treatments for that person. Sex therapy is as much an art as it is a science, just as hypnotherapy and psychotherapy are.

My aim in publishing this work is not to put you into rigid boxes as a therapist but to encourage you to expand your present skills so you are brave and prepared to grow. We not only learn hypnotherapeutic techniques, but they also teach us every day how to be better therapists.

Chapters: Throughout the chapters I report 40 cases from my clinics. Different techniques are shown with each case to teach you a wider repertoire of tools you might use to help your clients.

Some of these techniques might be used universally throughout sex therapy and hypnosis, or with clients experiencing difficulties other than reported here.

In parenthesis: In hypnotic scripts work you will find brackets (parentheses) which will contain notes on hypnotic and therapeutic techniques that I am using with that particular client.

Trance intentions: Here I show you the hypnotic and therapeutic intentions I formulated before I induced the official trance state or artificial somnambulism and whilst working within instant artificial somnambulism.

Appendix A: This is a collection of hypnotic and sex therapy techniques you might try with your clients who have similar problems to the cases that are referred to in the text.

In the main text I do not show you all these steps, only the ones I want you to learn most about in that case. You will find numbered references to items in appendix A within the text, relevant to those techniques.

Glossary: This is a simple glossary of hypnotic, sex therapy and psychotherapeutic phrases and their meanings that you might find useful in reading this work.

References List: Here are the references referred to in the text by chapter order. They consist of research found in a wide selection of databases and publications. Some are more recent, and some are classics and have stood the test of time.

Resources: This is a list of downloadable resources you can use in your clinic.

As a health professional, over time you will also need to seek up-to-date references and resources to flesh out your skills as knowledge and times change.

IMPORTANT NOTE ABOUT GRAMMAR AND PUNCTUATION:

The trance scripts I have included in this book do not follow typical rules of punctuation or grammar as unconscious communications are not literal and do not follow conscious grammar rules. Some communications run on with no full stops or commas. This is not a mistake but a deliberate device to convey hypnotic 'speech' as opposed to regular, everyday English speech.

You will find that some phrases are highlighted in bold which indicates emphatic tonal delivery. In other words, marked suggestions.

However, suggestions are also hidden in the non-bold markings as indirect suggestions to bypass conscious resistance, even though they may be direct suggestions.

METER AND DELIVERY TIMING

You will find '…' in the scripts and communications. This indicates timing breaks of around three seconds before the next delivery. The unconscious mind, like the conscious, needs time to process information to make cognitive and experiential changes. Co-ordinate these pauses with the client's breathing so suggestions are delivered on the out breath. This can be waived during bombardment delivery to cause confusion.

Treat this work like a meal with many courses: take your time, enjoy the journey and be prepared to try new dishes with an open mind and a sense of adventure. The journey is not just about changing your client's hypnotic experiences but yours as well.

1 The Sociology of Sex

Sex is a complex experience that involves physiology, mental state, emotional capacity, identity and social programming. There is no separation of these interwoven elements.

When it goes well, sex can be rewarding, beautiful, ecstatic and even a divine human experience. Its allure is so powerful that people will cross the globe and battle every human difficulty, just for one more night of passion.

If it goes wrong, it can be devastating, demoralising, humiliating, embarrassing and depressing. That can make the people involved deeply unhappy, resentful, angry, and even send them to the brink of self-destruction and wanting to end their lives.

We now know that the French 17th century philosopher Descartes (Mehta, 2011) was wrong and there is no real separation between mind and body. To take the Cartesian dualism stance trying to treat one without considering the other is pure fantasy not based on science.

Whilst Mesmer, Braid, Charcot, Bernheim, Erickson and many more left us vivid illustrations of miraculous hypnotic cures, they need to be viewed within the context of their time and social conditions (Gauld, 1992). Our advancements of knowledge of bio-functional medicine and identity formation must update our hypnotic approaches to treating the sexual issues our patients present with today.

Masters and Johnson (1966) described four basic phases of the sexual response:

1. Excitement (arousal) whether that be initially an innate physiological stimulus that gives rise to conscious interest or vice versa.
2. Plateau is the extended period of sexual activity.
3. Orgasm is the release of tension, ejaculation and climax.
4. Resolution is post-sex relaxation and feeling of satisfaction.

Whilst this model was originally based on the biological sexual response cycle, it can be broadened to encompass multiple influences that we will discuss later in this book.

The biological feedback loops within the body help form and determine the shape of the mind and experience. Psychological experience can also alter the physiological feedback loops, which must be considered when formulating hypnotic approaches for treating sexual problems and quality of sexual experience.

Sex is also cultural. It changes when we cross geography, culture, language, religion, beliefs, values, local laws, social conduct rules, upbringing, sexuality, family doctrine and personal historical experience.

Humans continually group together in cultures and sub-cultures, whether they be based on families, education, wealth, political belief, socio-economic status, counties, countries, continents, age groups, interests, religion or skin colour. All of these affect our perceptions of sex.

Also, those groups develop their own guidelines, beliefs, rules and restrictions, all influenced by the power brokers within those groups. Doctrine can become normalised very quickly and create positive and negative hallucinations within the individuals in those groups.

We don't just have sex but have sex according to what we believe it is or is not. That also changes throughout our life according to how we adjust our beliefs.

The internet has not been a universal educational leveller as many people may have restricted access, so finding information on sex, gender and sexuality can be limited.

To teach sexuality and sex experience as purely biological and psychological negates a large part of a person's social experience.

Those mistakes have been made before when women going through menopause were classified as hysterical. They were advised to have a myriad of strange treatments and their wombs and ovaries removed (Tasca, 2012). It was a misdiagnosis of a natural menopause, largely by male doctors.

Medicine tried to describe all intersex people as having a disorder of sex development (Lunberg, 2017). Gay, lesbian and bisexual people were listed in the Diagnostic and Statical Manual of Mental Disorders (DSM) as a having a mental disorder (Drescher, 2015). Trans and gender diverse people were also automatically listed as being mentally disturbed (Russo, 2017).

The very idea that people are exclusively heterosexual, gay, lesbian, or bisexual is a major fallacy, social construct and class system, similar to wealth and education.

Sexuality is as much learned as it is an innate instinct. We can see this from single-sex prison populations when sex between inmates becomes a convenience and choice (known colloquially as 'gay for the stay'). Government studies on these populations are generally biased in covering up such sexual activity because they choose to not understand how to research those populations (Lawton, 2022).

We can see how teenage girls in single-sex schools have crushes on other girls or female teachers, and experiment sexually with other students (Bumiller, 1997). Adolescent hormones are raging and when females are the major population, the biological need to form attachments can take over.

The same is seen in the history of boys' schools when boys have had exclusive sexual contact with other boys (Alvarez, 2005). Acknowledgment of those activities is generally buried by the schools to preserve their stilted public image.

Puberty-induced sexuality is suppressed in most cultures with legal ages for sex running from 12 in Angola to 21 in Bahrain. Most countries have battles between religious bodies to eliminate sex education and social reformers to promote it in schools.

It is clear from research that comprehensive early-age sex education reduces teenage pregnancies, sexually transmitted diseases, poverty, over-population, homophobia, intersexphobia and transphobia.

The United Nations Education, Science and Cultural Organization (2023) promotes the benefits of early-age comprehensive sex education but in reality, many religious schools continue to refuse to make it part of their curriculum.

Extreme right-wing religious groups still fight the provision of sex education in schools (Johnson, 2024). They labour under the delusion that not giving youngsters the full facts about sex keeps them safe from harm or from having sex. There is also the factor that scientific-based sex education challenges their Adam and Eve, or faith equivalent, model of the world.

These extreme right-wing groups also view people who are hypersexual or lifelong virgins as being maladjusted and in need of psychiatric help. Some people, however, are more sexually active and others may choose to be asexual.

When the Christian world engaged in colonisation, local sexual practices and knowledge were changed and destroyed. Natural regional practices of polygamy were outlawed in Africa and other countries (Becker, 2022).

India's knowledge of sexual, erotic practices – thousands of years' old – including male on male or female on female partnerships were made illegal. The British constrained everyday sexual interest to a purely heteronormative model. It has taken 70 years so far to disengage the sexual persecution laws that the British left behind.

Not only did the British change the legal system after invasion but the effects of occupation also profoundly changed social attitudes. When Indian independence happened in 1947 after 90 years of occupation, the British Raj were booted out, but thousands of years of sexual beliefs had been largely devasted.

For instance, in the Hindu religion sex can be considered a very spiritual experience where male and female are considered one before birth; then at birth the two are split, and sex is considered the spiritual reunification of the whole.

There is the Hindu god of erotic love, desire and pleasure, known as Kamadeva or Manmatha who is seen beside Rati, his female counterpart and consort. Rati is the goddess of love, carnal desire, lust, passion, and sexual pleasure whose name comes from the root meaning of sensual joy and desire.

We can compare this to Christianity where Mary, the Holy Mother of Jesus, Son of God, was desexualised into a virgin. The sexual power of the previous ancient Greek Aphrodite and Roman goddess Venus were stripped as men took over the religion in the second century AD. For 2000 years women were treated as chattels, possessions, and at times bought and sold for domestic convenience and male sexual pleasure, which disempowered them sexually (de Beauvoir, 2011).

Sex is used by religion as another social control mechanism. The Vatican makes decrees on what is acceptable sex and what is not. There is also an Islamic-produced guide to what sex is acceptable for Muslims. Wherever there is religion, there is doctrine about the must, should and ought-to around sexual practices. In linguistics we call these modal operators of necessity. In hypnotics they are governors, suggestions and direct commands to promote and contain behaviours.

The law also shapes people's sexual behaviours. Legal prohibitions on sex outside marriage, abortion, contraception, gay sex, the sex industry and gender identity can carry penalties such as losing your job, imprisonment, torture, commitment to a mental facility, and in some places, the death penalty.

At the very least, restricted non-normative sexual practices can lead to shaming, guilt, and excommunication where someone may lose connection with their family and social background.

On the other hand, the exultation of certain kinds of sex, usually heteronormative, can elevate and promote sexual experience and pleasure. In social psychology we call this 'normalising behaviours' and in social politics 'majority rule'.

Intra-cultural sex practices and guidelines are profoundly interconnected with other cultural practices. So the perceived threat to one practice can spark social paranoia about destablisation of the entire culture.

This can currently be seen in the US and Russia with Donald Trump and Vladimir Putin promoting social rejection of abortion, contraception and sex, gender and sexuality diverse equality (Haberman, 2022; Sperling, 2014)

In Arabia women are, for the most part, still treated as possessions, not individual citizens with their own full human rights (Sasson, 2010). They must cover themselves up in public, assume total modesty for fear they will tempt men sexually. In some places, if they engage in extra-martial affairs, they can be stoned to death.

The United Nations estimates there are around 5000 known honour killings of women and girls per year (Encyclopædia Britannica, n.d.). They are usually linked to religion, but they can also be committed in patriarchal societies, simply because a male believes a woman or girl has brought dishonour on the family. It can happen in different societies as well as places such as Saudi Arabia, Pakistan, and other countries ruled by religious fundamentalists. The assailant can be found not guilty in court in some countries and that the killing was justified.

In the UK Moore (2023) reported in The Guardian that less than 1% of reported rapes actually achieve convictions. The ordeal of going through a legal case and cross-examination in court is so traumatising for women that many drop the case.

In the US the Bureau of Justice Statistics (Sinozich & Langton, 2014) estimate that only 20% of students and 32% of non-students report sexual assault. In many countries women reporting rape or sexual assault can be framed as the criminal because it is assumed they tempted the man.

In some countries the law allows the rapist to marry their victim to avoid prosecution as a husband cannot legally rape his wife. This is to avoid the shame those women are assumed to bring or have brought on the family.

Modern masculinity has also come into crisis for many men as populations move more into cities due to industrialisation and the technological revolution (Williams, 2022). Feminism can be seen, particularly by the right wing, as a threat to the masculine, and thereby male sexual identity.

With the rise of the single-parent family, divorce, and separation from extended families, many males lack prominent male role models in their formative years.

In China the government announced a plan to teach traditional, prescriptive Chinese ideas of masculinity to boys at schools (Wang, 2021). Feminists commented that was out of line with a modern society as it had previously included violence and devaluing females.

In the West the rise of the right-wing reassertion of hegemonic masculinity can be seen through the misogynistic behaviour of figures such as Donald Trump and Jair Bolsonaro (Gordon, 2022).

We can see a parallel in Russia with Putin in public riding horseback, bare-chested for the press, flaunting his public masculine power image (Propper, 2022). Whilst world leaders made fun of him for blatantly promoting those images, they were themselves buying into stereotyping of male statesmen as only blue-collar workers.

Men can become confused around what masculinity is or is not, which constantly affects their self-confidence, sense of self-efficacy, and sexual performance.

In this book we will only touch lightly on sex and gender diversity, as it is a vast subject in and of itself and I cover it in my other works. Whilst at times it may cross over with sexuality, it needs special study and consideration that is beyond this book.

The common myth that sex and gender diversity is exclusively rooted in sexuality is an illusion and propagated by the right-wing media seeking to create panic and clickbait. Sensational stories of sex and gender diversity are often not an explosive sociological phenomenon, but marketing tricks to sell advertising to fearful and uneducated people.

Denying the need to supply younger people with real sexual facts is prejudice and based on paranoia around sexuality, not on the protection of the young. Younger people are sexual and engage in sex as we have around 12 million births from teenage pregnancies annually (World Health Organization, 2024).

As therapists we see the effects on people of confusion around sex, rooted in ignorance in their teenage years. It creates a lack of personal confidence and confusion that can later lead to lifelong sexual dysfunction.

We cannot consider identity politics without taking in age discrimination which pervades throughout our social structures. Again, this affects a person's sexual self-identification, engagement, and performance.

Older people can be desexualised in the public eye (Simpson, 2021). In a culture that prizes youth above experience or wisdom, to be called older often becomes a diminutive insult.

Although fecundity, fertility, stamina and libido can decline in older years, particularly over 50, many people continue to have a sexual life. Yet the media constantly engages in harming and mocking older people and describing them as having lost their looks or attractiveness.

This damages older people's self-perceptions and self-esteem and lowers their libido and sexual performance for fear of being seen as perverts for engaging in sex (Schaller, 2023).

Sex trafficking is a major world problem with millions of adults and minors falling victim every year, recorded in over 115 countries (Allan et al., 2023). It is hard to police because victims are afraid to come forward because of fear of retribution by their abusers.

Authorities are basically powerless to reduce the flow of victims who can be kept under lock and key for years, serving customers who often require unusual sexual services, including violence. Victims are usually naive, kidnapped, and include young children.

Incest is one of the biggest problems facing many sexual abuse victims presenting in therapy. In very rare cases incest can be consensual among adults but is generally rape or molestation through a cohesive, abusive, controlling, oppressive behaviour by the perpetrator (Courtois, 2010).

The abuse is two-fold because it involves sexual exploitation but also perceived betrayal from and of the family if the survivor speaks out. So the victim can find themselves empowered by speaking out, but disempowered by disclosing the secret that fractured the family. Families frequently try to hide the incest and can sacrifice the victim for the sake of family unity.

In considering sexual abuse we must also remember that this happens to male babies, boys, teenagers and adults as well as females (Douglas, 2018). It damages their integral sense of self and sexual performance.

We must also consider that women are sexual abusers of children, teenagers and adults as well (Elliot, 1994; Cortoni, 2017). Not only are they primary abusers but also can be involved in initiating male rape of victims. Women in families can hide and ignore sexual abuse of children in order to avoid having sex with their spouses.

So, sex is viewed differently everywhere by everyone all the time, and cookie-cutter therapy, hypnosis and hypnotherapy are not generally successful.

THE ART OF SEX AND SEX THERAPY

When we serve a client, we must all leave our own negative sexual perceptions behind. First and foremost, we need to be highly attuned observationalists and empirical data collectors, as we must tailor each therapy to the individual client's needs.

The majority of people looking for hypnotherapy for sexual health issues and problems will bring a host of negative gestalts with them. Those will be stacked up from biological to psychological, educational, sociological, environmental, and experiential.

That stacking is constantly changing and affected by exposure to new experiences, influences and their intra-personal dynamics and interpersonal interactions with the people around them.

Sex can be a positive, rewarding experience that depends on learning the art of sexual practices. Those learnings require education, practice, acceptance, and positive re-enforcement.

The evidence lies in sexual function and satisfaction. Happy people living low-stress lives, who have had a sex education, and have positive attitudes to sex, tend to have more satisfying sex lives and relationships (Wylie, 2010).

They are more engaged and present during lovemaking and intimate interpersonal relationships. This is regardless of whether those relationships are autonomous, male on female, female on female, male on male, bisexual or omnisexual.

The level of sexual satisfaction is also not exclusively dependent on whether those relationships are long term, a brief affair or a one-night stand.

Using hypnosis to help someone overcome sexual difficulty or elevate their sexual experience requires the clinician to train in sex therapy using hypnosis. Being a hypnotherapist with a limited knowledge of sex will lead to continual failures. You can only teach someone to drive a car if you yourself know how to drive a car.

It also requires us as therapists, to love sex and be excited about healthy, wholesome sexual practices. The client's unconscious and conscious perceptions of our attitudes towards sex will be continuous, from the moment they speak to us on the telephone, until the end of therapy.

General school education frequently has little to do with teaching life skills. It is designed to fit humans into the industrial complex, regardless of what political philosophy is in that country. In treating patients, we the professionals need to become highly knowledgeable on sexual practices.

As we have seen, families and religion also suppress that acquired knowledge, skills and exploration of sex in the younger and older generations.

If you are working with hypnosis and sex therapy, I find it always goes better when you take the attitude of sharing your knowledge, rather than taking a commanding, top-down approach.

No one is born with evolved lovemaking skills. We are born with biological sexual impulses that are initiated in the womb and start to be moulded before we can walk and talk.

Then at puberty when sex development hormones are boosted, sex drive is profoundly magnified. It is incredibly important at this developmental time for the teenager to know what is happening to them and how to channel that sex drive in safe and satisfying ways.

You may have experienced lack of knowledge around sex when younger. It is possible you may have had some sexual difficulties yourself. Try to imagine the highest level of empathy around sexuality, that you can develop now, to help your client.

The sex drive begins to dwindle after menopause and andropause. The libido becomes weaker but the desire to have sex may still be as strong. It is important for the therapist to be able to guide the client on how to maximise sexual experiences in older years.

Sexual impulse must never be confused with sexual skills, for one is innate and one acquired. High impulse does not override the need for sex education or the art of lovemaking, whether that is acquired knowledge or experiential.

My mother saw sex as a chore, something she had to do in a relationship and not something she wanted to do. She was brought up in a Victorian household where the word 'sex' was never mentioned or talked about. To mention it would have been considered completely inappropriate, vulgar and rude. So, she never got any early positive messages around sex and understood very little about lovemaking her entire life.

I was a teenager of the 1960s when sex became more talked about in society. However, I simply could not understand why sex education at school, when I was 14, only talked about what bunny rabbits did. Given that, in poverty, I had lived in a brothel and worked as the maid for a short time when I was 12, I found the whole educational curriculum bizarre.

For me sex became a self-motivated project at an early age. I read as extensively as I could on the subject. I talked freely and naturally about it, just as I would talk about the weather or any ordinary subject. I developed a positive attitude towards sex, so when I lost my virginity at 22, it was a wonderful experience.

As a person I know no shame or guilt around wholesome, consensual sex between adults. Therefore, that is the positive attitude towards sex that I take into the consulting room, plus my sex education and clinical skills, so clients pick up on that consciously and unconsciously.

I can honestly say that sex has been one of the great joys of my life. This is my private and public discourse around sex, so it creates the confidence in the clients that they are in safe, knowledgeable and non-judgemental care.

This puts people at ease, so they are free and safe to discuss sex and ask for help in a fully supported and respected way. I tell them they can tell me anything to enable me to help them. This lowers defence mechanisms and often I am the first person with whom they have discussed these issues.

Historically many cultures have had this positive, wholesome and educational attitude towards the art of sex and lovemaking.

We can see on the carvings of the 13th century Sun Temple of Konark, India, depictions of erotic images for the public to imitate and enhance their sex lives (Watts & Elisofon, 1971). There is even more explicit, graphic sex education on the walls of the temple that can be found in Madhya Pradesh in the town of Khajuraho that include men and women (Béguin, 2017).

The Ananga Ranga (stage of the the bodiless one) was written by Kalyanamalla or Kalyan Malla, the fifteenth or sixteenth century Indian poet. It is a Sanskrit manuscript of the art of love and sex and a marriage manual (Malla, 1885/2023).

Its philosophy is based on the many ways a man can satisfy his wife to solidify the relationship to keep the couple together. Its contents discuss allure, foreplay, types of men and women, arousal, creating an erotic atmosphere and sexual techniques, some of which were taken from the Karma Sutra.

It is important for Westerners to understand that such works and manuals are of pleasure, not base, mindless sex. Pleasure in lovemaking in India has been seen as a way to have a stable marriage, family, life and society.

There are cave paintings by Australian Aboriginal people in Arnhem Land in the country's north from around 28,000 years ago that depict genitals and pornography (Conway, 2012). What is fascinating is when I tried to view these images, Google had blocked and banned them.

Erotic Paleolithic cave paintings from 37,000 years ago can be found in Cussac, in the valley of the Dordogne, France (Lichfield, 2001).

What this depicts is that over time sex, art, education, the art of sex and sharing of sexual activity has been a perfectly natural human experience. Of course, this is only the art that has survived so it would be safe to assume that such recordings of sexual experience will go back to the beginning of human communication.

We can also see learned sexual social behaviour in chimpanzees who live in family groups. Dominant males have sexual privileges above all other males. Younger, non-dominant males learn to divert their sexual behaviours by having sex with outliers from the group to keep them safe from attack as much as possible from the alpha males (Boehm, 2021).

We, like chimpanzees, are primates and share 96% of our DNA so we have many of the same biological urges, including sex drives, even though we may have different social orders (Suntsova, 2020).

What this shows us is the human sex drive is highly controlled and even at times excused by social and cultural norms. For us as therapists we have to educate ourselves around those cultural and legal nuances that affect our clients' sexual experiences. Unless we do that, we are going into a session unaware of many of the variables that may be causing the client's sexual dysfunction.

It is clear that the art of sex in a society is as much a learned behaviour as it is a natural biological drive. Social norms and examples within human societies shape our experience of sex from our earliest biological, cognitive, emotional, educational and experiential experiences.

SEXUAL IMPULSE AMPLIFICATION AND SUPPRESSION

As with all human experience, suppression or elevation of sexual expression affects engagement, performance, and pleasure. Repetitive exposure to a wide range of stimuli at an early age and during adulthood imprints our cognitive gestalts that affect our everyday sex lives and fractionates them.

Those stimuli create and recreate the sexual trances we are living at a deep, unconscious and conscious level. They become automatic behaviours, reactions and experiences.

The more repetitive the stimuli, the more entrenched our sexual thoughts, initiations and responses become. They are permitted and constrained and altered by Freud's concept of the super ego part of our psyche that regulates sexual impulses and behaviours (Freud, 1964).

This super ego regulation mechanism, however, is frequently dysregulated. During sex, like during eating, our natural, everyday defensive behaviours can be suspended or we place reduced attention on them. This means at those times we become more vulnerable.

When we are vulnerable, a single stimulus has the power to dramatically shape our psyche with longer-lasting effects. It can create sexual desires, fetishes, obsessions and phobias. Often the person has no conscious awareness of those sex impulse alterations or constraints, even if they have been sexually functional or dysfunctional for a long time.

Psychoanalysis, of course, is the basis of uncovering the root causes of behaviours, bringing the knowledge into conscious awareness. The problem that occurs is that we have so many subpersonalities (parts). What is allowed to become conscious by all those parts can be restrained by the individual interests of each part of the psyche.

So intra-psychic conflict can break out and healthy sexual development does not mature or regresses to cause sexual dysfunction. However, intra-psychic conflict is natural, for we have so many needs and each impulse, desire and aspiration is always vying to become the main focus.

Therapy is always as much a negotiation between our unconscious and conscious needs and fulfilment as it is the evolution of skills that enables the individual to have a rewarding sex life.

The language of sex is as much sociological as it is linguistic. If a client does not have that language, they are unable to recognise their experience. They may experience intra-psychic conflict and conscious distress but have not yet learnt to voice their problem or good sexual experiences.

If we as therapists do not have a comprehensive language of sexuality, therapy can become disastrous, because it descends into the unknowing trying to guide the unknowing.

Whilst in this book I am discussing my observations of and techniques with hypnosis and sex therapy, I am neither teaching you to be a sex therapist nor a hypnotherapist. You must learn those clinical skills if you treat sexual problems.

This book comes with and educates with the presupposition that you have studied or are studying both fields and are seeking to expand your knowledge on sex therapy and hypnosis.

I have said sex therapy is a vast field, so it requires you, the clinician, to have a vast knowledge of sexual practices and dysfunctions, far beyond a sterile clinical environment and basic training.

I have spent a great deal of time and working life with people in the sex industry, as well as sex and gender diverse, gay, lesbian and bisexual, BDSM, cosplay, religious and many other cultures. So, a lot of my education around sexuality has been as much outside the therapy room, on the street, as it has been academic.

I have also had a lot of sex during my life of many different kinds in different parts of the world in different cultures. Two husbands and one wife later, I never nailed my sexual identity to be anything other than fluid.

Part of my work is also as a systemic couples and family therapist, as well as an individual psychotherapist. It is important to help people with their sexuality within the context of their life journey and relationships, wherever possible, to preserve any social structure that they may need.

Being trained as a clinical hypnotherapist and medical hypnotist, I use hypnosis every day in my practice. Even if I am treating a physical disorder or disease, it is likely I will add some hypnotic treatment, even if minimal, to assist bringing the body back into homeostasis.

What accompanies every sexual dysfunction is stress, anxiety and often depression around the problem, which hypnosis can help alleviate. So, it is wise for you to be a psychotherapist as well as a hypnotherapist and to undergo training in sex therapy. You will frequently need to be treating adjunct problems that a client presents with.

There is no one or handful of hypnotic techniques and phenomena that can be applied universally to all sexual health problems or performance. The infinite range of sexual experiences are so vast, so I do not teach rote therapy here.

The vast scope of sexual issues presenting to sex therapists would take many volumes to even cover the basics. People are individuals and require individual solutions. I use many solutions to tip the scales so the client can enjoy sex.

This work is not a directory of magic, hypnotic solutions that can be used with the vast scope of individuals. Neither is it a theoretical doctrine, chapter and verse. This work is simply myself, as a clinician and researcher, sharing with you, the professional, some of the cases I have worked with in my hypnotherapy clinic over more than 30 years, and the way I guided those clients to a better sex life.

2 Physiological Contributors of Sexual Experience

Experiencing sex begins with the physiological formation and performance of your body. Even though humans, like other creatures, can have a range of body types, such as male, female and intersex variants, and everyone's body operates differently, there are basic principles.

As psychosexual therapists we must be fully aware of the physical contributory concomitants in sexology. In using hypnosis with sexual dysfunction or elevation of the sexual experience, we need to be fully educated on the biomechanics of sex and sexuality.

GENES

Some genetic sex variants can be hereditary, due to mutations that happen preconception, developmental mutations, or are activated due to the cascading effects of other genes on the body.

Harden (2014) discusses how genetic variations affect the onset of adolescent sexual development and behaviour. This can even vary between identical twins. Consequently, it affects the individual's sexual experiences and confidence.

Gene variants of sex development and performance affect the testes, ovaries, ovotestis, adrenal gland, endocrine system, and brain. Further gene variation affects strength and conductivity and size of the pudendal nerve, vagus nerve, urinary nerve, or spinal cord, hypothalamic pituitary/adrenal/

(HPA) axis, multi-organ performance and intracellular metabolism.

Gene variations can also affect the sensitivity to sex hormones by the receptors on the surface of cells. Sex binding globulin hormone (SBGH) that transports sex hormones can be less effective in some people due to genetic variance.

Interference of a healthy sexual response to stimuli can happen at different stages of life due to genetic damage, chromosomal malfunction or damage to the telomeres at the end of the genes.

There are two groups of people with genetic variants for us to consider. The first are those sex developmental variations such as Klinefelter's, congenital adrenal hyperplasia, androgyne insensitivity syndrome, Down's syndrome, multiple Y and X syndrome and many others (Witchel, 2018).

The second group is those with bifunctional genetic variation such as rs5186, rs1800795, rs1799983 and rs1800629 in AGTR1, IL6, NOS3 and TNFA genes in diabetes (Shoily, 2021), MTHFR in folate metabolism (Raghubeer, 2021), SAM in methylation (Li, 2021), CYP11A1, CYP11B2, CYP17A1, CYP19A1, CYP1A1, CYP21A2, CYP3A7 in polycystic ovaries syndrome (Ajmal, 2019) and many more.

As more everyday genetic testing becomes readily available in clinics, we can consider a greater number of functional genetic anomalies, their effects, and use of targeted medicine for the individual.

The question for hypnotists is, "Can hypnotic interference into genetically predisposed physiological failure of the sexual response cycle be effective?" In other words, "Can hypnosis override physiological failure?"

The answer is always formulated on an individual basis, what the variation is, its effects and how it impacts that person.

The dilemma for the hypnotist who is not trained in biological medicine, and does not understand the effects of genetic anomalies, is that they may be working in the dark.

The automatic presumption of a psychosomatic sex response cycle failure may be incorrect, and the sexual dysfunction may have a physical etiology that hypnosis cannot ameliorate.

For the first groups, which give rise to primary sexual dysfunction, there is little sex therapists can do for mechanical sexual performance, so therapy needs to be based around better education of sexual pleasure.

In the second group, with secondary conditions and lost biological function, hypnotherapy can sometimes help rectify the problems. Here, as this physiological dysfunction is being addressed medically, hypnotherapy can help restore sexual confidence.

Most hypnotherapists, psychiatrists, psychologists, psychotherapists, counsellors, and social workers using hypnosis rely on family doctors to screen patients. But those GPs rarely have the knowledge, experience, skills, time, money or resources to screen for a raft of genetic markers that will interfere with the sex response cycle.

It can better to work with biofunctional medicine or naturopathic practitioners who specialise in treating those patients with genetic variations.

ENDOCRINE INFLUENCES

Many hormones contribute to a healthy sexual response. Let me qualify here by saying I regard a heathy sexual response (libido and performance) as one that is satisfactory to the individual, not society in general.

The sexual response only sometimes begins with the ability to focus the attention on sex, whether that response be consciously or unconsciously initiated.

The infant boy with an erection in the womb or during nappy change can be driven by a full bladder. As the baby grows, he may consciously explore his own genitals, seeking sex stimulation and the pleasure response.

Shaming and parental over-regulation of this behaviour by installing guilt can set up psychological blockages and can cause erectile dysfunction and male anorgasmia later in life.

The teenage boy who wakes up with a spontaneous erection in the morning or who has experienced night emissions is not necessarily driven by sexual fantasy, but by the surge of testosterone at puberty.

The less researched area of female infant sexual arousal can be governed by social regulators that see sexual arousal in females as socially unacceptable, risky behaviours. So young females are often told girls do not do that as it is a sign of being an immoral female.

This shaming and negative psychological regulators can initiate cortisol and catecholamines that send the child into the fight or flight response by the suggestion that such things are dangerous. So that association may stay with the person for life in certain cases.

Cortisol produced by the adrenal glands during stress and the fight or flight response generally gives rise to anxiety and lowers the sex response (Hamilton, 2008). This lowers testosterone, oestrogen, serotonin, and post-orgasm or ejaculation dopamine, which is all present in a normal, healthy sexual response.

High cortisol is associated with high thyroid stimulating hormone, restricting conversion of thyroxine (T4) into the active triiodothyronine (T3), which leaves the person tired and disinterested in sex (Walter, 2012.)

Repeated exposure to stress can interfere with the hypothalamus/pituitary/adrenal (HPA) axis and there is a reduction in the production of sex hormones in the gonads (Helmreich, 2005).

However, in cases of sadomasochism and submissive/dominant role-playing, the submissives' fear can raise cortisol and initiate an elevated sexual response.

Cortisol interference also affects the production of melatonin, the sleep hormone, which leads to tiredness, exhaustion, anxiety, depression, mental health issues, sexual dysfunction and lowering of the sex response (Kobori, 2009).

Although a study in gay and bisexual men showed sex could be more frequent during tiredness, it seemed to be associated with poor decision-making (Millar, 2018). However, Juster et al. (2015), found that higher levels of cortisol in gay and lesbian populations did not necessarily modulate the sex response. This was probably due to the accommodation of socio-cultural factors when those populations lived in a more threatening environment.

We can, however, see in male war combat veterans with post-traumatic stress disorders that there is a higher incidence of erectile dysfunction than those without PTSD (Cosgrove, 2002). It can also be observed that adult survivors of childhood sexual abuse who experience PTSD have higher levels of sexual dysfunction (Gewirtz-Maydan & Lahav, 2020).

At puberty the adenohypophysis (anterior pituitary) begins to secrete gonadotropin-releasing hormones, luteinising hormone (LH) and follicle stimulating hormone (FSH) which elevates the body's level of testosterone, oestrogen and progesterone in females (Lee et al., 2020). LH and FSH are elevated at puberty for females to commence menses and at menopause they become extremely elevated, whilst progesterone, oestrogen and testosterone decrease.

In males at puberty LH and FSH become more elevated as testosterone rises, whilst at andropause, along with human growth hormone, they are more irregular and testosterone decreases (Pincus, 1996).

The decline in sex hormones with ageing decreases gonadal size and efficiency and the SRC in both males and females.

We can see that medications such as Viagra (Sildenafil citrate) and similar drugs increase arterial dilation and volume of fluid in the blood, and therefore engorgement of the genitals (Dhaliwal & Gupta, 2023). However, when psychological blocks to sexual experiences are in place, the nocebo effect can happen and those drugs fail to work.

Some women have sexual desire that fluctuates extensively and is linked to their ovulation and menstruation cycle (Guillermo, 2010). Many women do not track their menstrual cycles, are unclear about when they ovulate and do not track their mood changes.

The sexual desire and response cycle can be affected by sex hormone suppression with the use of contraceptive pills which tend to make many women put on weight and they feel less sexually attractive. Low SRC may also be a sign of a pituitary tumour, disease, or gonadal dysfunction in both sexes.

Fernández-Carrasco et al., (2020) found differing sexual desire during pregnancy for women. Couples may reduce their sexual desire to accommodate the difficulties women experience during pregnancy, particularly in the third trimester. Fuchs et al., (2019) found, however, that some women can experience increased sexual desire during the second trimester. This, of course, is all relative to quality of life, socio-economic and cultural influences.

During pregnancy, hormones remodel a woman's brain (Barba-Muller, 2018). Childbirth changes a woman, and the oestrogen and progesterone levels drop. The neural re-development often changes the personality from an independent individual to being a maternal caregiver. The sudden drop in oestrogen and progesterone can also give rise to postpartum depression, personality changes and reduced sex drive.

The loss of sex hormones in women can cause profound physical and mental changes. It can create vaginal dryness and shrinkage, causing discomfort during sex and lowering of the sex drive. For some women there is a loss of temperature control, which sometimes causes hot sweats for decades. There can be a loss in breast volume, a tendency to put on weight, insomnia, loss of energy, and irritability.

In allopathic medicine perimenopause is seen as the intermittent cessation of menstruation, and menopause as no ovulation and menstruation for one year. From a naturopathic perspective perimenopause is better understood as starting in a woman's thirties, as her fertility declines and pregnancies become less viable.

Some relief can be provided for transition from fertility to post-menopause through progesterone and oestrogen supplementations. Women who may be predisposed to the genetic risk of oestrogen-induced breast cancer may choose to use naturopathic supplementation and herbs.

Testosterone therapy of around 1 gram per day for women who still have ovaries has been used to restore a woman's sex drive, sometimes with oestrogen and progesterone. The research to support this is, however, vague at best.

Women who undergo bilateral oophorectomy are depleted of oestrogens, progesterone and testosterone. It is more logical to prescribe testosterone and oestrogen together in these cases (Cappelletti & Wallen, 2016). Whether these are synthetic hormones or bioidentical depends on the patient and prescribing practitioner, but both may elevate the risk of cancer.

Andropause is often seen as a medical mystery and wholly under-researched. It is also not set at a specific age, although some researchers classify it as 40-60, but it is very individual (Mousavi, 2018). There is testicular shrinkage, lower testosterone, increased erectile failure, premature ejaculation and decline in libido from 30 years old onwards. We must remember that for many men their sexual peak is in their early twenties. Despite this, fecundity (fertility) in some men can remain into the nineties.

Rajfer (2000) reported that men with low testosterone experienced erectile dysfunction or premature ejaculation, mainly being associated with hypogonadism. Some of those men reported better erectile function when administered exogenous testosterone, but not all. For some men there may also be sex binding globulin hormone (SBGH) issues where testosterone is not transported properly into cells. Even though testosterone and SBG hormones can be high, there may be SBGH failure or cell receptor failure to recognise testosterone.

There are also men with normal blood panel testosterone levels who reported better erectile function with testosterone supplementation. Even though testosterone raises libido, exogenous supplementation is often seen as controversial within medicine, because of the fear of higher cardiovascular disease. However, a study reported in The Lancet by Tran et al. (2024) found no difference in major cardiovascular events between men who had supplementation and those who did not, except for the possible occurrence of atrial fibrillation.

For both men and women low libido can be associated with low DHEA-S and supplementation has shown increased levels of energy (El-Sakka, 2018; Panjari, 2009). DHEA-S is a steroid prohormone that raises testosterone and decreases up to tenfold with age.

Obesity with a body mass index (BMI) above 25 causes the excess adipose tissue to create oestrogens that counteract the levels of androgens, and can lower sex drive and function (Moon, 2019; Mozafari, 2015). Weight loss has clearly been identified with improved sex drive and performance.

Anorexia has also been associated with lowered sex drive and amenorrhea, in women (Pinheiro, 2011). In men starvation and malnutrition-induced hypogonadism results in lower sex drive and androgens as the body shuts down (Skolnick, 2017).

Hypothyroidism and Hashimoto's disease elevates thyroid stimulating hormone (TSH) when the thyroid is not working sufficiently. A failure of thyroxine (T4) being converted into triiodothyronine (T3) to give energy reduces sex drive (Gabrielson et al., 2019). The greater problem I see in practice is undiagnosed hypothyroidism when the TSH levels state normal on lab tests, but the clinical presentation is clearly thyroid insufficiency.

It is important to remember when using hypnosis in this field that simply changing the person from norepinephrine (noradrenaline) alertness activation to parasympathetic activation is not a hypnotic cure. Being less anxious does not necessarily in and of itself cure the fear of sex, premature ejaculation, vaginismus, and other issues.

With all people presenting with sexual dysfunction, I order a full blood panel including all sex-related hormones, glucose, thyroid, and adrenal hormones. This is particularly relevant in older people whose sex hormones may be in decline. In younger people with primary sex response failure, I also order panels to discover if there has been a failure to produce enough sex hormones to initiate the sex response cycle.

MEDICATION SIDE EFFECTS

Many antidepressants also suppress sex hormones in both men and women (Higgins, 2010). Whilst this is a listed side effect, prescribers constantly fail to warn patients this may happen. They may even be restrained by their associations or government registration boards from mentioning that to patients in case the patient decides not to take the medication.

Other medications that suppress sex hormones and lower the sex response include antipsychotics (Park, 2012), antihistamines (Mondillo, 2018), anticonvulsants such as phenytoin (Dilantin) or carbamazepine (Tegretol) (Singh, 2015), opioid and synthetic opioids such as hydrocodone/acetaminophen (Vicodin), oxycodone (OxyContin), or oxycodone hydrochloride (Percocet) (Brike, 2019), and statins particularly contribute towards erectile dysfunction (Kostis, 2019).

Since radiation can never be precise, it often damages other tissues, organs and cells as well as the targeted area (Majeed, 2022). This can include imaging diagnostics techniques as well.

Chemotherapy damages tissue and cellular function and can lead to sexual failure and infertility in many people (van Basten, 2000; Hernández-Blanquisett, 2022).

This is particularly prevalent in children and damages the ability to produce human growth hormone in many of these children who then experience failed sex development (Chow, 2007).

PHYSIOLOGICAL FAILURE AND DAMAGE

Developmental failures or tissue damage can inhibit the sex response cycle or the ability to follow through on the cycle. It is important in screening the client's history that any such contributory factors are recorded. In the first group of genetic variations there may be failure to grow sex organs, such as an absence or under-development of testicles, ovaries, penis, vagina, or breasts. This, at times, creates a partial or complete inactivation of the sex response cycle.

Congenital sex developmental difference can create Peyronie's disease, absence of vas deferens, deviated or contorted vagina muscles, absences of or partial absence of vagina, pudendal or urinary nerve entrapment, gonadal insufficiency or damage, brain damage or tumour, spinal deformities and pituitary gland insufficiency.

People who experience major physiological trauma, pain, loss of limb, disfigurement, burns, loss of or damage to organs, heart attack, stroke, brain injury, or nerve injury can experience a reduced sex response (Connell, 2014).

This lowered Quality of Life (QOL) not only results in lowered biological and physiological function, but also in severe damage to sexual confidence. The problem here, however, is that many recovery programs do not include sexual rehabilitation. In some countries no psychological rehabilitations are offered post-trauma, leaving the individuals, couples, and families without the skills to adjust to their new situation.

Medical and surgical treatments can also damage sex organs and production of sex hormones. Radiation treatment for any kind of cancer, particularly prostate cancer, can damage the ability to produce a sex response (Ramirex-Fort, 2020).

Prostatectomy surgery is notorious for severing nerves that initiate an erection. Even with modern microsurgical techniques there is still a risk of complete nerve severance, giving rise to permanent erectile dysfunction.

Brain and spinal surgery, direct trauma, childbirth, chronic constipation, excessive cycling, and prolonged sitting can all damage the quality of signal passing thought the pudendal nerve to the genitals (Kaur et al., 2023). At times this can cause pudendal neuralgia and chronic pain and can make having sex unbearably painful.

One of the common causes of loss of sexual function is heart surgery (Foruzan-Nia, 2011). In a study of 279 men, with a mean age of 55, 76.4% experienced impotence, premature ejaculation, and decreased or loss of libido 12 weeks post-surgery. Only 20.1% experienced sexual dysfunction before surgery.

Pelvic floor dysfunction (PFD) includes pelvic organ prolapse, urinary, bowel and sexual dysfunction, after women have given birth (Mahoney, 2023). Vaginal canal childbirth can result in the pudendal nerve being stretched, whether it is after the first or subsequent births. The nerve can contract back but for some women it does not. Pudendal nerve damage can also occur during a cesarean section delivery where it is permanently severed.

DISEASE AND INFECTION

Bacteria, viruses, parasites, and nematodes all contribute to sexual dysfunction. The damage can occur in any system of the body depending on the infection. Health and homeostasis require all the body's systems to work together and be balanced.

Ghosh & Klein (2017) discussed how viral infections such as human immunodeficiency virus (HIV)-1, vesicular stomatitis virus (VSV), hantavirus (Seoul virus), influenza virus (H1N1), hepatitis C virus, Theiler's murine encephalomyelitis virus (TMEV), herpes simplex virus (HSV-1) and coxsackievirus, all affect sex gene expression or gamete preconception and during intrauterine development.

Although the studies are not yet in, in clinical practice we see patients with Long Covid that initiates a lower sex drive. There is a direct symptom parallel to the lowered sex drive in chronic fatigue syndrome (CFS). Covid infection randomly and unpredictably damages many organs and areas of the body and nervous system, which gives rise to damage to the sex response cycle and QOL. The same can be seen in Covid vaccine damage (Fraiman et al., 2022).

Bacterial infections in sexually transmitted diseases such as chlamydia, gonorrhoea, and syphilis give rise to irritation of the genitals and can cause infertility, mental derangement, and death. Some are now antibiotic-resistant infections (Rubin, 2020).

I have also seen cases of hospitalised necrotising fasciitis that has eaten away and devastated the genitalia and led to considerable loss of sexual function and suicidality (Windsor, 2022).

MEDICAL TREATMENTS

In some people medications can help but since they are formulated for the universal patient and do not consider the individual's physiology, they often fail.

Erectile dysfunction (ED) phosphodiesterase type 5 inhibitor medications such as Sildenafil (Viagra) (lasting around four hours), Vardenafil Avanafil (Stendra) (lasting around five hours), Avanafil (Stendra) (lasting around six hours) and Tadalafil (Cialis) (lasting around 36 hours and activating when the person desires sex), can be useful in helping with erections (Krzastek, 2019).

Side-effects can include sensitivity to light, muscle aches, heart palpitations, heartburn, nose bleeding, flushed skin, problems falling asleep, tingling in the arms, feet, legs, or hands, numbness in the arms, feet, legs, or hands, headache, diarrhoea, heartburn, trouble differentiating between colours such as blue and green, seeing a blue tinge on objects, and visual distortion.

The problem with these medications is that they should not be used in people with high blood pressure, cardiovascular disease, angina, arrhythmia, history of heart attack, risk of heart attack or kidney issues, nitrate or alpha blocker medications, or people drinking grapefruit juice or alcohol. Family doctors frequently do not screen before prescribing. As mentioned earlier these drugs do not work for some men due to unknown reasons or the nocebo effect.

The use of penile pump devices has also been used for ED over the years, where a chamber is placed over the penis area and a pump creates a vacuum which draws blood from the body into the penis (Lin, 2013). Generally, men do not like to use it as it can be cumbersome and embarrassing for them during sex.

There are intracavernous penis self-injection medications such as Caverject, Trimix (prostaglandin, papaverine, and phentolamine), Bimix (papaverine and phentolamine), and Quadmix (prostaglandin, papaverine, phentolamine, and either atropine or forskolin) (Lidawi, 2022). These vasodilate the vessels, creating an erection but can create pain, bleeding, soreness and, at times, priapism (where the penis remains erect for hours without stimulation or after sex has ended).

Penile prosthesis insertion devices were first used in 1973 and have been used for total biological ED. They can either be flexible rods that can bend the penis into an erect position, or inflatable with a small pressure pump inserted under the skin. Whilst researchers have recently reported a 90% satisfaction rate in patients, such devices are prone to infection and functional failure (Rodriguex, 2017).

Viagra has been used off-label in the US to treat female sexual interest/arousal disorder (FSAID). Two drugs were approved by the Food and Drug Administration (FDA) for women: Vyleesi (bremelanotide) is injected into the thigh or stomach up to 45 minutes before sex and can last for 24 hours (US Food and Drug Administration, 2019).

Addyi (filbanserin) is a pill for pre-menopausal women taken nightly that can take up to eight weeks to show results (US Food and Drug Administration, 2024). It should not be taken by women who have liver conditions, take the contraceptive pill, are using CYP3A4 inhibitors, drink alcohol or are nursing mothers. It can cause severe hypotension, fainting and can interfere with other medications.

Side effects can be nausea, vomiting, flushing, hot flushes, skin irritation, rash, headache, flu-like symptoms, fatigue, dizziness, darkening of the skin, hyperpigmentation on the gums, face and breasts, high blood pressure, decreased heart rate and tingling.

NATUROPATHIC APPROACHES

Naturopathic medicine differs considerably from allopathic approaches. In allopathic medicine mono-chemicals are generally used to alter or suppress the body's functions. In naturopathic approaches we aim to support and balance the body's functions so nature can effect a remedy.

There is room for both approaches in sex therapy according to the short- and long-term need of the patients. Sometimes the approaches can work in tandem, but sometimes they may be opposing, and the patient needs to decide which direction they may wish to choose.

The enemy of vascular inflammation and occlusions (blockages) are satatured fats (Hall, 2009). Penile and clitoral engorgement are dependent on good blood flow in major and micro vessels. Without reservation I place all my sex therapy clients on a wholefood plant-based diet, as evidence shows it can also raise sex binding globulin hormone (SBGH) and testosterone levels (Allen, 2000). It lowers blood pressure, triglycerides, LDL and oestrogen in men, often creating leaner body mass (Allen, 2000).

Evidence shows that vitamin D deficiency contributes towards erectile dysfunction (Crafa, 2023). It is suggested that low blood serum levels are the problem, but we have to remember that lab results do not represent the therapeutic levels needed, particularly in older people. Since low vitamin D is also indicated in anxiety and depression, I would prescribe 5000iu twice a week or more.

We can see that low vitamin B12 and folate causes hyperhomocystinuria, vascular dysfunction and impairment of nitric oxide sensitivity (Haloul, 2020). I would prescribe 5000mcg B12 once or twice a week.

In cases where an MTHFR genetic test comes back with an MTHFR C677T or MTHFR A1298C variant for folate process deficiencies, I would prescribe 500mcgs L-5-Meythylfolate daily with 30 mgs B6 (Lombardo et al., 2010). Even if results came back negative, I would prescribe a vitamin B complex twice a week minimum, and more frequently in anxiety and depression. There is a need, however, to keep an eye on B6 levels as they may become over-elevated which can temporarily cause loss of feeling in the extremities.

Zinc supplementation seems to have increased ejaculatory latency and sexual competence (Besong et al., 2023). It seems in the experimental groups that supplementation also led to elevated prolactin (PRL) and testosterone. In post-menopausal women it was found that zinc supplementation significantly improved sexual desire, arousal, orgasm (Nia, 2021). I would supplement 50mgs per day but would keep an eye on copper levels to make sure they do not go too low.

A multi-vitamin can be used three times a week to support general health but the practitioner must again be careful if prescribing B6 that the patient is not being double dosed, and levels become too high.

Particularly in patients older than 40 I will add 250mgs nicotinamide adenine dinucleotide (B3 supplement) daily to prevent the reduction of NAD with age (Radenkovic, 2020). Its effects are to increase vitality.

I would always prescribe Vitamin C 3000mgs liposomal for antioxidant effects, to reduce oxidative stress and increase blood flow. It also tones and strengthens vessel walls (Morellie, 2020). Since as humans we cannot produce or store it, ingestion daily is our only source of therapeutic levels.

Aerobic, resistance and stretching exercise is essential in sexual function. It raises circulating DHEA, serotonin, SBGH, and endorphins, increases stress tolerance to psychosocial stressors, and lowers cortisol levels, anxiety and depression (Caplin, 2021). What is equally important is that the body's oxygen levels are being elevated.

When a herbalist prescribes herbs, every case is different, so the formulation must be specifically for the patient, not a patient self-prescribing off-the-shelf formulations. What is also different about herbs is that they have complex chemical compositions so they may be treating more than one problem at once.

Many herbs have been found to contain PDE5 inhibitors, including Kaempferia parviflora (ginger root) (Temkitthawon, 2011), Epimedium brevicornum Maxim (horny goat weed) (Ganapathy, 2021), Ginkgo biloba (Ginko), Eurycoma longifolia

Jack (Longjack) and Vitis vinifera L. (Grapevine), Punica granatum (Pomegranate), Pausinystalia johimbe (Yohimbe). Withania somnifera (Ashwagandha) is an adaptogenic that helps balance the body's systems. Arginine taken with those herbs also increases their effectiveness.

These herbs have been in the Materia medica and used for thousands of years, and scientific analysis has now validated their usefulness in ED and female genital engorgement.

In menopause and menstrual irregularities we use herbs such as Actaea racemose (black snake root), Glycyrrhiza glabra (Liquorice), Dong quai (Angelica sinensis) known as female ginseng, Vitex agnus castus (chastetree), Dioscorea villosa (wild yam), Oenothera biennis (evening primrose), Ginkgo biloba (ginkgo,) Panax ginseng (ginseng), Piper methysticum (kava), Valeriana officinalis (valerian), Leonurus cardiaca (motherwort), St. John's Wort Hypericum perforatum (St. John's Wort) (Geller, 2006).

Vitex agnus castus (Chastetree), Dioscorea villosa (Wild yam), and Oenothera biennis (Evening primrose) are generally prescribed in premenstrual syndrome (PMS) and when a woman is having problems getting pregnant.

What non-herbalist researchers need to understand about the use of herbal medicine is that we will make a mixture from four to five herbs for a treatment, with one herb supporting the action of another to restore sexual function.

Hair mineral analysis can check mineral levels to profile mineral imbalance, heavy metal poisoning, low lithium and low iodine (Choi, 2019). Standard blood serum profiles only check levels at the present time whilst tissue analyses tell us what has been happening over the preceeding months.

I may also order a genetic profile test and gut analysis to check for any dysbiosis and unexpected genetic variations. It is important to always support general biofunctional health and supplement when necessary.

It is further important to remember in naturopathic approaches that we are treating the whole patient and treating different contributory factors to the problem at the same time, thereby maximising the results.

In naturopathic approaches we are also focused on the mind and body link. This segues perfectly to the core subject of this work of using hypnosis with sexual dysfunction and elevation of sexual experience to change the mind and the body to install or reinvigorate sexual function.

As sex therapists we need to understand this biological background in client history-taking to define the difference between biological dysfunction and psychosomatic failure of the SRC. Failure to study this background can mean the hypnotist is simply stumbling around in the dark, making ineffective and indiscriminate suggestions.

Of course you can only prescribe supplements and/or herbs if you are trained as a naturopath or medical herbalist. Otherwise, it is important to refer clients to these specialists for those purposes and work in collaboration with them.

3 The Individual Psychology of Sex

The psychology of sex is fluid and influenced by sociological, biological, familial, environmental, relational and experiential forces. For every individual the confluence of these influences initiates, fails to initiate or blocks the sex response cycle.

So, no one absolute theory applies to everyone, and reductionism fails to work in sex therapy, just the same as no one trance induction is successful with everyone.

ALTERNATIVES TO THE SEX RESPONSE CYCLE THEORY

It is important to acknowledge here that sex does not follow one single pattern or theory. Whilst Masters and Johnson's (1966) excitement, plateau, orgasm and resolution stages are often used for expressing the sexual experience, they are not exclusive.

Foucault in his work *The History of Sexuality* (1978/1990) examines the differences between the desire for sex and the pleasure of sex, noting how from the 17th to the 20th century the Western world suppressed the concept of sexual pleasure.

Masters and Johnson's work was an examination of sexual behaviour, whilst Foucault's deconstruction of desire and pleasure was an instruction manual.

It is through modern-day erotica, and the field of sex therapy that we now understand that sex does not have to follow only the four-stage model that ends in orgasm.

In fact, for many people, sexual pleasure does not end in orgasm or may not have an extended plateau period. For others it does not even include a sexual act but simply the consideration of or fantasising about erotic experience.

The explosion of the visibility of queer (non-heteronormative) sexuality has forced the exploration of sexual pleasure wide open in the West and the emerging Eastern Block (Fejes, 2008; Fejes & Balogh, 2013). Unfortunately, despite human rights commitments in those areas, this has caused, at the time of writing, a misogynistic backlash as patriarchy perceives that growth of knowledge around sex as a threat to its dominance.

Many theories of human sexuality have emerged. However, as Foucault warned, in making a science of sex, we are in danger of focusing solely on the functioning of sexuality and not increasing pleasure.

EDUCATION

A person's sex psychology (how a person's mind works in relation to sex) is at times genetically innate, as well as being due to their education and experience. All contribute towards their sex experience and the gestalts they bring with them to therapy. As sex therapists we need to endeavour to investigate all those influences.

Even when the biological sex impulse, stimuli and drive are strong, they can be disabled by a lack of knowledge, fear around sexual contact or previous sexual experiences with the self and others. The client's education around sex is often taken for granted by therapists. However, many parents hardly ever mention sex in the home.

A Onepole survey of 2000 parents in the US, with children between five and 18 years of age, reported in the *New York Post*

(Lefroy, 2022), found that 20% of parents would not talk to their offspring about sex, and 60% of those parents admitted they were raised to think that talking about sex was taboo.

Religious schools run by conservative Christians, Muslims, or Hassidic Jews can ban sex education altogether. This not only leaves the growing person with little knowledge, but also implants into their unconscious mind the idea that sex is sinful or bad. This has been shown to damage the sex response cycle (Krule, 2016; Slominski, 2020; Smerecnik, 2010).

This particularly affects women, gay, lesbian, bisexual, intersex, sex diverse, trans, gender fluid and sex non-specific identified people. If you are not taught that sex with yourself and others would be positive and wholesome, but instead shameful, then your sex response can be damaged.

THE DIFFERENCE BETWEEN ASSOCIATION AND ATTACHMENTS

An association is a loose and flexible connective relationship between two or more experiences. One may have an association with certain beliefs, values, likes and dislikes, or people, but not be strongly attached to them. You often do not know, consciously, that you are operating many associations unconsciously, which drive your thoughts and actions.

Attachments are stronger connections in your relationships to others. They form according to the influences of your family of origin, relationships, life history, learnings (or lack of them), and can be strong. Many people who have experienced negative associations with sex and sexual identity may be unable to form positive attachments with other people emotionally and sexually.

Sexual experiences that have strong associations to pleasure or perceived benefits may also set up attachments to certain people, sexual practices, and objects as with fetishism. With repetitive or heightened sensory exposure, those attachments may become lifelong, until the trance is interrupted.

POSITIVE ASSOCIATION TO SEX AND SEXUAL IDENTITY

For the ideal sexual experience, the person needs to have a good association with the sex act and their own sexual identity. Walker (2023) surveyed 78 people on what for them made good sex and the answers were distilled down to orgasm, an emotional component, and chemistry/connection. I caveat this with the usual set of cultural filters and individuals' concept of what is an ideal sexual experience.

Since sexual self-identity is set generally very early in life in most people, positive re-enforcement by others leads to good sexual confidence and satisfaction. Law (2012) finds that positive re-enforcement in youth development programs creates higher levels of success and life satisfaction.

Good associations with sexual acts promote positive attachments generally. Khoury and Findlay (2014) found in an online survey of 125 people between 18-65, that anxious individuals and those with a lower Quality of Life (QOL) score showed lower levels of sexual satisfaction.

What they also found was those with a higher level of QOL score showed better ability to communicate about and during sex. Therefore, it is not just the sexual act and positive sexual self-identity, but also a lack of repression around discussing sex that leads to higher levels of sexual satisfaction.

NEGATIVE ASSOCIATION TO SEX AND SEXUAL IDENTITY

As professionals we should never dismiss the profound influence in a client's psyche to negative associations with their sex and sexual identity. It can happen at any age, anywhere, in any environment and last a lifetime.

First-year female college students in the US completed monthly assessments of their sexual behaviours and their positive and negative effects (Wesche, 2019). It was found they had more negative associations during months they engaged in intercourse as opposed to other sexual behaviours. The implications by the authors were that these young women would have benefited from sexual education earlier.

Little research has been done around male negative association to sex and sexual identity, except in the field of gay males and men experiencing minority stress (Bruce, Harper & Bauermeister, 2015). In my clinical experience, much of the heterosexual male negative associations with sex are based in religious extremism that is centred around creationist theory.

In a meta-analysis of studies Decou (2017) identified connections between social reactions to disclosure of sexual assault and psychological distress. It was suggested that assault-related shame was one driving force behind unresolved PTSD.

Saevik (2023) found that sexual desire was reduced and repressed by emotional regulators due to social shaming around sexual identity and gender. Whilst it is possible to experience sexual desire and sexual shame at the same time, emotions always suppressed or increased libido and levels of sexual pleasure.

WOMEN AND GIRLS' SEXUAL IDENTITY

It was the feminist Simone de Beauvoir (1949/2015) that said, 'One is not born, but rather becomes, a woman'. There is a great truth in that, as everything we experience contributes towards our life experiences and identity.

Women in nearly all societies are often seen as having less value. We generally do not earn as much as men or hold as many key positions. And due to child-rearing duties we often put our careers on hold.

Financially disadvantaged or single mothers' daily struggle to pay the rent and put food on the table can be stressful, and, at times, exhausting. As a mother you are often a 24-hour carer for the children, which, to some, seems a relentless task.

These changes can lead to high levels of stress that raises cortisol and reduces the sex drive. If the woman is struggling, she can also be reluctant to engage in sex due to the fear of getting pregnant again and worsening her social and economic situation.

Commercialisation of female body images through the media and fashion industry's stereotyping of being young, white, beautiful and slim damages the average woman's sexual self-image. Unconsciously we can carry those comparatives to ourselves around with us and have an underlying, nagging sense of ourselves being less worthy or attractive.

Some women may never have had or now do not have a positive body self-image and sense of their own sexual power and self-determination. In many cultures women having those things is shameful and considered dangerous, because it would be interpreted as being morally bankrupt.

Layer those experiences with a lack of comprehensive education around sexuality and we can have a fearful woman, who has trouble connecting with her body and enjoying a healthy sex life.

EARLY NEGATIVE SEXUAL EXPERIENCE IN FEMALES

Women are generally and naturally more affected by emotions. For females, losing their virginity can lead to good emotional memories or poor ones. Young women are continually judged by their sexual value and availability for sex with men.

They get double messages in that they are supposed to be chaste (maintain virginal purity) in many cultures, but then they are suddenly supposed to become available for male sexual pleasure and producing children.

Women are being valued by their looks, sexual availability, and ability to produce children. These often seem to be tests of her value as a human being. If she does not conform, she is frequently rejected by men or society. If she is told she fails one of these measures, it can scar her sexual self-esteem, so she shuts down her sexual response cycle.

Sexual assault, rape and inappropriate advances towards females are some of the biggest reasons why women shut down sexually. Statistically rape is one of the most under-reported crimes. The National Sexual Violence Resource Center in the US (2015), reported that one in five women compared to one in 71 men were raped.

One in 10 rapes were found to be by intimate partners. Very few of these crimes are ever reported. Most women know that they will often not be believed. The ordeal of going through a trial can be equally, if not more traumatising, creating complex PTSD.

MEN AND BOYS' SEXUAL IDENTITY

Males are highly competitive for the most part. They are generally physically stronger, driven by testosterone surges, and often the major breadwinners under great pressure and stress to compete in the job marketplace.

Industrialisation has tended to rob adolescent males of adult male mentoring around relationships and sex with others. Reeves (2022) finds lack of good sex and relationship education at school, absent fathers, and estrangement from core family members often creates an identity crisis in many males today. As feminism rises in the West, masculine studies fail to keep up with the need to sit men in their strengths.

Displacement of thousands of years of male dominance of the sexes has left many men with an existential crisis of being around their masculinity. Whilst Joel (2019) discusses the shaping of the male brain away from the default female form, it is important for us to consider the influences of childhood and adolescent sexual development on the formation of male sexuality.

Whilst some men have high levels of testosterone and are naturally more sexually active, many men are more affected by environmental factors that shape their sexual confidence. Sexuality is never solely determined by physiology.

EARLY NEGATIVE SEXUAL EXPERIENCES IN MALES

Poor early male sexual experiences can instill a deep unconscious phobia or guilt during sexual interactions. The male may even be desperately consciously wanting to have a good sexual experience, but unconsciously lacks self-esteem, leading to poor and disappointing first sexual experiences.

This creates protective mental defence mechanisms associated with sex, and he associates it with danger, so it cancels or reduces the sex response. This includes the sex stimulus or progression to the plateau, orgasm or resolution stages.

We can see this in men who had poor first intercourse experiences and afterwards developed erectile dysfunction or premature ejaculation. Such unsatisfactory sexual performance can remain for life, because the man does not understand what has happened or know that he can get help.

Anthropologists also found that cross-cultural male fear of sex with women can derive from inter-tribal warfare, population pressure, confusion around sexual identity or an over-exaggerated Oedipus complex (Ember, 1978).

THE CONSEQUENCES OF SEXUAL ASSAULT

Women who have been raped can go into the freeze response during sex, simply becoming a passive vessel. Dhawan & Haggard (2023) report how the freeze response is a standard self-protective mechanism during rape. Women may later reject sexual advances or fake orgasm to satisfy their partners and buy into their own self-deprecating belief that sex is only something to satisfy men.

The effects of sexual assault on men are profoundly under-studied. Petersen (2011), in a systematic review of studies, found male victims of sexual assault reported psychological, sexual, and interpersonal problems in relationships, similar to those in women. What also can happen, post-assault, is that it has a profound effect on their identity as a whole, confident male, leaving them feeling less than a man.

Sexual assault, molestation and inappropriate sexual advances in childhood can change the brain and set up abnormal neurobiological responses to sex. It frequently amounts to post traumatic stress disorder (PTSD), generalised anxiety disorder (GAD), bipolar affective disorder (BPAD) and a wide range of mental psychopathologies (De Bellis, 2014).

Later in life, trauma due to sexual assault, physical or mental abuse, threats, bullying or major life traumas and stressors can also change the structure of the brain (Xi et al., 2022).

In treating sexual difficulties that arise from those traumas, a therapist must also help the client process those traumas. The sexual disorder cannot generally be ameliorated if the trauma is still active because it is interfering with the sexual response cycle.

SEXUAL DOMINATORS

Sexual dominators are predatory. They are not the same as those who are the top in voluntary and consensual BDSM relationships. They are predatory, manipulative, and have no social conscience. These personalities can be narcissistic, passive aggressive, coercive, sociopathic, psychopathic, persistently violent, and serial rapists.

The introduction of laws around coercive behaviours in different parts of the world particularly focuses on protecting the vulnerability of women against predatory dominators. Mahon (2020) focuses on the lack of criminality around violence in families and its detrimental consequences, which includes a person shutting down sexually. It is also not always women that are the victim. When we take a full mental health history we need to bear in mind that previous abuse may never have been fully processed (see downloadable form in Resources section).

People who have been under the control of sexual dominators have frequently experienced sexual abuse, violence, and are constantly exposed to detrimental isolation and controlling behaviours. They can be left with a deep sense of fear, anxiety, depression, and trauma, and can have a damaged sex drive and attachment problems.

LEVELS OF CONNECTION DURING SEX

As sex therapists one of the dangers that can happen in practice is that we become very monodirectional in the way we approach solutions to poor sexual satisfaction. We are constantly bombarded by academics, professional associations, colleges, government health funding, insurance companies and laws telling us we have to only follow science-based approaches, known as the gold standard. We can end up just dealing in pathologies and cures alone, leaving the client bereft of many ways of deepening sexual connections.

Whilst we can use science-informed approaches, we also have to consider all the levels that people connect in their sexual encounters, as every person is different.

The base sex connection that seems to be more prevalent when a person is young is the physical level, when hormones are high, and orgasm often is the ultimate goal. As we age and sex hormones diminish, that physical pull can become less powerful.

We emotionally connect to others through sex. During and after sex and orgasm, as oxytocin rises, we get the sense of being emotionally connected to the people we are having sex with, which gives rise to empathy and often love.

Relationships also offer us another way to connect. From a psychodynamic perspective, when we date, live with someone, partner, marry or have children with others, a form of contractual mating and bonding emerges. It can create a deeper or diminished sexual connection depending on what each partner brings to the relationship.

Our social guidelines, rules, values, beliefs, and permissibilities further filter the kinds of connections we can have with others. Someone may become attractive if they have similar psychological and cultural filters to ourselves or exciting because they buck the normal social standard and are considered a little risqué.

For many of us there can also be a large spiritual element during sex. The kinds of ecstatic physical and emotional experiences are akin to the kind of highs experienced during religious encounters. When both collide, it can heighten the sexual experience.

Part of our job as sex therapists is to help the client stack those positive levels of connections in more long-term relationships during sex to give greater satisfaction.

Even in short-term sexual encounters, the stacking of those connections can lead to a lifelong connection with other people.

AGEING AND SEXUAL IDENTITY

As women age they experience lower levels of sex hormones, and breasts, knees, stomach and facial wrinkles surrender to gravity. In a commercialised, youth-centric culture, we can frequently be considered beyond our use-by date and sexually unattractive.

Men too are seen as less sexually attractive as they lose strength, hair, and teeth. Men tend to suffer from greater levels of loneliness and depression as they get older, particularly around loss of purpose in life, which can lead to depression (Neville, 2018). They may still want sex, but the libido is depressed by reduced mental health.

The social attitude towards older people in and of itself damages our sense of deserving sex and being beautiful. While a 90-year-old male billionaire dating a 25-year-old woman is considered smart and successful, a poor 60-year-old woman dating a 30-year-old man is considered tragic. So, misogyny can also play into this demeaning of older people.

In an industrial society, lack of connection to family and loneliness is also a major mental health problem. This impacts and limits older people's libido, sexual desire, and relationships.

THE BODY KNOWS AND REMEMBERS

Our dual aspect of mind and body both have memories. We have behavioural memories where we do the same things again and again, and that behaviour has become automatic. It becomes the trance we are living in. In hypnosis, via suggestion or negotiation with the unconscious, we as hypnotists can help the client install new behaviours, values, beliefs and expectations around sex, and eradicate unwanted ones.

We also have muscle memory that is normally completely out of our conscious awareness, such as walking, running, swimming, or riding a bicycle. Due to trauma or negative experiences, these muscle memories can interfere with our conscious intentions and thoughts during sexual encounters.

As far back as the early 1990s, Foa (1993) reported successful reduction of the PTSD muscular rigidity fight response in patients who were raped, by beginning treatment with deep muscle relaxation exercises. The clinicians were reprogramming muscle memory. When using this in hypnosis it is more powerful because it can induce hypnotic muscular flaccidity by suggestion, stopping defensive muscle reactions to sex. It becomes an interrupter pattern, and suddenly the client has another option other than defensive muscular tension that spoils sex for them.

Dolezal & Lyons (2017) discuss how shame is dramatically under-researched. The body also remembers sexual response failures. If you have an early or later life disastrous sexual encounter, you can experience shame and embarrassment when you think about or engage in sex in the future. This creates a phobia for future sex and/or the thought of sex. The person physically moves into the flight response, cortisol rises, testosterone declines, and the sexual response cycle is interrupted as the body seizes. Regular exercise can help break this pattern (Brownlee, 2005).

The body even has auto-suggestion mechanisms to re-enforce or weaken mechanical functions. It is a physical self-fulfilling prophecy that becomes out of conscious control.

We know this from how athletes build body memory, which is an extreme example of how humans and animals physically self-program. Sharples (2023) in the *American Journal of Physiology* showed how skeletal muscle memory can be primed by early positive encounters. The muscles can have both positive and negative memories.

It is a feedback loop where neurology programs muscles and muscles program neurology and thoughts. We have various sources for this theory in hypnosis. We can see the increase of blood flow by suggestion in trance or even the waking state (Bhatt, 2017). A reduction in blood flow can also be achieved by hypnotic suggestion (Clawson, 2011).

There is more than 200 years of data on the production of anaesthesia and analgesia in hypnosis (Wobst, 2007). In Neuro Linguistic Programming the practice of manipulating sensory submodalities can lead to somatic hyposensitivity or hypersensitivity.

Erickson (1980) reported a case of sexual sensory relocation in a woman who was paraplegic. She was hypnotically induced to have an orgasm through sensory experiences in her nipples, taking a memory from one part of the body and inducing a replication of the sensation in another part.

His experimentation and clinical practice of using sensory alteration and relocation was born out of his own personal hypnotic alteration of pain due to polio.

HYPNOTIC PHYSIOLOGICAL MANIPULATIONS

Depression contributes towards lack of libido, thereby cancelling the sex response cycle. Yapko (2013) demonstrates treating depression with hypnotic techniques as opposed to medications.

I always classify anxiety as a different condition from depression. Whilst they can coexist, and may have crossover treatment approaches, generally I find they need to be treated separately. Both depression and anxiety are major interrupters of sexual arousal and poor performance. Gurgevich (2007) shows us treatment for anxiety with medical hypnosis is effective, and Yapko shows us the same for depression.

Whilst we know hormones such as cortisol, oxytocin, serotonin, and endorphins can be manipulated by hypnosis (Kasos, 2018), there is no real valid evidence that testosterone can be boosted by hypnosis. However, it is clear the hypnotic reduction of cortisol can help allow sex hormone levels rise to the individual's natural levels.

The case for cortisol and oestrogen is more complex. Cortisol can suppress oestrogen, but increased oestrogen can also raise cortisol. Since both cortisol and oestrogen can depress testosterone and the sex response cycle, increasing libido in women is not exclusively about raising testosterone levels.

Wood (2009) shows us that in perimenopause and menopause cortisol levels can rise, depressing sex hormones. So lifting the sex drive may need to be more about hypnotic behavioural training and self-exploration to raise oxytocin than exclusively sex hormone manipulation.

Males can also experience high testosterone and cortisol at the same time and fully experience the sex response cycle, but in general cortisol is reduced at the beginning of the sex response cycle (Rahardjo, 2023).

Wong (2016) found in sex offenders that there was no difference in testosterone levels between offenders and non-offenders. Glenn (2011), however, found that there is higher cortisol to testosterone levels in psychopathy.

Victims of sexual assault were found to initially have higher levels of cortisol post-assault, but later developed lower levels than the average person, and disturbances to the hypothalamus/pituitary/adrenal (HPA) axis. Trickett (2011) and Scardino (2014) reviewed how hypnosis can be used to balance the HPA axis, and restore homeostasis, reducing irregularities in cortisol.

Here we must err on the side of science and evidence-informed treatment. If an individual has a genetic variance or medical condition that creates low testosterone, no amount of hypnosis is going to raise the levels. To lead a client to believe that it might be possible is clinical negligence, because failure will further damage the client's sense of sexual self-efficacy and mental wellbeing.

What does this mean to us as hypnotists working with sexual function and dysfunction?

It is easy to deduce that there can never be one gold standard hypnotic approach or script to apply to everyone in sex therapy. Since sexual dysfunction can arise from individual biology, psychology, anxiety, depression, PTSD and psychopathology, treatment must be custom-designed for that specific person.

Many times, I have heard from hypnotists how they produce hypnotic phenomena and then use a singular hypnotic technique to resolve sexual difficulties. It is rather like saying that a surgeon will use one scalpel for all surgery.

I believe, as I have stated many times, that all hypnotherapists need to be trained as psychotherapists to handle the client's psychodynamics to lead them to resolution. This includes sex therapists, who for a large part, act as psychosexual therapists. Everyone's map of the world is different. Their sex map is also different so every solution must be different.

The clues to formulating that treatment come from the client's medical, mental, and life history. The dysfunction lies in their body and stories, so we must constantly watch, listen, and observe what is happening to them and how our treatment affects them.

SCREENING

As I teach my students, screening needs to be 95% of what we do in clinical practice, which enables us, as clinicians, to target the 5% treatment as accurate and motivating for that specific client. This includes constant observation and questioning of the client to find out how treatment is progressing.

Simply reading scripts out of a book to the client will not produce consistent results and frequently no results at all in sexual function. Our treatment must be based on all the information we have gathered from the client and any external reports.

Hypnotherapy is the oldest psychotherapy we know of, but still we need to understand psychodynamic and behavioural therapies. This might not be the case in medical hypnosis, but it carries a caution that having a degree in medicine does not automatically qualify someone to practise hypnosis legally or effectively.

When manipulating a client's psychological and emotional state, it is imperative to be able to tell the difference between conscious and unconscious reporting and motivation. What the client says is not necessarily what they mean or are motivated to carry out, and as clinicians we must understand the difference.

Sex therapy and hypnosis is not waving a watch in front the of client's face and hoping for the best. It is a cascade of therapeutic and remedial techniques.

A full medical screening and history-taking must be carried out in all cases to screen for metabolic or disease-state dysfunctions. This must include blood profiles.

I urge caution here because many lab reports show normal levels of hormones, disregarding that these are not necessarily therapeutic levels of hormones. The medical establishment is frequently reticent to supplement testosterone or boost thyroid function when higher levels can often be efficacious, of course on a case-by-case basis.

Are we working solely psychologically or psycho-biologically?

What we are doing as hypnotists is using hypnosis in resolving sexual dysfunction and improving people's sex lives. We are manipulating physiology.

We are working psycho-biologically because we are attempting to manipulate a biological function. Sex experiences are physiological, psychological, emotional, social and a myriad of other aspects depending on the individual.

The body speaks all the way through vital signs, muscular activation, and body language. We must pay attention to this language to help the client create sexual resolution.

TEST AND MEASURE

As hypnotists, all treatments applied through hypnotic techniques need to be tested, as much as is ethically permittable, within the intra-hypnotic state and post-hypnosis for evaluating results. Even if that is testing using psycho-imaginary future pacing.

Sometimes you may use a Likert 1-10 (1 being low and 10 being high) subjective rating scale with clients where they can report the satisfaction and effectiveness of results. Whilst this can be useful in anaesthesia or analgesia, I do not recommend it in other hypnotic experiences with sex therapy. The danger is that a client can be discouraged unless they get immediate high levels of satisfaction.

Observation of body language and linguistic analysis are far more telling of what the client is experiencing. We need to look for congruence or incongruence between what the client says and what the client's body, face and breathing are telling us.

What the client says is useful in screening for self-defeating or self-supporting thoughts and behaviours. There is frequently a difference between the client's surface language and their unconscious intention. To get results, we need to help the client have congruency in their body, face, breathing, surface language and intended communication.

We need to offer constant suggestions to induce congruence in every single communication we have with the client in official hypnosis and artificial somnambulism. As hypnotists we need to be using suggestion in all our communications.

DEPTH OF THE HYPNOSIS

In some ways the depth of hypnosis and effectiveness of hypnotic work is a misnomer unless in hypno-anaesthesia and analgesia. Change can take place at every level for every person, and the depth of hypnosis and response to suggestion is different. I will demonstrate different levels of depth throughout this book, as I show you some of my cases.

Academic researchers also always use hypnotisability scales which again is a misnomer in clinical practice because they were composited in an artificial, experimental, laboratory environment. Everyone is hypnotisable with the right technique that will suit them. At times we don't even have to call it hypnosis.

In reading this chapter you can now see why I support the idea that you also need to have psychotherapy training when dealing with psychosomatic sexual dysfunction. We need to understand the psychodynamic workings of the client's mind in order to create the correct suggestions for sexual motivation and function.

COMPLIANCE AND COSTING

One of the issues we always face as clinicians is what the client can tolerate and afford. Many clients seeking hypnosis for sexual dysfunction are seeking a miracle cure. They do not understand the complexity of sexual dysfunction that may be affecting them.

Certainly, they may have the preconceived idea that the hypnotist will change their sex response cycle without them having to do anything themselves. They may have tried many other avenues of failed treatments that depended solely on one single solution.

It is important for the hypnotist to be honest and explain that the client must also take responsibility for making other appropriate changes.

Clients can come with the idea that, just because the treatment may be hypnosis, they do not have to spend additional money on making the necessary changes themselves.

To create effective change, right at the beginning of therapy we, as hypnotists, need to create a contract with the client that they will comply with all changes that are requested. All my clients are required to sign a contract that they will follow my instructions, including all homework between sessions (see downloadable contracts in Resources).

What people say, driven by their emotional distress, is not always what they will comply to later. When they have a copy of a contract, which they can see visually, to take away with them, it gives a higher level of transparency, trust, and compliance. I will not treat people who do not sign the contract.

CREATING EXPECTATION

The placebo factor is a large part of the hypnotherapeutic process. Our job is to help the client set their mind to the expectation of success. However, we must be careful not to create false hope and over-promise what might not be achievable.

I take a full medical and mental health history, ask for any recent reports, blood tests or specialist letters to be brought to the first session. I order tests I think may be relevant. If a psychiatrist is treating the person, I require a referral letter as a matter of professional courtesy and legality. The client is also asked to inform their family doctor of treatment. Remember, you cannot contact any of those professionals without the client's permission.

I do not see clients who are being treated by other psychologists, psychotherapists, counsellors or naturopaths. Multiple clinicians at the same time creates confusion. Compliance to one therapist's treatments often undoes what another is doing. It is a case of too many cooks in the kitchen.

As a therapist, if you are not qualified in allopathic medicine or clinical naturopathy, you need to co-ordinate with a biofunctional medicine practitioner and sometimes a urologist or gynaecologist.

I lead my client into a journey of exploration. I begin with:

Tracie: "What would you like to achieve?"

The therapist is not the client so whilst we can guide them, we need to check back that the shopping list of goals they create satisfies *their* needs, not ours.

Tracie: "So how does the shopping list feel in your gut as you read it?"

Tracie: "If you achieved that list, would therapy have worked for you?"

As with any therapy, I create a safety anchor (stimulus/response trigger).

> Tracie: "When you hear my voice you can be aware of an instant deep sense of safety."

As noted earlier, what is frequently missing from sex therapy, which can become obsessed with pathologisation, is freedom to talk about fantasies, desire, lust, pleasure, joy, thrills and the love of sex. We will explore these later in this work.

4 Sex and Hypnosis: The Research

Since the subjects of sex and hypnosis are so expansive, here I shall simply profile some research to authenticate its use. It is not possible to deal with all the sexual dysfunctions in this volume, but I include some of the common ones to help you be aware of the clinical scope you may need to deal with in this field. For some areas of sexology and the use of hypnosis, there is no research at all. In subsequent chapters I shall highlight further research.

First, we must define what hypnosis is and is not, which is always an interesting exploration. Here I am not going to discuss the theories of hetero-hypnosis but look at hypnotic altered states influencing the change of participants' experiences.

This, of course, can become vague when we also include instant artificial somnambulism, without an official hypnotic induction, which we use in a clinical setting, and I use in every session.

Certainly, we cannot rely on experimental hypnosis for a definition because that takes place in an artificial environment. It therefore creates experimental and situational bias and does not necessarily translate into clinical practice. The comparative is akin to in-vitro and in-vivo scientific investigation, and the first frequently does not translate into the second. Though sometimes, we glean some knowledge from those results.

How far back in history can we go to find hypnotic influence around sexual experiences?

If we regard hypnosis as concentrated and focused attention, we can go back to ancient Egyptian, Greek, Roman and Pagan times (Gauld, 2012). Avicenna, a Persian physician, wrote about the trance state in 1027 (Hassan, 2014). In more recent history we note the work of Mesmer, Braid, Bernheim, Liébeault, Charcot, Hall, Erickson and many more.

When we look at hypnotic influence on sexual practices we need to go back to ancient Pagan religions when the divine power was female-led. These religions were based around fertility, and sex rituals during the full moon, which called for an altered state. This was prevalent in the bronze age, early Greece, and Minoan Crete period with the marriage of Indo-European cultures, which were basically matriarchal (Thomas, 1973).

As mentioned earlier, this socially perceived hypnotic sexual power of women and goddess worship was later considered threatening to many men. In the second century AD, early Christian male power brokers banished goddess worship and converted her into the sexless Virgin Mary, which filtered through to Islam.

The Bible, written by men, then invents cautionary tales of the dangers of marginalised women's sexuality by inventing Mary Magdalene, who was portrayed as being a loose woman. The tale progresses by her abandoning her sexuality and serving a male god – a perfect example of hypnotic governors. The Catholic church then takes over hypnotic influence, using prayer, around women's sexuality by creating chastity until marriage for women or the threat of hellfire (The Holy Bible: King James Version version, 1991; Wood, 2019).

Sex and hypnotic influences were perceived together before modern science invented the discipline of clinical hypnosis. For us as clinicians, hypnosis can be a magnifying influence when wielded in our communications to alter the client's experience. This complies with Spanos's (1996) social learning theory of hypnotic phenomena.

Further, it could be the self-hypnosis we teach to our clients to control their own experience. We use the words 'hypnosis' and 'trance' to validate that process when needed.

The first prominent, reported controversial case of hypnosis and sexuality in recent history was noted by Josef Breuer in the case of Anna O (real name Bertha Pappenheim). He treated her from 1880 to 1882. During a hypnotic altered state she revealed incidents of trauma she suffered. Sigmund Freud, who worked with Breur, but never treated Anna O, believed that an Electra complex and incestuous sexual fantasies she had towards her father were the cause of her symptoms (McLeod, 2024).

In 1884 the Czynski trial became notable in Germany, when a baroness was hypnotised by a lay hypnotist, who then seduced her whilst he was still married to his wife and convinced the woman to fraudulently marry him. At the same time the novel *Trilby* was published about an abusive lay hypnotist who convinced the main character, a young woman called Trilby O'Ferrall, to do whatever he said (du Maurier, 1922.) So, for a while faith in hypnosis was damaged. In the public's eye hypnosis was associated with sexual abuse.

As far back as 1980, Brown reported the validity of utilising hypnosis in sex therapy. The author stated five particular strategies to be effective: (1) as a diagnostic tool, (2) to improve self-confidence, (3) as an adjunct to behaviour therapy, (4) for the direct removal of symptoms, and (5) to facilitate the resolution of neurotic conflicts.

SEXUAL AROUSAL

It is not surprising to us as hypnotists that hypnosis can raise sexual arousal. Kumalasari (2020), in a meta-analysis of hypnosis and sexual arousal, observed that it can increase excitement by 2.16 times.

For us as hypnotists, who can use fractionation daily, Kumalasari's increase seems very small, when in clinic with the right therapy and suggestions, sexual interest can be initiated, multiplied many times and actually restored.

Clearly what is happening here is one of the basic principles of Kundalini and sex therapy which is bringing the person's attention into the present time, and taking them out of the fight or flight response.

Focused attention aids every stage of the SRC. If you are thinking about your shopping list or repairing your car during sex, you are distracted. Whilst distraction is used by some hypnotists to lengthen the plateau stage of SRC, it reduces intimacy and lowers the pleasure response.

CONFUSION AROUND SEX EDUCATION

Hayley (2010) reported that Milton Erickson had many cases where he treated people with sexual health problems. These were frequently around inappropriate attitudes to sex, excessive modesty or incompatibility of sexual partners.

Erickson, using family therapy and couples therapy, along with sex education and hypnosis, assisted in the client's alteration of interpersonal dynamics through solution-focused therapy. Much of his work was also around sensory alteration of the sexual response cycle and manipulation of the perception of modalities and submodalities. This allowed clients to decrease or increase sexual sensory experiences in many parts of the body, including their physical levels of sex sensations, as well as the location of those sensations.

He used these techniques hypnotically with clients experiencing premature ejaculation, retarded ejaculation, vaginismus, anorgasmia, and failure to experience sexual desire.

In the early 1970s the feminist Betty Dodson held masturbation workshops for women in New York that helped them get in touch with their bodies. She still held them until she was nearly 90 years of age (Weiss, 2018).

What both Erickson and Dodson did in teaching about sexuality is a perfectly natural and wholesome, human experience.

PREMATURE EJACULATION (PE)

Sexuality and hypnosis is a poorly researched area, mainly due to the difficulties in running randomised, controlled trials. Psychotherapy, CBT combined with SSRIs is frequently used (Yang, 2023). The side effects from those drugs, however, can at times, be too difficult for many patients to cope with and sometimes creates erectile problems (Anagha, 2021). This also largely ignores sex education and sex therapy.

Erickson (1982) treated a young man who experienced premature ejaculation (ejaculation praecox) over several sessions of psychotherapy and hypnosis. The man had no problem achieving and maintaining an erection, even after ejaculation, but tended to ejaculate prior to intercourse.

Erickson used metaphor laced with post-hypnotic suggestions, in his indirect delivery style, for a delay of ejaculation for half an hour after the commencement of intercourse. These suggestions were repeated again and again in different forms at different times.

Psychotherapeutically he was treating the man's neurosis and desensitising him to the fear of sexual performance. This resulted in a psychodynamic change and the man being able to engage in satisfactory intercourse, without immediately ejaculating.

The etiology of PE is complex, multifactorial, physiological, psychological, emotional, social, and driven by relationship dynamics. Classification for the cause of ED generally comes down to epidemiological symptomatology, which is generally ejaculation before one minute of intercourse (Saitz, 2016).

Unfortunately, that narrow classification creates victims out of many of our male clients who are simply confused and afraid of what sex for them could be like. If we as therapists buy into that falsehood, instead of treating all cases individually, we are practising anti-therapy.

Like the reduction of hypnotic anaesthesia when chemical anaesthesia was discovered, the treatments of psychogenic PE and other psychological sexual problems has become overshadowed by pharmaceutical companies' drug marketing. The problem is that this primary chemical-based approach does not deal with the psychological reasons behind PE. Any chemical relief such as lomipramine, fluoxetine, paroxetine, dapoxetine and sertraline can be short term, and have frequent risks of side effects. Also, these drugs are not necessarily approved for treating PE, but they are frequently prescribed off-label for this purpose.

ERECTILE DYSFUNCTION (ED)

Rosso et al. (2016) examined the application of Ericksonian hypnosis in erectile function and QOL, post-nerve sparing prostatectomy. Participants were administered a 30-minute hypnosis session twice a month for nine months, against a control group who did not have hypnosis. The results of the preliminary study show neither group recovered complete erectile function, but hypnosis can speed up recovery and restoration of QOL.

What the study did not consider, however, was the variability of surgical outcomes and functional erectile failure post-prostatectomy. It is rare in such cases to have full recovery and in some cases, men may have no erectile recovery at all. My experience is surgeons are frequently not truthful with patients about the outcome of such surgery.

Crasilneck & Hall (1985) regarded erectile function as largely involuntary, mentioning that erections can even occur in paraplegics with complete transection of the spinal cord. They maintained that no conscious awareness comes into play during intercourse. Yet they maintained that the use of psychotherapy and hypnosis could produce successful outcomes.

In 1982 Crasilneck reported a study of 100 men receiving hypnotherapy for psychogenic erectile dysfunction, declaring that 87 received relief and full erectile restoration. His mode of treatment was hypnotic, uncovering the root of the problem, ego strengthening and creating new self-image techniques.

What we clearly see from tantric sex training is that conscious control can be exercised over erectile function, timing, ejaculation and intensity of orgasm (Richardson, 2003). This concept, however, challenges our Western authoritarian medical system's foundation, because it empowers the client, not the clinician.

Hypnotically in treating psychogenic ED we do well to remember the formula – unconscious unknowing, conscious unknowing, conscious knowing, unconscious knowing and conscious awareness. Just like learning to walk.

VAGINISMUS

Fuchs (1980), reported in the *American Journal of Obstetrics and Gynecology* hypnotic desensitisation to help a patient with vaginismus. The strategy was based on relaxation and avoidance of anxiety. The approach taken was to use an imaginary comfortable sexual experience rehearsal strategy, during office visits with hypnosis, and to teach the patient to duplicate that during actual sex with a partner.

During the home self-hypnosis state, first a finger, then more fingers were inserted into the vagina. Then, progressive introduction of dilators of increasing sizes to stretch the vagina to get the patient used to intercourse.

Fuchs found that between 1965 and 1975, 71 women were treated with this method. Results seem high with no relapses after five years. The problem with the study was that there was no differentiation of the kinds of vaginismus the women suffered from so it was not possible to determine why failure rates occurred.

Al-Sughayir (2005) compared the success of treatment for vaginismus with hypnotic techniques versus behaviour therapy. The sample was 36 women, assigned into two groups, attending the out-patient psychiatry clinic at King Abdul-Aziz University Hospital in Riyadh, Saudi Arabia, between 1999-2003.

A female psychologist treated the women. Whilst all women eventually achieved intercourse it was found that those treated with hypnotherapy achieved results faster. Hypnotherapy was more effective in reducing the women's sex-related anxiety about intercourse. An interesting measurement taken was also the husband's level of satisfaction with intercourse, which seems to demonstrate women's position in that society.

RECOVERY FROM RAPE

Rocha (2016) recounts a case of using hypnosis and eye movement desensitisation and reprocessing (EMDR) used with a female rape and kidnapping victim, who experienced PTSD. The symptoms were panic attacks, crying, and sadness, in a climate of constant social fear.

In the first four sessions EMDR was used, and hypnosis in the second to ninth sessions to control emotional abreaction and strengthen self-esteem. The client reported a significant decrease in anxiety attacks and stress levels, along with improvements in general wellbeing, tranquility, optimism, self-esteem, and resilience. Control of PTSD was achieved.

RECOVERY FROM CHILDHOOD SEXUAL ABUSE

In Hodder-Fleming and Gow's (2005) study, participants were interviewed about triggers for memory retrieval of childhood sexual abuse during hypnosis. Participants stated that they were not triggered to remember childhood sexual abuse during hypnosis and therapy. This is contrary to some studies that cite hypnosis as potentially dangerous when treating childhood sexual abuse.

Poon (2007) reported the treating of a 33-year-old Chinese woman, who suffered affect dysregulation and chronic trauma symptoms due to childhood sexual abuse by a relative. Hypnosis was used to ground and stabilise the client. A three-phase treatment was employed, consisting of training on affect management, strengthening the ego and re-processing the trauma. The client reported a significant reduction in trauma symptoms. Later, Poon (2009) reported four cases of women treated by the same method.

ADULT SEXUAL ASSAULT

Hypnosis has been used in recovery from adult sexual assault for many years. Spiegel & Spiegel (1989) commented that auto dissociative hypnotic phenomena are used during a sexual assault as a form of defence mechanism due to the presenting trauma.

In the treatment of ensuing PTSD, hypnosis and suggestions can help the person restructure their memories and experiences. Spiegel suggests reviewing the memories with greater hypnotic control as a process of desensitisation, weakening the trigger for traumatic emotional recall in the present time. This included the use of the split screen technique.

The split screen technique is used in different ways: Firstly to put a moving picture on one side, and a still picture on the other. This can help to teach the person to deal with one part of a memory at a time, to reduce overwhelm (Leavitt, 1991). Secondly it can also be used in a comparative way with one movie of the person not coping and another with the person coping in a whole new, resourceful way.

It is often used in forensic hypnotic memory recovery techniques by playing the movie on one side and each still on the other. Slowing down a movie gives more detail to recover perceived facts about a crime.

The research into using hypnosis with rape victims is sparce to say the least. From a feminist perspective, controlled trials would be unethical. When grant money and economic power to research rape goes to men, it is another form of economic violation. Academia and clinical medicine are also male-dominated, so again it is another form of social and human rights violation. So in using hypnosis with female rape victims, it is highly recommended to involve female professionals.

The factors that interact with therapy for rape recovery are physical, mental, emotional, economic, social, familial, cultural, linguistic, religious, and legal (Asadi et al., 2023). Therapeutic techniques for cancelling trauma alone do not empower rape survivors, particularly if there are multiple incidents and further threats of rape. In fact, this strategy may put the person in further danger.

You cannot treat a female rape victim without being an educated feminist, whether you are female, male or other, because you would be violating the woman by assuming the dominant top dog position.

Is this statement radical?

No, these are feminist statements, and anti-appropriation of the rape narrative by non-feminists. Many times, I have heard hypnotists talk about curing people who suffer from rape trauma, without understanding the process of female empowerment.

Chivers-Wilson (2006) stated, "A better appreciation of the biopsychosocial repercussions of sexual assault will aid in developing a more holistic and individualised therapy to help alleviate the physical and emotional pain following the trauma of rape."

There are so many hypnotic methods to aid women recovering from trauma and PTSD, but unless they are applied from a feminist empowerment perspective, they will have limited use in helping women recover from the trauma of rape.

There is so little research on the use of hypnosis and males recovering from sexual abuse. This reflects men's and boys' fear of seeking therapy for such issues and fear of disclosure.

When males encounter sexual assault, the loss of control can be devastating to the male ego and their sense of male identity, particularly when penetrative acts have taken place. It can instill a great sense of not being safe in the world.

Men do not generally want to talk about what happened and they can bottle up their distress inside for decades. Men are expected to take care of themselves and be strong in society and the family around them. Post-assault they can have a sense of failure to protect themselves and shame that somehow they let it happen to them.

We can see the sex offender Reynhard Sinaga (Halliday, 2020) was convicted of 159 offences of drugging and assaulting men, including 136 cases of rape, in Manchester, UK, between 2015 and 2017. Police believed that he probably had more than 206 victims, many of whom they could not identify, as many did not want to come forward or be identified.

In addition, the perception of hypnosis somehow being a way of surrendering personal power to another, frightens many men who have been abused and who feel vulnerable.

In later chapters I report cases of men who successfully recovered from sexual abuse with hypnotherapy to go on and live their lives.

HYPNOSIS WITH SEX OFFENDERS

Cooney (1999) reported the use of hypnotherapy in prison groups, and probationary follow-up programs for sex offenders. The hypnotherapy seemed to be an adjunct within a counselling setting to uncover motivation for offenders to release unrecognised emotions, combined with cognitive awareness, using CBT and offence relapse prevention therapy.

One of the major problems with Cooney's paper is that it seemed to lump all sex offenders into the same category, the 'sex offender' per se. As sex therapists though, we know that sexually motivated behaviour arises due to many psychological drivers.

Aigner (2008) shows us that brain abnormalities exist in some sex offenders, but not all. Hucker and Bain (1997) report elevated androgen levels in many sex offenders, but also in violent offenders not of a sexual nature. In some sex offenders, researchers found there were associations with genetic variations (Langstrom et al., 2015).

Ward et al. (1995) proposed that sex offenders have attachment issues where they are unable to experience empathy within intimacy, thereby they objectify people as sexual objects. Social learning theory proposed that if they were sexually abused (Burton, 2003), they are more likely to be sex offenders. Considering the number of people abused as a child, these studies can likely suffer from selection bias because participants are drawn from convicted sex offenders.

I have found that no one therapy fits all in working with sex offenders. Certainly, early learning experiences and modelling can normalise sexual aggression. There are also those who came from wholesome, supportive, loving backgrounds. Therefore physiological, psychological, and sociological factors can contribute to abusive sexual behaviour. This leads me to believe that cognitive awareness alone does not change that behaviour in or out of hypnosis.

FORENSIC SEX CRIME VICTIM RECALL

Hypnosis has also been used in forensic hypnosis over the years in the investigation of rape and sexual molestation crimes (McConkey, 1987). Whilst modern surveillance and investigation techniques have made tracking criminals far more efficient, there are times when a sole witness recall can be the key to catching an offender, which can be aided by hypnosis.

There must be a warning here, however, that in most countries there are insufficient police officers (O'Connell, 2024), who are under so much pressure they often do not follow up on or take crimes of a sexual nature seriously.

Also, the witness's expectations about hypnosis can produce false memories. Hypnotically-retrieved memory can undergo challenges in court for reliability, so it should never be used as a main source of evidence, simply as a fact recall prompt, and even then, sometimes the courts reject that evidence.

We must also consider victim trauma, since the hypnotic process must take place early in the reporting of crime to give the best recall and chance of catching the sexual offender. Passing time can produce accommodating changed memories as the person tries to process the trauma.

In any such forensic hypnotic recall, the police must be involved to direct the investigation. As the hypnotist we must always put the wellbeing of the hypnotised witness over and above every other consideration.

SEX CRIME WITNESS TRAUMA

Police first responder trauma to sex crimes is a well documented and researched area, which at times leads to secondary traumatic stress (STS), lower QOL and PTSD (Bryant, 2021). This not only affects the first responder but also their families, relationships, social circles, and their own sex lives. Frontline emergency workers seem to be affected by STS and when under-treated it can lead to suicidation (WA Police Union, 2023).

Those working with internet child pornography (Catanese, 2010) and being constantly exposed to horrific abusive images and videos can begin to become cynical. They may lose empathy and begin to shut down emotionally, often becoming unavailable in relationships. Some police forces rotate those staff out of those positions, but staff shortages and the need to follow through an investigation can trap many officers in constant exposure far beyond where they are able to cope.

This STS can also affect a wide variety of medical staff and health professionals, including therapists. If you are dealing with violent sexual attacks and torture, child abuse, bestiality, or snuff pornography, it can affect you at deep unconscious levels, no matter who you are. You can lose faith in human nature, become depressed and lose interest in sex.

My own experience in dealing with fatigued police officers is that contributory factors including long working hours, high caseloads, plus the trauma, often leads to persistent depression and PTSD.

Here treatment always begins with getting the person to step away from the work, having physical and time distance from that material. Then I use hypnotic treatment to process the PTSD, and last of all we address their own sexual health issues, which have frequently been affected.

TRANSFERENCE

Transference is an issue hypnotists need to be aware and careful of when dealing with a client's issues around sex. This can be an accident and not necessarily intentional. Corey et al. (2023) discusses the issues of ethics in helping professions, warning that we must all be vigilant about what a client may bring to sessions, purposefully or accidentally.

Sex is such an intimate experience and when relief for sexual problems is achieved, it can release a high level of serotonin, endorphins and oxytocin, stimulated by thoughts of the therapist who helped the patient. Sometime clients are so pleased that they project onto that therapist a kind of hero status that can give rise to sexual attachment.

I remember one case of a man for whom I helped restore erectile function and by the third session he was telling me how sexually attractive he found me and that he fantasised about having sex with me. Gently, I explained to him what transference was, how it could occur in therapy, and how we practised clear boundaries to protect him as the client. I altered the hypnosis to steer him towards other erotic stimuli during the excitement stage of the SRC.

If this ever happens to you, document it, and take supervision immediately, so there is never any ethical confusion around what happened and what you did.

FALSE MEMORIES

One can never consider sex and hypnosis without considering false memory syndrome. The occurrence of false memories and their frequency are unpredictable. All memories are false as they serve the purposes of a present time, dominating the executive personality and subpersonalities.

It is important, particularly in hypnotic regression, to inform a client that all memories are false and reconstructions. They may be real, and they may not be, and hypnotic-induced memories are not considered reliable in court of law.

Dittburner (1993) stated that depth of amnesia is positively correlated with alien abduction and childhood abuse. I could not disagree more. Amnesia serves a purpose and screens memories to protect the executive central personality from information it is unable to process. Amnesia frequently fractures, and memories or perceived memories, may come flooding into consciousness. Consequently this releases disturbing memories of trauma from the past.

Hambleton (2002) warns us that pressure, inappropriate suggestions, and coercion from a hypnotist can produce false memories and dangerous complications as the client tries to facilitate the therapist's agenda. In regression, whilst recovering memories, we must always remain neutral, use simple, comprehendible suggestions, and facilitate in a supportive way what the client needs to disclose.

There are many reasons a person experiences amnesia for early sexual experiences. It is important for us as hypnotists to respect the executive function of their mind and allow the client to deal with only what they can tolerate at the present time.

Otgaar (2013), in investigating spontaneous memories, showed that incorrect memories can occur both in children and adults. They may be initiated by incidental sensory experience or communications, or they can be unconsciously provoked fabrications.

What is interesting about this report is that the experimenters say they were not doing any therapy but were simply using hypnotic induction and reawakening.

This demonstrates two possible phenomena. Firstly, repressed memories can emerge in hypnosis when therapeutic suggestions are not being used. For some reason that participant now believes they can handle that information and process that material, so amnesia for the events is broken.

Secondly, people produce false memories to facilitate psychological, emotional and defensive needs, for reasons they may not know consciously, and we as therapists may not know or do not have the time to observe.

In therapy, particularly sex therapy, it is paramount that we, as much as possible, continually check for congruencies of what the client is telling us, by subtle cross-questioning and observation.

A client may not intend to mislead us, tell us an incorrect history or misdescribe what has happened or is happening to them. They may, however, only be able to communicate within the bounds or the gestalts of their present perceptions.

SPONTANEOUS ABREACTIONS

Spontaneous hypnotic abreactions happen at times in therapy. Hlywa (2008) talked about spontaneous and purposeful abreactions that need to be handled with care.

Some of sex therapy is about dealing with and reliving trauma. This means that at times there is a sudden psycho-dynamic shift in the client out of their conscious awareness, and memories burst into conscious awareness. At that time, the client may be unable to understand what is happening to them and they may be confused, highly defensive and at times aggressive.

This is why I always encourage all therapists to put a safety anchor in at the beginning of all therapy to be able to trigger when this happens. Not only can it bring a client back to a sense of safety, but also continually triggering it can allow the client time to process the material that may be consciously new to them. The trauma must be resolved by the end of the session, the client taken out of trance and intra-psychic fissures where the trauma escaped into consciousness sealed.

Always ensure your client is out of the trauma state as they leave your clinic. Failure to do so can lead to psychotic decompression, when war breaks out between the subpersonalities, and the client loses major coping mechanisms, which can lead to suicidal ideation.

What can research teach us?

I have only showed a small amount and breadth here of the research around sex therapy and the use of therapeutic hypnosis together. Without doubt the research shows the long history of its use and value within clinical settings.

The soft sciences are always thwarted with pitfalls when it comes to quantitative research because, for the greater part, we are measuring subjective experiences, which cannot be statistically observed on an individual basis.

With hypnosis and sex therapy, the incidental variables are so wild and specific to the hypnotist and participant that they cannot be standardised and controlled. Every hypnotist and trance experience are different, just as the elements of every sexual experience are constantly changing.

This leaves us with qualitative reporting by hypnotists and participants themselves, and both are subject to reporter bias, and much minutiae cannot be externally measured or validated.

The breadth of that reporting is also vastly different due to varied methodologies used. Hypnotists use different inductions at different times in therapy. Many have no training in sex therapy at all, simply rely on a hypnotic cure-all technique and approach, sometimes in one single session, with no follow-up.

Many reporting hypnotists, medical and non-medical, fail to consider biofunctional disorders, order the appropriate tests or consult with other specialists. The patient is being treated for what is presumed to be psychogenic sexual dysfunction, when in fact there may be at times a biological cause to their distress.

We can certainly learn different approaches to hypnosis and sex therapy from previous reporting hypnotists. However, to do justice to the patient, an accompanying physical and biological approach can aid recovery and make the difference between success or failure.

We must use the research to defend the use of hypnosis in this area. From the hounding of Franz Anton Mesmer and Milton Erickson to the rise of the almighty pharmaceutical industry, there are always attacks on hypnosis. So, pass on the research to the colleagues you work with to validate the treatments you provide.

Having said that, research methodology supports the Western concept of reductionist medicine, with a name, pill and technique to fix all the separate human ills. This can end up with 10 unco-ordinated specialists trying to fix one specific ailment at a time, and the client carrying the burden of something always being wrong with them.

In working in sex therapy, we must remember the whole person is greater than their parts. We are not just treating one condition, but the whole person, because it is the whole person that is experiencing sex, not just their penis, vagina, breasts or any other part of their body and mind.

Briken (2020), in reporting a German study, found that 33.4% of men and 43.4% of women had one or more sexual problems in the past year. I believe the ICD 10 (2022) under-reported sexual dysfunction.

The average person with sexual health problems never seeks professional help and does not appear in the statistics. They are too embarrassed to raise the issues with healthcare professionals, or they simply deprioritise sex within their life criteria of needs.

The mass failure of sex education in society means many people are not prepared for their sex lives when they happen (United Nations, 2024). They glean their ideas about sex either from religion, pornography or the internet, none of which is generally resourceful.

What this means is sex can seem trepidatious from the outset and when things go wrong, people are terrified. Most people do not know what a sex therapist does or that there is such a professional, so they suffer in silence.

Havnevik (2023), in Norway, reported a therapy dropout rate of around 25.3%, with clients having poor social support showing a higher rate. This was in a country with universal health coverage.

When we factor in global poverty, social attitudes to sex, absence of health fund refunds or state health support, lack of practitioner experience, economic pressures, religious suppression, embarrassment around sex, and parallel psychopathology, sexual health can get neglected.

What this means is the probable dropout and absence rates for those who could benefit from sex therapy is likely much higher, and I would venture to predict more than 50%.

For us as sex therapists and hypnotists, we do well to hone our skills and make every dollar of the client's money count. There is research and training out there – enjoy it.

5 The Application of Hypnosis in Sex Therapy

For those of us who are highly trained in the application of hypnosis and use it every day in our clinical practice, we understand the power of hypnotic techniques to motivate and change clients.

That change can be physiological, psychological, behavioural, and emotional. Thousands of pieces of research and clinical evidence point to this conclusion.

Some clinicians and experimenters have the opinion that a clinician should not treat a condition with hypnosis that they cannot treat without it, which is naive. Hypnotherapy can be the variable that changes the equation and effectiveness of treatment that would not happen without its use. That is why it has been used therapeutically for thousands of years.

Furthermore, many clinicians and experimenters who simply dabble in hypnosis, and do not use it daily, often do not have the skills or experience to use it effectively.

Having said this, when it comes to the application of hypnosis to sex therapy, a clinician needs to amass a background in sex therapy to be effective. Whether you are a student or seasoned professional, you do need to have an understanding of biology, psychology and sex, not just the use of hypnosis.

We are dealing with all three elements in working with sexual health issues. As we saw earlier in this book, sexual failure is a complex dynamic with many different and sometimes concurrent causes, which need to be investigated.

If you are not medically trained, you need to be working in co-ordination with other appropriate professionals. Quite often, however, those professionals can fail to spot or understand sexual issues, so, it is important to make yourself fully conversant with the problems you are dealing with.

Research is the key. Take as much time as you can to research the condition, consider studies and make yourself familiar with the treatments that other clinicians have used.

THE SEXUAL IDENTITY HYPNOTIC CLUSTERS

Freud identified the libido energy as the biological sex drive and pleasures and positioned it as part of the id (biological driving forces). This steered sex away from moral choices towards the medical and psychological perspective. His early work was, of course, dissecting brains for the neurologist and hypnotist Charcot in Paris, which coloured his view.

The psychoanalytic perspective that libido can be blocked or tilted out of balance by various psychological complexes and syndromes also stems from Charcot's perspective that hypnotic behaviour is pathological (Freud, 1922/2010).

Sexual arousal and plateau stages of the SRC are indeed hypnotic behaviours that lead to the third stages of orgasm or ejaculation. They are hypnotic, trance-like states because there is focused concentration to the exclusion of external distraction, to a greater or lesser degree.

Where Freud's theory partly falls down is that it was specific to social attitudes of the time. The oppression of and lack of education around sex of that historical period was absent from his causation theory.

The quest of psychoanalysis is to make all the unconscious conscious as a form of cognitive awareness cure but it neglects the fact that as humans we are constantly in different trances that frequently cannot be broken by conscious, critical thinking. Those trances become behavioural and autonomous, operating with competing psychodynamic demands.

These are hypnotic clusters of concomitant trances that make up our sexual experiences including the physical, psychological, emotional, the innate sexual libido, sex education, familial and social influences, fear, joy and accumulated experiences and expectations.

Providing the physical element is working, we can begin to influence the other concomitants as sex therapists and hypnotherapists. In some cases when interference in the SRC is due to the failure of homeostasis, we may also be able to help to alter the course of physiology via hypnotic and psychotherapeutic therapy.

SEXUALITY IDENTITY MAP

Our sexual identity is both separate and connected to our general identity as a person. How we see and perceive ourselves and how others see us affects our sex drive. It creates our own personal sexual identity map.

Our sense of how happy and adjusted we are with our general physical and sexual anatomy influences our sex drive, promoting or blocking the libido. As human beings we are constantly comparing ourselves and our physiology against those we come into contact with.

Kedia (2014) reviews how we constantly judge others and compare ourselves to them. It is an automatic survival mechanism where we judge if we are in danger or if there are opportunities for food or mating:

> *'Are they bigger, smaller, more powerful, weaker, more or less classically good-looking, or more or less physically attractive?'*

This can inflate or deflate our libido and sense of physical sexual worthiness. It becomes our trance of physical sexual readiness.

Our gender identity is an accumulation of how we perceive ourselves in the male/female social continuum:

> *'Are we man enough? Woman enough? Or other enough?'*

> *'Do we have peer status, or will we be rejected for not matching up to common idealistic perceptions of gender expression?'*

> *'Do our sexual preferences match those of a potential partner?'*

> *'Do we like the same sexual practices, or will they think I'm odd or stupid and reject me?'*

Added to that are life experiences, fears and expectations that are not always conscious. Therefore, hypnotic regression is the best way to retrieve these, as it bypasses conscious, critical thinking and defence mechanisms.

Most of the time regression is not necessary and we can effect behaviour and emotional change simply by suggestion, but there are times we need to regress the person to find the root cause of the problem.

THE FRAGILITY OF SEXUAL IDENTITY

Our sexual identity is fragile and can be damaged easily by life experiences, our lack of perceived adequacy or other people's negative reactions to us.

In sex therapy we sometimes find that a single negative incident or comment by someone else has been internalised into the client's unconscious and becomes a self-fulfilling prophetic trance. The client acts it out autonomously over and over again. When the negative comment sets up a trance, the damage becomes compounded.

X said, 'I'm fat and not sexy.'

Y said, 'I had a small penis and am a wimp.'

Z said 'X made fun of my breasts.'

People don't share with others that their sense of sexual sufficiency is low. They get caught in the game of 'not wanting to be thought of as being less than'. This also happens in therapy when clients purposely withhold information.

Sakaluk et al. (2020) conducted a meta-analysis research review of the connection between self-esteem and sexual health. Not only did it find a strong association between self-esteem and sexual health, but also that those with low self-esteem may be more at risk of unsafe promiscuity.

Generally, psychiatrists, therapists and family doctors do not have the time or skills to help the client break that trance and replace it with sexual adequacy self-suggestion. Hypnotists carry out this kind of gestalt replacement fast every day in our work.

THE WILLINGNESS TO CHANGE

Of all the people I have seen with sexual problems, those who have the highest motivation to change get the best results. However, many deprioritise sex within the criteria of needs in their life journey, so do not do as well.

Some people simply have low sex drives. Others are bound up in a web of religious or social constructions around sex that causes them to ignore or suppress their sex drive.

Verrastro (2020) found that most healthcare professionals do not discuss sexual issues with service users. Most staff (86%) were found to be poorly trained and most (94%) were unlikely to discuss sexual issues with their patients. This lack of interest in and knowledge about sexual issues can demotivate service users from seeking further help.

Life pressures of trying to pay rent, mortgage, medical bills, and other financial commitments can leave people tired, drained, and exhausted. They are just trying to survive an everyday, over-stimulated industrial society. The dinosaurs we face today are the 40-hour-plus working week and lack of contact with nature, so we can remain in a constant sense of neurosis and anxiety, where we have no energy left for sex.

When a client contacts us with a willingness and desire to change, as hypnotists our first communication needs to be our first suggestion:

"Let's see what we can do for you."

People frequently ask for success rates and guarantees, neither of which we can offer because of the complexity of presentation and the need for individual treatment. Plus, in many places such a statement would be illegal.

THE INFLUENCE OF CO-PATHOLOGIES

As mentioned earlier there tends to be a much higher level of mental and emotional disturbance in those presenting themselves for sex therapy. People who experience sexual insufficiency can become anxious, depressed, aggressive, angry, self-destructive, and even suicidal.

Defar (2023) found those with mental illness experience declining health-related quality of life. A feedback loop of negative mental experience and negative sexual experience can pull people into an ever-increasing trance of unhappiness, reducing their health-related quality of life (HRQOL).

In sex therapy we frequently find underlying mental and emotional problems that need to be treated.

THE USE OF HYPNOTIC PHENOMENA

Hypnotic phenomena such as artificial somnambulism, dis-association, catalepsy, arm levitation, positive and negative hallucination, anaesthesia, analgesia, hypersensitivity, hypo-sensitivity, amnesia, hypermnesia, regression, and time distor-tion are essential abilities for hypnotists. This is alongside the ability to produce altered physical functioning and emotional and mental states (Erickson, 1980).

These phenomena are not in themselves treatments but they support and accelerate treatment objectives, as well as at times being used as validators of the trance state.

It is important not to use them indiscriminately to exhibit hypnotic prowess. They are powerful and should be used with caution, as the client needs to feel assisted, not dominated, which could cause a defence mechanism to kick in and give rise to resistance.

These hypnotic phenomena must also always be attributed to the client's unconscious ability and power. This way we are re-enforcing self-efficacy. I would say something like: "See how clever and powerful your unconscious mind is in the way it can hold your hand in midair like that for 10 minutes. Isn't that amazing? And of course, that very smart unconscious of yours can also help you in enjoying good sex."

We all owe a great deal to Milton Erickson (Rossi et al., 2010) for his breadth of research and work in hypnotic phenomena and its use in medical hypnosis and psychotherapy.

THE HYPNOTIST'S DELUSION AROUND DIRECT SUGGESTION

Unfortunately, too many hypnosis schools teach a few inductions, and then provide a series of scripts for the client's problems. Ultimately this fails a great deal of the time.

Let us go back to Hull (2002) and his hypnotic recordings that people sat and listened to go into trance, which contained only direct suggestions. This was very much in the vein of Charcot's authoritarian style.

Direct suggestions do have a use in self-help programs. They can succeed some of the time, but in sex therapy, the problems are more complex, being physical, psychological, emotional and even social.

Therefore, complex approaches are needed because we may be activating several corrections all at the same time. Sex therapy needs multiple foci.

It is clear Erickson understood this, and did not do just hypnosis, but did hypno-psychotherapy. What most people see when they watch videos of Erickson is an older man dispensing sage advice. If you look more carefully, however, you see that he is constantly monitoring the client, and with that information, formulating individual psychodynamic treatments that are delivered by hypnotherapy.

To use hypnosis in sex therapy we first need to be a sexual dysfunction problem solver.

INVOLVING PARTNERS IN SEX THERAPY

Most people turn up for therapy for sexual health issues alone. They are frequently too embarrassed to bring their partner along with them. At times they do not even disclose to their partner that they are having therapy for those issues.

There is a popular idea in sex therapy that the partners should be present to create a supportive sexual environment between them, but it is just that – a popular idea. For most clients, solo therapy is what is needed.

When both partners are in the room, intra-relationship issues and conflicts can spill over into the session, putting the client into resistance, where rapport can be lost. In fact, at times, it can make the situation worse for the client, as the session turns into couples therapy.

In some cases, the partner's behaviour may be a part of the problem that pushes the client into sexual dysfunction. The partner can also try to use the material from the session as leverage at home to negotiate for their nonsexual needs.

Sadikaj (2016) notes that over-dominant behaviour in partnerships can lead to low quality of relationships. This also follows through in the therapy room and can affect the quality of therapy and its outcomes.

If there are times when I do think about having the partner invited into one of the client's sessions, I will suggest it, but I never force the issue.

PATIENT COMPLIANCE

Patient compliance is vital and without it, results will not happen. Life gets in the way of people's dedication to homework or following through with medical tests and other activities.

When elements of treatment are missed out and neglected, or people do not turn up for their appointment, treatment failure occurs.

I say to clients, "I'm happy to help you and you will need to follow everything I ask you to do. Do we have an agreement?"

In the public health system, there is a much higher rate of people simply not turning up for appointments (Byrne, 2021). They forget, become unmotivated, or deprioritise the need for help.

In private practice I only take clients with sexual health problems on packages because I want to know that they are doing the work I ask of them, and that the person is committed to moving forward. They get reminders and cannot change their appointments less than seven days in advance. If they miss an appointment, they are charged for it, and if they miss two appointments, they lose all their credits. This system has given me maximum client compliance and better treatment outcomes. Money motivates, but the fear of losing money motivates more.

Remember, hypnosis is about suggested compliance. Our job as hypnotists is to do everything to get clients to comply with those suggestions. What it also does is guarantee that the client has the funds to continue treatment through to resolution.

DROPOUT RATES

Willis (2020) found a dropout rate of 20.6% in couples therapy. Hanevik (2023) reported a dropout rate of therapy around 25.3%, with older clients more likely to stay in therapy, along with people who have had access to higher education and have social support.

Because there is a higher level of mental health issues in sex therapy, the dropout rates are higher, although no one has really reported any study that gives clear indications.

My own experience is that dropout rates can be high if the therapist is not managing the patients.

Reasons for dropout:

- Mental difficulties
- Physical illnesses
- Addiction
- Unstable family and social support
- Economic instability
- Poor time management
- Unrealistic expectations of what therapy can provide
- Interference in therapy by partner and family
- Failure to carry out tasks between sessions
- Other professionals making disparaging remarks about hypnosis

Therapists must proactively employ strategies to reduce dropout rates, not just in sex therapy, but also in all the work we do.

FAILURE RATE

Here we have to address both the areas of hypnosis and sex therapy. Failure rate in hypnotherapy is such an interesting calculation to consider in both clinical and experimental hypnosis.

First, experimental hypnosis takes place in different circumstances from clinical applications. It tends to be prescriptive to control the variables, and for most of the time, cannot be applicable to clinical work.

In clinical work as hypnotherapists, we allow unexpected variables and deal with them as they arise. We may even paradoxically utilise them as they arise to tailor the hypnotherapy to that individual client. This way we reduce failure of hypnosis and hypnotherapy. Therefore the success rates of the hypnotherapy part of our treatment of psychogenic problems can be high.

Lazar (2011) looked at the variables that promoted hypnotic and hypnotherapeutic failure techniques, strategies or the therapist's reactions that are inappropriate for that treatment. Today we tend to talk more about what techniques we can use to achieve therapeutic goals rather than about a dichotomous success or failure rate.

The same cannot be said for sex therapy as many sexually dysfunctional clients have physical problems beyond the scope of hypnotherapy, even though they think hypnosis might fix them.

Sex therapy in and of itself often fails for the reasons stated in the previous section. By the time we see people seeking hypnosis for sexual difficulties they have often already been to several healthcare professionals who could not help them. They can arrive with the underlying belief that this is just another therapy that will fail. They have become professional patients who know so much about their failures and are buying into the gestalt that they cannot be fixed.

To avoid high failure rates, it is necessary to screen clients carefully to assess whether the problem is truly psychological. I do not accept most clients who approach me for hypnosis and sex therapy if it is clear to me the problem is beyond hypnosis, or if they are not prepared to undergo physical treatment if necessary.

If you are not a nurse, doctor or naturopath, you need to refer the physical aspects of treatment to the appropriate professionals, and you can never ignore their presence. Whilst in this book I present some of my successful cases, there were 10 times more people I did not accept for hypnosis and sex therapy.

THE USE OF THE TANTRA

Sex in the Western world has been commercialised. Hu (2020) looks at how sex has been used in advertising to move product. This pervades every part of our lives, so we become over-saturated and disconnected from the intimacy and beauty of sexual interactions.

In many cultures, sex has been demonised. And in some cultures, talking about sex is not permitted. Where the client lives, and their cultural norms will determine what hypnotic suggestions they will accept.

Just like fast food, many people attempt to have fast sex that can be unsatisfying and dysfunctional. Here I am not talking about a sudden, hormone-driven liaison or the passions of youth. What I am alluding to is the time-poor and attention-starved average person who finds survival in a modern world stressful.

Sexual experiences change for people over time, and relationships change too. Nothing is static, nothing stays the same, including sex. For clients to enjoy a good sex life, we need to be teachers of sex, so the client can follow the basic ways of the Tantra.

In the Western world people's goal of sex is ejaculation for men and the illusive orgasm for many women. Sex needs to be much more and be a way of deeply connecting with the other person. In the Eastern yogic Tantric tradition, the goal of sex is connection. It is the weaving of the many elements of attention, focus and pleasure during sex (the word 'Tantra' in Sanskrit means 'to weave together.'). Some gurus refer to Tantra as the technology of living, thereby the technology of how to do sex satisfactorily.

Sex takes time and consideration, not discounting a quicky with your lover. There is a difference, however, between hurried sex and putting time to one side to make love with your partner. It is about taking time to connect, talk, play, kiss, stroke, fondle, play games, worship, be adventurous, be adored and have fun during that special space put aside for sex and lovemaking.

It is about relaxing together so each partner feels safe, worthy, special, unhurried and that their needs are met too. Sex lasts longer when there are intermittent periods of relaxation to facilitate multiple orgasms and orgasms without ejaculation.

Part of being a sex therapist is teaching people how to breathe during sex and to control their flow of energy. None of us are born with the skills of a seasoned lover, we simply emerge from the womb with a libido.

We have a huge advantage here as hypnotists in that we already deal in altered states of awareness, self-efficacy and expectations.

I do give a warning here as there are people teaching Tantra, who whilst they acknowledge the anima and animus in all of us, only teach a male/female binary model of sexual correctness. There are even practitioners who see nipple play, attention on the clitoris or even orgasm as a distraction from the goal of connection.

THE SEX THERAPY CONTRACT

We are in an age of nuisance lawsuits, complaint boards, the Me Too movement, and a vicious media that uses any story it can as clickbait. Any complaint against you by a client does not need to be true or valid to ruin your career.

When a complaint is made of a sexual nature, government officials can sell that information to the media and do. I have seen this happen several times with practitioners. Gossip and sex stories sell. The media only has to say 'alleged complaints' in an article to make a lot of money out of online advertising and clickbait.

People coming to see us with sexual issues are often deeply afraid and at times paranoid. It is possible they may misinterpret your intentions and the course of the therapy.

For these reasons I advise practitioners to have a special sex therapy contract, separate from your ordinary therapeutic contract, which states you will be helping the client with sexual health issues. The client signs the contract, declaring that they are fully aware therapy will involve dealing with sexual issues and that the therapist will be giving hypnotic suggestions of a sexual nature (You can download a sample form from the Resources section at the back of this book).

Then the client gets a copy of that contract. This is to keep both the client and the therapist safe and everyone fully informed of what will take place in therapy (O'Keefe, 2008).

Many therapists think they should not use contracts as they break rapport and trust, when in fact it creates transparency. Not to do so in sex therapy puts your client, you, your business, reputation, and your family at risk of potential legal actions.

SAFE SEX

Whilst advising safe sex may seem obvious in helping clients with their sex lives, most clinicians never mention the need. There are different reasons for this happening.

The clinician may be too embarrassed and do not think it is their job to get into such intimate details during consultations. They may have religious beliefs that they presume the client shares about no sex before marriage and prohibition on adultery.

The client often does not disclose that they are having unsafe sex and not using condoms or dental dams when having non-partner sex. They purposefully withhold that information from the therapist.

There are clients who are not educated about the dangers of STI transmission including HIV, chlamydia, antibiotic-resistant gonorrhea or syphilis. This can often be the case with people who are takingly PrEP: they can be deluded that because HIV transmission becomes low, their sexual activities are safe.

It is our duty in helping people with sexual issues that we do have these detailed conversations with clients. Infection can lead to sterility and, in some cases, death.

Garcia (2023) reviewed guidelines for clinicians in tackling the issues of STIs with patients and clients. It is essential for those involved in using hypnosis and sexual health problems to understand these guidelines.

LEGAL SITUATION

Your legal situation as a therapist depends on where you practise. In different countries, states, and cultures, there are various laws around providing therapy and discussing sex-related issues with your clients. The same situation exists with hypnosis, hypnotherapy, and psychotherapy. So, we must be careful around practising legally.

For instance, in Iran it can be difficult to provide advice around birth control and safe sex. In Indonesia a therapist must be careful in giving advice because the client could be arrested for breaking the morality law. In Texas and red neck states in the US, advocating for clients on trans issues as a therapist can lead to you being attacked by the local community. In the US certain states have licensing laws for practitioners to be able carry out therapy. In France some uninformed medics are still trying to frame hypnosis as potentially hazardous, which is left over from the banishment of Mesmer.

In my state of New South Wales, Australia, psychotherapists, hypnotherapists, naturopaths and sex therapists must abide by the guidelines of the Health Care Complaints Commission (2023). I have known therapists be struck off because the Commission did not think their sex advice was efficacious.

Whilst you may have practice insurance, the regular habit of insurance companies is to make a payment out to the client rather than support a legal battle to clear your name of wrongdoing.

According to Walker (2011) there has been clear evidence that large, highly profitable pharmaceutical companies have invested in attacking non-allopathic medicine and therapies. The profits of drug companies run into the hundreds of billions. In 2023, industry body The Pharmaceutical Research and Manufacturers of America (PhRMA) and two other organisations launched a lawsuit against the US government to defend their profits (Wingrove, 2023) by blocking the enforcement of a program that gives Medicare the power to negotiate drug prices. We can see how a patient might be coerced into taking drugs for sexual health problems when therapy may be more suitable for that case.

FULL DISCLOSURE AROUND THE USE OF HYPNOSIS IN SEX THERAPY

Hypnosis, in and of itself, is not a treatment for sexual health problems. Unfortunately, many hypnotists lead clients to believe that is the case. This is misleading and an indication that the therapist does not understand sex therapy.

There is also no one sex therapy. Researchers including Assalian (2013) have positioned it as behavioural and cognitive as well as psychodynamic and educational intervention, underpinned by medical investigation. I have found it useful to scavenge techniques from medicine, psychotherapy, cultural sexual practices, sex workers, and my own life experience of having had a large amount of sex with both men and women.

Just as hypnotists collect different kinds of hypnotic techniques, so do sex therapists. This means the kind of sex therapy you practise is dependent on your collected studies, knowledge, skills, and experience.

I further have never been coy about self-disclosure with clients. To be so would give the impression that I do not think of sex as something quite natural and wholesome.

Your unconscious communication discloses to the client your attitude towards sex. The client's unconscious picks up all those signals, influencing the outcomes of your hypnotically applied treatments.

RECORD KEEPING

Where I practise, we must legally keep a patient's record for 15 years, and if we die, these records must be securely preserved until the time expires.

Some practitioners choose not to keep their client records electronically and still use paper. Data breaches are standard in most medical record systems today (Seh, 2020). Hackers can hold data to ransom and if you find they have all your clients' records, you may have to pay a large fee to unlock that data. You must also inform the client there has been a security breach and must inform every past client and patient. Plus, legally you can be prosecuted for not keeping the records safe.

We find ourselves in a bind of having to keep those records secure, and managing the financial cost of doing that, which can be considerable if you are in private practice.

People come to me with the deepest private sexual health issues that they would never wish other people to know about. In a breach of data, the press will pay high fees for those records. When someone is well known, that fee can be even greater. That information being published can ruin our client's life.

Sometimes clients ask me to write court reports about the problems they experienced and for which they have been treated. Here it is essential to redact all information that is not relevant to the case. My records may even be subpoenaed and again I heavily redact. The law has no business digging for information on clients that is not specific to a particular legal case.

LEGAL REPORTING OBLIGATION

This is always a gray area. Certainly, if a child, animal, or other person is being sexually, physically, or mentally abused, we may be required by law to report this to the local authority. The definition of abuse is, however, different in all parts of the world so we must deal with different legal consequences.

We must refer to our professional codes of practice but also consider the moral obligations we have to the clients and those who may be being abused.

In cases of historical rape or abuse that is not presently happening, we must be careful about whether we have any reporting obligations at all. This is particularly relevant when disclosing may put the client or the abused person in danger.

At times we walk a fine line between client care, legal and moral obligations, and protection of our practice. Whilst supervision is useful, we also must be careful that any disclosure does not put our supervisor in danger.

Grace (2020) reviews the, at times, highly complex task of psychologists making moral decisions in therapy. And there can be times when those moral decisions are not strictly in line with the law, particularly when the law is out of date or oppressive of human rights.

6   Absence of Sexual Desire

In looking at the absence of sexual desire, we must first differentiate libido from lust.

Libido is the physiological driving force to create, seek and engage in sexual experiences. This is a biological driver like hunger, thirst, and the urge to seek safety.

Sexual desire, often referred to as lust, is driven by psychological, emotional, social, and cultural quests for sexual fulfilment (Calabrò et al., 2019).

The two are not the same. They may be present simultaneously, but not necessarily. As both individually drive the need for sex, one can exist when the other is not present.

People are physically driven by their libido to have sex, even when cultural and psychological governors kill their sexual desire by framing it as wrong and forbidden. Others with low testosterone or Androgen Insensitivity Syndrome (AIS) can have a high and persistent desire for sex, whilst not having high testosterone-driven libidos.

We must be careful of not entering into theoretical exclusivity here in presuming both must be present for the sex drive to be activated.

There are people who have no or low sexual libido or desire for a myriad of physiological and psychological reasons at different times of their lives, or for the whole of their lives. There are also those who make a conscious choice to be asexual, not engaging in sexual activity at all.

It is important, in males particularly, to distinguish between an absence of the desire for sex and the inability to experience penile arousal. Some people who do not want sex may still experience libido, but it does not translate into sexual activity. Others may have the absence of libido and desire.

Whilst Frankenbach (2022) found that males have a greater sex drive than females, this cannot be applied universally. The complexity of sex drive, much of which we still do not understand, means that we must consider every individual according to their physiological, endocrinological, psychological, emotional, experiential, sociological, spiritual, and historical parameters.

Fereydooni (2022) clinically trialled the use of cognitive hypnosis at the Babolsar Eltiam psychological clinic in Iran with 11 women who complained of low sexual desire, over 11 sessions, each lasting 90 minutes. The participants were measured against a control group who received no intervention on the Sex Desire Scale and Enrich Marital Satisfaction Scale. The experimental group reported a marked increased level of sexual and marital satisfaction.

Hypnotic suggestion and psychodynamic development can only activate the kind of sex drive that the body and the unconscious mind allows or is capable of initiating.

Whilst with hypnotherapy we can activate certain psychological processes, as well as physiological functions, we must be careful not to raise a client's false hopes. Framing sexual expectations as an absolute can give rise to shaming, guilt and pathologisation around the absence of sexual competency. Whilst for most of us sexuality is an integral part of health and wellbeing, it is not the case for everyone.

CASE STUDY: MARIA

Maria: "I'm 42, been married for three years and I've have never had sex."

Tracie: "And why do you think that is?"

Maria: "I just don't want sex. I've never wanted sex. I didn't promise him sex when we got married and he's now very angry. I'm Roman Catholic so can't get divorced, but I'm fed-up with his complaining."

Tracie: "Thank you for telling me that information Maria. I'm a little confused (transderivational search by proxy) to begin with what do you want from therapy? Wondering what you want from coming here today."

Maria: "I don't know. You're the therapist (resistance to engaging in self-reflection). What should I do?"

Tracie: "Well as a Catholic, do you remember your wedding ceremony and the priest talking (using her religion to activate transderivational search) about the union of a man and woman? What do you think that means? Are you aware, procreation is part of the Catholic marriage contract?" (interrogative overload)

Maria: "I know that, but I don't feel like it. My mother told me 'Don't do it if you don't have to?'" (spontaneous regression)

Tracie: "Well you're here so your mother must have had sex at least once. You tell me you have four brothers and two sisters, so that makes a minimum of seven times. If she didn't like sex that much, you as the last child, wouldn't have been born (challenging her mother's statement). If you've never had sex, how do you know you don't like it? Why did you get married? What is it about sex you don't like?" (interrogative overloading)

Maria: "I lived with my mother, and she died. The house was sold, and I didn't have anywhere to live. He asked me to marry him, and I said yes."

Tracie: "You're telling me four things. Firstly, you deceived your husband when you married him by not intending to have sex. Secondly, you say you're a good Catholic, but you're breaking the Catholic marriage contract. Thirdly your mother told you not to have sex, but she had seven children. And finally, you say you don't like sex, but you have never tried it. (Challenging her incongruency). What do you want from therapy?"

If we fail to challenge our client's incongruencies and delusions, we reinforce their false reality and compound their problems.

Maria: "I want you to help me stop my husband asking for sex."

Tracie: "That would be unethical of me. He's not my patient. I would be supporting you breaking your marriage vows. And I would be confirming your mother's silly statement, 'Don't do sex unless you have to'. She may have loved you, but that was a terrible thing to tell a young woman. It was destructive. It really hurt you and prevented you

seeing sex as a natural and enjoyable activity for
a husband and wife. If you want help with sex for
you, that I can help you with. Or if you want help
dealing with your husband, that I can help you
with." (Hobson's choice)

The session ended there after one hour. I cut the session short and sent her away for a month to think about what I had said to her. Also, to talk to her priest and tell him what I had said and then she returned for the second session.

Tracie: "So what have you decided over the past month?"

Maria: "I suppose I might try sex once to see what it's like."

She has now given permission to engage in sex therapy, indicating she has reconsidered her mother's advice.

Her sexual identity clusters were due to what her mother told her, being a good girl, not risking being a bad girl by having sex, not taking a risk and having sex, not seeing herself as a sexual woman, lying is okay to get out of sex and she had an association between sex and danger.

Trance intentions

1. Artificial somnambulistic trance induction.
2. Lowering her resistance to sex.
3. Connecting her to her physical body.
4. Allowing her religious virtue by having sex.
5. Associating sex with affection.
6. Maturing her self-image to being a sexual woman.
7. Desensitising her to sexual experiences.
8. Teaching her to build physical sexual pleasure.

Now I don't want you to do sex too soon (she will have sex at some stage but not immediately, allowing limited resistance)... in fact I absolutely don't want you to do sex until you... **educate yourself about sex** (direct suggestion for sex education, inferred suggestion that at some point she will have sex)...**you learn sex like you learn to drive** (simile suggestion) ...you're going to read some books on sex (post-hypnotic suggestion)...instruction manuals just like you read computer manuals (normalising sex education)...**and as you become more knowledgeable and confident** (contingent suggestion)...you know what you're doing during sex (putting control in her hands)...you know when and how you will make love (associating sex with affection)...**try small things to begin with like petting and fondling** (chunking down to make it easier)...close your eyes and go inside and relax (official trance induction)...it's clear your husband finds you very attractive (playing to her self-worth)...it's clear he wants to make love to you (associating sex with her being desirable)... **take things slowly** (giving her control)...just focus on enjoying being beautiful and desired...you create that feeling within you in your mind (Ki+, emotive driver)...seeing yourself as a full woman (Vi+, indirect suggestion for sexual maturity)... saying to yourself...**I'm beautiful...I am sexually desirable... I'm Aphrodite** (Ai+, self-affirmations, building sexual self-esteem)...as a woman it's nice to experience those thoughts and feel good (attaching Ki+ to the affirmations, mind mechanics)... **they make you feel special** (Ki+, post-hypnotic suggestion)... slowly each time you try sex a little more (presupposition there will be many times)...of course this is all in the Catholic code (enlisting the superego)...**doing what is perfectly natural for a man and woman**...sex being a gift from God (using her religious adherence to override her mother's negative messages around sex)...the body is sacred and revered...**with all its pleasures** (indirect suggestion to include sex in pleasures)...a pleasurable touch on your skin (Ke+, silent suggestion)...stroking your nipples...a touch on your clitoris (desensitising her to sexual and erotic experiences)...**you can enjoy those good things** (permissive suggestion to enjoy sexual experiences)...it's okay to have good sexual experiences (deprogramming imbibed negative messages about sex, giving her permission to enjoy sex)...even the smallest pleasure can be good (throwing the net wide to catch small pleasures)...**each pleasure can add to the next** (stacking sexual pleasure, fractionation)...you and your husband creating your marriage (buying into the Catholic commitment)...just as God intended a man and woman to enjoy (using religion as a lever for change)...just as god intended you to enjoy...seeing (Vi+)...hearing Ai+)...feeling (Ki+ & Ke+), (initiating physical pleasure and connection to her body)...**yourself as a beautiful happy sexual woman** (direct suggestion for change)

Maria reported that she had never had a libido. Her blood tests also showed elevated luteinising hormone and sex binding globulin hormone, indicating perimenopause. She had not married for love, but because her mother had died, the house was sold, the proceeds were distributed between all the offspring, and she had nowhere to live.

Her mother's negative attitude towards sex and her comments about not doing it unless you had to also served to suppress Maria's libido and install a governor that prohibited sexual excitement. The way to create sexual desire from within her was to find the levers that bypassed that anti-sex governor, such as Catholic commitment, keeping her marriage together.

This was then co-ordinated with remapping her self-perceptions to become a sexual woman by using her religious beliefs to cause a behavioural adjustment (see Appendix A, item 1).

She and her husband made an agreement to have sex once a month. When asked how it was for her, she said, "It's not too bad and okay sometimes." That was what she could experience, so that was the end of therapy as she had adjusted to her marriage.

CASE STUDY: KIJANI

This was a 30-year-old PTSD survivor who had lost most of his family when young and been brought up in an orphanage. He was an immigrant, working in a government facility. English was his second language.

Tracie: *"Tell me Kijani, how can we help you?"*

Kijani: *"I've to check everything twice, sometimes three times. I had to do that, so they don't shoot me. They shoot anyone you know. They were good people in the orphanage, but once someone came to shoot us there, and I hid under the bed."*

Tracie: *"Thank you for telling me and that must have been very scary for you as a child."*

Kijani: *"Sometimes at night I think the soldiers will come and shoot. If they shoot me, I won't feel it."*

Tracie: *"You've been through a lot in your life (acknowledging his distress)...it must have been very frightening for the children...you're safe now today (time-specific safety anchor)...here...you're safe now in my office (locational-specific safety anchor)...you're safe...when you hear my voice in your mind...always." (re-enforcing the safety anchors, global suggestion)*

It was clear Kijani had complex PTSD. He had counselling through the refugee services when coming into the country as a political refugee. He did not understand his PTSD at that time as he was still running towards a better life. He had also spent three years in a brutal detention centre for arrivals while applying for political asylum.

Kijani: "I won't feel it. I won't feel anything. If I hit my hand with hammer, I don't feel it. There's a woman from my country. I want to marry her. I can't feel sex for her."

Tracie: "Have you felt sex for anyone else?"

Kijani: "I don't feel."

As far back as hypnotist Pierre Janet (Craparo, 2019) in the 19th and 20th century, his theory of trauma-induced dissociation enlightens us. But we must be careful here, in using the theory, not to get drawn into overly protracted psychoanalysis.

We also now consider the fight/flight response as extended to include the freeze response (Noordewier, 2020), where dissociation often occurs in response to perceived physical, psychological and social threats. A person uses a defence mechanism to buffer against trauma, psychologically and emotionally, by leaving their body as they shut down. This can lead to psychosomatic self-induced anaesthesia, the blocking and reduction of neurological sensations, emotional unavailability, and the cancellation of the sex response cycle (Bird, 2021).

PTSD is a continuous, repetitive self-retraumatisation by recalling psychological, emotional, and physical traumas, creating prolonged dissociation. For some people this includes episodic or continuous anxiety, anaesthesia, catalepsy, hysterical paralysis, and derealisation. Whilst it is a protective self-defence mechanism against attack, unless processed, the person can remain in a state of dissociation permanently.

> Tracie: *"Would you like to feel? Would that be okay for you to feel sex? Ca c'est bien (is that good)? Tu sais ce sentiment que parfois le sexe est autorisé (You know that feeling sex sometimes is allowed)?"* (bombardment questions, confusion, language change [his dead mother, who he adored and who he lived with before his trauma, was French], the language change creates regression to a safer time, trance induction)

He has already indicated, "I can't feel sex for her", meaning he wants to feel sex.

> Kijani: *"Are you trying to hypnotise me?"*

> Tracie: *"Who said I was only trying (ratifying an altered state)…you're sitting safe in my office and… you came to me for help…you came to me for hypnosis…**I help people with safe sex feelings** (establishing authority, two statements and an indirect suggestion, fractionating the safety anchor)…I also help people overcome childhood trauma…so we have work to do (creating an alliance)…**let's begin as my fees are expensive** (call to action)…and you want as much as you can get for your money (leverage)…**close your eyes…** there is a good woman waiting for you…you're lucky (disrupting self-victimisation)…let's not keep her waiting"* (motivation)

I first treated him for PTSD over four months. In most cases it is pointless trying to treat a sex problem when the PTSD is still vehemently active as it will interfere with the sex therapy. Part of the work was reassociating him into his body, and only then did we begin to do sex therapy, or so he thought.

I used Kijani's OCD to help him become diligent in his therapeutic actions, a form of paradoxical redirection of symptoms.

His sexual identity clusters were attached to his PTSD. He remained in a constant state of alert, alarm, fear, and dissociation. He associated sex and physical sensations with letting down his guard and being vulnerable, so his sense of sexual development had been halted.

Trance intentions

1. Creating self-efficacy.
2. Arm levitation induction for open eye artificial somnambulism.
3. Trance ratification.
4. Memory recall for kinaesthetic resources.
5. Validating autonomic functions.
6. Reassociation to sexual feeling in his body.

You have come such a long way in your life (distancing from his original country and past trauma, locational disassociation)...a hero of your own journey (acknowledging successful survival)...you know my office is safe (locational safety anchor, Ki+)...**concentrate on your right hand and look at it** (law of focused attention, instant artificial somnambulism)...just your right hand...every time you breathe in...a little bit of air comes underneath the right hand...**and it slowly lifts into the air** (intra-hypnotic suggestion)…one breath at a time (chunking, arm levitation)…a little higher each time (4 to 5 minutes silence whilst we watch the hand rise)….**that's right your unconscious mind knows what to do** (somnambulistic trance ratification)… just let it happen (instruction to the whole mind)…you know what to do…**now it's eye level you can let it rest in mid air and look at it** (catalepsy)…you can know that is one of the hands that helped you grow up… one of the hands that helped you get to my office (acknowledging his survival mechanism)…**that hand felt when it rang the telephone number for my office** (stacking memories of feeling in the hand)…your unconscious mind can remember…you know how to feel…you know how to feel the ground beneath your feet…and put one foot in front of the other when you walk (drawing attention to and validating autonomic function)…**you know how to feel safety in my office** (fractionating the safety anchor)…it's safe to feel other parts of your body too whilst you are in a trance (maintaining artificial somnambulism, allowing him to reassociate into his body whilst the fight/flight/freeze response is cancelled by the safety anchor and hypnotic state)…**you will feel in any part of your body when you want to** (direct suggestion)…that good woman is waiting for you to have a good life (leverage)…**you will have a good sex feeling in your body** (direct suggestion, post-hypnotic suggestion for reassociation)…will you wake up first or your hand? (trance ratification)

In my book *Inspiration for Survive and Prosper* (O'Keefe, 2013) I talk about how trauma recovery has three stages: survival, transformation and prosper. Dissociation is linked to being stuck in the survival stage, and our job as hypnotists is moving the client forward to transformation, then to living in prosperity, living the full life experience in the body and mind.

Hypnotically, working with instant artificial somnambulism allows us to talk to both the unconscious mind and conscious awareness at the same time during reassociation. Inducing catalepsy cancels the ability of the body to enter the fight or flight response. Memory retrieval of physical competence allowed Kijani's unconscious mind to bear witness that he did feel and that it was safe to do so, making the freeze response redundant. Therefore, his unconscious mind was forced to renegotiate the perception that he had no feeling.

As part of physical reassociation into the body for a traumatised person, the unconscious mind is always forced into unconscious parts negotiation, integration and resolution. We were cancelling the autosuggested disassociation, PTSD-induced anaesthesia and nerve-blocking (see Appendix A, item 2).

Kijani was instructed to journal every day all his physical activities and what he had felt in order to perform tasks. Over four further sessions he was able to accept that he did feel, and it was safe to do so, even around sexual desire and pleasure. The couple got married and he carried on with his life, including a sex life.

CASE STUDY: NORMA

When I asked 36-year-old Norma, of Asian descent, on the telephone, at the time of booking, if she saw any other healthcare professionals, she told me she was regularly seeing a psychiatrist. For professional courtesy and legal compliance, I asked for a referral from her psychiatrist.

Her history was one of being diagnosed as schizophrenic when she was 13 years old, constantly in and out of psychiatric wards, and heavily medicated with antipsychotics. Only when she was 35 was she finally diagnosed with polycystic ovary syndrome (PCOS), and extremely high levels of testosterone and cortisol (Doretto, 2020).

No other previous healthcare professional had tested her before her new family doctor, but it was clear from her constant acne, facial and back hirsutism, and obesity that she was hormonally dysregulated (Shamim et al., 2022). She was started on metformin and spironolactone through her GP to regulate glucose metabolism and testosterone, and her psychosis receded. It was clear she had been misdiagnosed for over two decades, but unfortunately it was hard for her to come off the antipsychotics and the psychiatrist did not want her to do so.

In many cases obesity reduces the sex drive (Abdelsamea, 2023) as high adipose tissue produces excess oestrogen which suppresses testosterone. Testosterone and oestrogen regulation increases and decreases the sex drive in women (Cappelletti & Wallen, 2016). However, Montejo (2021) shows that antipsychotics can cause sexual dysfunction regardless of hormone levels.

Norma reported she had never had a sex drive, which, with her medical history and medication issues, was hardly surprising. Over the past year she had lost 30 kilos, her acne had subdued but not cleared due to her fast-food diet, and she now thought she should a have sex drive. She was practising restricted eating.

> Norma: *"You see, I've never had sex. I never felt like it. It's been so hard coping with everything. I hate being on antipsychotics. It's like I'm living in a goldfish bowl. I want to come off them."*

> Tracie: *"I hear you Norma (few professionals had really listened to her). I can see it has been hard for you.*

You've pushed through a lot and come through it all." (time shifting, the reduction of problems by ego strengthening her ability to overcome her difficulties)

Norma: *"I just want to be normal like everyone else and have a boyfriend."*

Tracie: *"That sounds reasonable, but for the moment, I would rather you focused on taking special care of yourself...**you know you deserve that don't you** (interrogative suggestion)...I think we really must get the PCOS totally under control to begin with. Are you up for that?"*

Norma: *"If that would help me, I'll do it. My sister will help me. She always does."*

Since a relative (her sister, who had no mental health issues, and was paying her fees) was available, we could make a treatment plan that was likely to succeed.

1. I put her on a strict wholefood plant-based diet, 70% raw.
2. Do not eat after 6.00pm.
3. Since she lived on welfare benefits, she was able to get a cheap membership at her local authority gym for three visits a week at 6.00am, and shopped at the local market.
4. Every day she had two green smoothies with cinnamon which helps regulate glucose.
5. Multi vitamin daily.
6. B complex daily.
7. B3 500mgs 2 x a day.
8. Vitamin C 1000mg 2 x a day.

9. Vitamin D 5000iu 3 x a week.
10. Vitamin E 400iu 3 x a week.
11. Vitamin B12 5000mgs 1 x a week.
12. Nicotinamide adenine dinucleotide (NAD) 250 mgs mornings.
13. Lithium orotate 10mg 2 x a day.
14. Gymnem sylvestre leaf 600mgs daily.
15. Turmeric 1000mgs a day.
16. Magnesium 250 mgs at night three times a week
17. Probiotic (*L. reuteri* DSM 17938 and *L. reuteri* ATCC PTA 6475) daily.
18. Flaxseed oil daily.
19. Attending a community centre 3 x week.
20. Sleep 9 hours per night.
21. Go to bed at the same time every day as it gets dark, and get up at the same time.
22. No caffeine, alcohol, smoking, or recreational drugs.
23. Daily hypnosis on a weight loss program.

The sister, who she lived with, organised and maintained the whole schedule. In fact, what happened would not have been possible without the dedicated care of the sister. Reluctantly the psychiatrist agreed to slowly withdraw her from antipsychotics over a period of six months. In the end he was so resistant that she changed psychiatrists.

One year later she had lost a further 40 kilos, with no acne, was off antipsychotic medication, and her testosterone and cortisol were down to normal ranges. We tried her off the lithium orotate (in conjunction with her psychiatrist) and she seemed stable.

I always start with patients by getting them to focus on their health and be as fit as possible in all sexual disorders when they have the ability to improve their health (see Appendix A, item 3).

Norma: "So I think I'm now ready for sex."

Tracie: "How do you know?"

Norma: "I feel different. I'm a different person. I've changed, as my sister keeps telling me. I put on a dress and feel attractive now. It's like I can see me, and I look sexy."

Tracie: "How does that feel?" (resource mining)

Norma: "Different. People aren't telling me what to do all the time and I've signed up for a sewing course. I can make my own decisions. And I've decided I'm ready for sex, but I am quite nervous about it."

Tracie: "Look Norma, I would like you to try an exercise to raise your sexual energy and good feelings...you do it before sex...are you up for that."

Norma: "Oh yes please."

Sexual energy breath trance

Become really present now in your body and mind...close your eyes...this breathing raises serotonin, dopamine, and oxytocin...**the good feeling hormone**s...it also reduces cortisol the worry hormone and allows your testosterone to get you sexy...**you get double benefits** (motivating statement)... keep your mouth closed and smile really wide and naturally (body and face language activate neurology)...breathe really deeply and purposefully all the way in through your nose in one second...and all the way out through your nose only in one second for the exhale…keep repeating for one minute…keep your shoulders down…feel your body filling with oxygen…see and feel your body filling with sexual energy…**feeling your sexual energy rising**

Since the person is smiling wide at the same time as breathing, it stops the breath becoming a panic breath and cancels cortisol. It is important to guide the client to a natural relaxed smile with their mouth closed, not a forced smile (see Appendix A, item 4). If there is a severe nasal blockage, they can exhale through the mouth.

Also monitor the client's shoulders and coach them to keep them down, as when they rise, it takes the body into the fight or flight response. Smiling activates energy and pleasure hormones. Couples can use this breathing with their eyes open, staring into each other's eyes, whilst smiling at each other to raise sexual energy. The breathing can also be used to raise sexual energy during sex.

Do not use this breathing technique with someone who is actively schizophrenic, paranoid, manic or anxious as it can over-stimulate them. It is important to treat those conditions first in most cases.

Norma was misdiagnosed with schizophrenia when she started her menses, when in fact she had PCOS. Under the guidance of the healthcare professionals, she bought into that diagnosis and constantly took antipsychotics that suppressed her libido and sense of a sexual self.

She had associated herself with being a person who could not have sex. It was not that her sexual clusters had caused a nocebo effect for the SRC, but that the antipsychotics subdued the arousal stage. As she got control of her body, the libido started to emerge.

Trance intentions

1. Creating and encouraging autonomy.
2. Dissipating resistance.
3. Encouraging sexual fantasies.
4. Installing boundaries around sexual interactions.
5. Equating sex with enjoyment.
6. Initiating the arousal stage of the SRC.

Alright close your eyes and be safe…go deep…deep…deep inside yourself (she was already practised at going into trance)… to the centre of your mind (bypassing conscious resistance)… **that you make very very safe so safe** (it was important to aid self-efficacy)…you got this Norma…I'm not telling you what to do (initiating independence)…you don't have to want sex (law of reverse effect, allowing resistance)…**you have sex…when… you want sex** (direct suggestion)…you can feel sexy without having sex (Ki+ & Ke+)…you can look sexy without having sex (Vi+ & Ke+)…you can sound sexy without having sex (Ai+ & Ae+, stacking sex sensory experiences, mind mechanics)… **you can experience all those things stronger when you come to sex** (fractionation)…only you decide when you want sex (installing boundaries around sex availability)…your body… your life your choice…**you're in control** (building on her existing journey)…sex can be such a good experience for you (post-hypnotic suggestion, modal operator of possibility)… **you having fun in charge of your body** (associating sex with pleasure)…an adventure of exploration (all-encompassing suggestion for discovering sex)...**sex can be fun** (overriding the fear and anxiety response)…of course sex begins in your mind…you can think about sex (permissive suggestion)... **and thinking about how sex builds excitement in your body** (initiating physical sexual excitement, stage 1 SRC, and as she is already thinking about sex, intra-hypnotic and post-hypnotic suggestion)…always when it's right for you (silent suggestion)… it's good to be a strong sexual woman (giving her ownership of her sexuality)…**you can decide when and with whom you have sex soon** (presumption sex will take place in the near future)

A woman with Norma's history can be fragile and prey to sexual, emotional, manipulative, predatory dominators. Since she had no dating or sexual history or experience, it was paramount that along with suggesting sexual excitement, to also install boundaries around sex to keep her safe.

I saw Norma from time to time to review her health. She entered a relationship and had sex which she learned to enjoy. Her lover was also sexually inexperienced, so I encouraged them to embark on the exciting journey of sexual discovery together.

CASE STUDY: EDWARD (AKA TED)

Ted: *"People call me Ted or Teddy. My grandmother would never call me 'Edward' as she thought it was a stuffy name, so Ted or Teddy caught on."*

He was a small man of slight stature, quietly spoken, with cultured manners, in his mid-30, who lived alone. His blood tests showed low testosterone, and he had smooth skin, and a full head of hair with no discernable beard line. He worked on a telephone customer service helpline for a major manufacturer.

Tracie: *"What do you need help with, Ted?"*

Ted: *"I've never been sexually active. I know my penis and testicles are much smaller than the majority of men. I had to have human growth hormone injections to grow my height, but I never want stuff put into my body again. I hated showers at school with the other boys. People thought I was gay, but I'm just not sexual."*

Whilst being smaller in stature, with underdeveloped genitals, it also seemed likely that his testosterone was not converting well into dihydrotestosterone to effect full masculinisation.

Tracie: *"And how can we help you?" (whilst we listen attentively to people's stories, it is important not to allow them to rest in a distressed state).*

Ted: *"Everyone keeps asking me when I'm getting married. I come from that sort of family. I've never dated before, so you'd think they'd get the message by now."*

Tracie: *"Do you like being alone? Is there anyone you have been close to? How can we help you?" (triple bombardment questions, creating transderivational search, inducing trance-like states through confusion)*

Ted: *"There is a woman, who's really a friend I work with, who is divorced with a 10-year-old boy. She's like a friend. We all go for picnics and to the cinema. I'm teaching the boy to play chess. He's quite good."*

Tracie: *"Interesting how you preface that with 'who's really a friend'."*

Ted: *"Well she is. Her ex-husband was a bully, so she says she feels safe with me as a friend."*

Tracie: *"So how can we help you today?"*

Ted: *"I don't know really. I was just sort of wondering if I'm blocking the relationship developing into anything else, as the possible sex part terrifies me."*

The parapraxis "wondering" was a precursor to desire. It was an indication that he was considering that sex might be a possibility, but in his future. By putting the statement about sex terrifying him as the second statement, it indicates that he is open to conquering that fear.

One hundred and twenty years after Freud's proposal on parapraxis, Poscheschnik (2022) considers that listening to a client's unconscious mis-speaking and word placement tells us the state of unconscious conflicts.

From a hypnotic point of view, each word the client says not only tells us the trance they are living and levels of resistance, but also how open they are to altering those trances.

Ted also told me in his statement, "I hated showers at school with the other boys", that the origin of his lack of sexual experience was fear of interpersonal relations. He was afraid of being judged for his size, so his unconscious set up a defence mechanism to protect him by not entering relationships.

Tracie: *"Can I teach you something...tell me if...it's okay for you? (hidden suggestion)...would you like to learn something?" (bombardment questions, cognitive overload, trance deepener, by conceding to one, he commits to all three)*

Ted: *"Alright."*

Ted associated his lack of adventures into sex with his small stature and genitals. His sexual clusters all hung on the teasing he received from the boys at school when he was young, which positioned him as 'less than'.

Trance intentions

1. Instant artificial somnambulism.
2. Affirming his unconscious mind is dominating control of his body.
3. Create a resourceful part for negotiating interpersonal relationships.
4. Reclassifying sex as an impulse that operates without cognitive interference.
5. Validating his existing ability to already have meaningful interpersonal relationships.

I want you to sit back in the chair...I'm going to take your left hand and place it...face up...in front of you in mid air to your left...**your unconscious mind can help it rest there** (direct suggestion, artificial somnambulism deepener, catalepsy)... the ancient Greeks had three kinds of love (psycho-imaginary engagement)...in this upturned hand you can put Agape which means...**respect**... **friendship**...**caring**...**kindness** (I was pointing towards the content of the upturned left hand with my index finger, and nodding 'yes' towards it with my head and eyes looking in that direction)...in this hand (moving the upturned hand to directly in front of him in mid air)...is Eros which is...**sex**...**romance**...**passion** (igniting eros and libido)... it has no brain and is just impulse...in this right hand is Philia (I joined the right upturned cataleptic hand to the artificial somnambulistic tableaux before his face)...**which means blood connection** (drawing attention to the possible relevance of that to him)...it's a **spouse**...**brother**...**sister**...**parent**...**cousin**...

wife...partner...best friend (information overload, causing trance deepening)...tell me which one is the...**most important in a relationship** (loaded question, illusion of choice, direct visual suggestion because I looked towards the space where the left hand contained Agape)

Ted:	*"This one." (he moved his left hand to the left, minimal literal response due to being in trance)*
Tracie:	*"Why?"*
Ted:	*"Friendship most important thing."*
Tracie:	*"Exactly...sex and passion comes and goes...when relationships go through difficult times...and all relationships do at some stage...you can always depend on...**friendship...respect...kindness...caring**...is that okay for you...do you like that?"*
Ted:	*"Yes." (literal monosyllabic answer)*
Tracie:	*"Would that be comfortable for you in a relationship?"*
Ted:	*"Yes."*
Tracie:	*"Do you have that safe order of things in your friendship with your lady friend? Is friendship the main part of the relationship? Is that comfortable for you?" (interrogative overload)*
Ted:	*"Yes."*

Here we are desensitising him to the fear of sex by changing the focus of the relationship to Agape. This was done using a cataleptic hand experience for redefining the importance of sex in partnerships (see Appendix A, item 5).

It is important for the client to build on the resources they already have. To have confronted his fear of sex head on would have run the risk of increasing resistance. He did not indicate that he wanted to get married and had said, "Everyone keeps asking me when I'm getting married." indicating he was tired of and annoyed by the question. He had good, respectful manners so that was his strength to build on to overcome the fear of sex. He said, "She's like a friend", which indicated they were using Agape as their primary love communication and language.

We must listen to every single communication a client utters, using transformational grammar analysis for detecting surface and deep meaning (Ouhalla, 1994). At the same time we need to analyse their body language (Pease, 2017) to see if their verbal language and body language are congruent. It is also important to consider those analyses through the lenses of their family, social and cultural understanding to avoid observer bias.

I sent Ted away with the task of having a conversation with the woman to see if they were interested in a deeper friendship, which might or might not lead to a relationship. He did not physically withdraw, wince, or protest at the request, and in fact he seemed quite relaxed and reservedly enthusiastic.

Some clients need permission from others to change their behaviours. They have locked themselves in a cage or are perceiving themselves as limited and insufficient. Sometimes they need a little push to move forward.

He returned one month later saying they had decided they would like to get to know each other better to see whether it might lead somewhere. After more sessions, around how to run relationships, he declared he was ready to perhaps give sex a try.

Trance intentions

1. Self-validation.
2. Perceiving his body as pleasurable and whole.
3. Associating physical touch with pleasure.
4. Framing the relationship as safe.
5. Encourage proactive lovemaking with being more than intercourse.
6. Expanding his perceptions for what sex involves.
7. Initiating the arousal stage of the SRC.
8. Encouraging open communication around sex.

Alright let yourself be comfortable in that chair again with your eyes closed …safe in my office…you already know we don't do judgment here…**we value individuality** (the plural inclusive, creating therapeutic alliance)…some people have one foot bigger than the other…or leg longer than the other…everyone is different…**doesn't that make for an interesting world** (interrogative truism)…your body is a vessel of pleasure… the taste of strawberries… sound of Mozart…**you enjoying a tender caress** (direct suggestion, post-hypnotic suggestion)… it's so good to be you (silent suggestion)…it's good to have a lady friend…someone you can enjoy life's pleasures with…**a person you can feel comfortable with around sex** (inferred meaning for safety)…and of course you can provide the same experience for her (taking him out of self-consciousness and into altruism)…so many different kinds of sexual pleasure you can give to a woman…**you can enjoy the art of sexual pleasure giving and receiving** (permissive suggestion, turning sex into a two-way interaction)…caressing erogenous zones… cunnilingus…partner masturbation…playing with sex toys… and intercourse…**so many sexual pleasures you can both** enjoy (future pacing sexual success, implied mutual sexual satisfaction)…sex of course is like a tour of the world…there are so many places you can go…fun to explore sex isn't it (interrogative elicitation of commitment)…**how exciting for you to embark on this journey** (suggestion for commencing the sex response cycle)…having the time to have sexual fun together (associating sex with fun and coupling)…privacy to enjoy your sex life (he had complained about other people's intrusion on whether he was in a relationship or not)…**how exciting for you and your friend to embark on this journey together** (suggestion for relationship inclusivity)…creating your erotic individual and mutual sex maps…communication is the key…**talking to each other about what you like and what you need**…then trying that out.

I had previously got Ted to read sexual techniques books. I also got him to read *The Big Book of Sex Toys* (Taormino, 2009). He had disclosed to the woman that he had a micro penis and they had been shopping together for sex toys, including a strap-on dildo.

It took them another month to arrange for her son to stay with his grandparents so they could have sex for the first time. He reported it went much better than he had expected, and he was excited to continue to have sex as their relationship grew.

Here I used the cross-fertilisation of sensory pleasure technique (see Appendix A, item 6). If a person can have sensory, positive kinaesthetic experiences, it is possible to suggest that these pleasures can happen in other circumstances.

In hypnotically igniting the sex response cycle, when libido has failed, suggestions can be used to create the placebo affect around sex to motivate desire.

7 Erectile Dysfunction

It is estimated that 30% of the male population experiences erectile dysfunction (ED) (Gerbild et al., 2018). ED can be primary (no erections ever achieved) or secondary (history of erections then a sudden or progressive failure).

This figure increases dramatically to 50% of men aged 40 to 70 years of age, with 10% experiencing complete ED (Patel, 2012). It was found that only 20% of those had psychological causes, leaving 80% with physiological causes.

Male testosterone levels peak around 17 to 19 years of age. They can remain high for another decade but begin to decline after the age of 30. The decline in erectile function in older males is generally secondary hypogonadism due to ageing. In working with men with erectile failure, the best time to get them to have sex is first thing in the morning when their daily testosterone levels are at their highest.

The International Index of Erectile Function (IIEF) (Neijenhuijs, K. et al., 2019) is a self-reporting questionnaire that is used, generally in research, to measure erectile function. It contains 15 items with a short version of five items and whilst it may be useful in research studies, I believe it is counterproductive in clinical practice. It is far better to let the client unfold their story during the consultations. As with many psychotherapeutic interventions, more information is revealed when the therapist does not pathologise the client.

It is clear that ED is mainly related to declining testosterone in men. Research, however, found that it is complex and not possible to associate ED solely with declining testosterone in all cases (Rajfer, 2000).

Etiology can include hypothyroidism, benign prostate hyperplasia, primary or secondary hypogonadism, low sex binding globulin hormone, low luteinising hormone, low prolactin, low DHEA, partial Androgen Insensitivity Syndrome, Klinefelter's disorder, low vitamin B12, low vitamin D, excess oestrogen, hypertension, pituitary tumours, infection, testicular cancer, other organ cancers and physical trauma (Leslie & Sooriyamoorthy, 2023).

Other contributors include MTHFR folate processing failure, adrenal dysfunction, glucose dysregulation, obesity, heavy metal poisoning, post-viral fatigue, high LDL cholesterol and triglycerides, cardiovascular disease, stroke, myocardial infarction, vascular collapse and occlusion, physical trauma, smoking, drug addiction, chronic alcoholism, in some cases low alcohol use, iatrogenic drug complications, and organ failure.

Certainly, many men experience increased libido and erectile function during testosterone supplementation. But this treatment is not effective universally. There is also a rebound effect that can happen with supplementation in that it can reduce testicular function, causing secondary hypogonadism, and run the risk of polycythemia, peripheral edema, cardiac and hepatic dysfunction (Osterberg, 2014).

We know that the hormone vasopressin constricts penile vessels that control flow of blood into the penis and return it to a flaccid state post-erection (Ückert et al., 2020). Yet there are other hormonal and neurological controls involved that we do not yet understand or know whether they restrict blood flow into the penis in the first place.

We do, however, know that oxytocin may be involved in the relaxation of the penile vessels to allow engorgement (Melis, 2021). Unfortunately, a lot of research has been done on animals, which negates the effects of complex social interactions in humans and falls into the realm of quack science, as well as being highly unethical.

What this means for hypnotists is that reducing alarm hormones such as cortisol and catecholamines, and increasing hormones such as oxytocin, serotonin and endorphins likely makes clients more susceptible to suggestion for resolving psychogenic ED. If it feels good to have sex, the body and mind are more receptive to its physiological sex performance requirements.

From a mental perspective ED can occur during chronic or short-term anxiety, particularly anxiety around sexual performance, depression, post-traumatic stress disorder, bipolar episodes, borderline personality disorder, schizophrenia and dissociative disorders, confusion and distress around sex, gender and sexuality issues, religiosity, and cultural or familial restrictive beliefs around sex. Treatment is often and best approached from a physiological and psychological paradigm (Dewitte, 2021).

Etiology gets majorly more complex when resolved physiological dysfunction has left behind a psychological interference with the sex response cycle. In these cases, for males, phobias around sexual interaction can develop, being associated with all their past or some potential future sexual encounters (Zheng, 2021). A psychological loop can occur where the physiological and psychological failure of the SRC constantly links back to the other.

One of the major problems for men seeking help for ED is that they generally visit their family doctor first. Unfortunately, the majority of family doctors know very little about sex practices, so give the patient the wrong or inadequate advice (Sadovsky, 2002). To get them out of the office, after an inadequate six-minute consultation, they typically prescribe anti-depressants or drugs such as Viagra or Cialis, without appropriate testing. In many cases these are completely the wrong approaches and lead to a deeper sense of shame and depression when they do not work.

Drugs such as anti-depressants can increase ED. If the cause is psychosomatic, the nocebo effect can block the effects of erectile restoration drugs. This leaves men completely disillusioned, and they resign themselves to the belief that the problem can never be helped. Up to 25% of men are suffering from ED due to the side effects of prescription drugs, and unfortunately doctors do not warn patients that could happen (Leslie & Sooriyamoorthy, 2023).

This means that treatment must be multifactorial. Many hypnotists, with no training in clinical medicine or sexology, are advertising a cure for erectile dysfunction, which ultimately fails because there has been no physiological screening. What this does is damage the patient further.

The physiological causes must be ruled out before proceeding with hypnosis. Further complications arise in that many patients cannot afford to do the medical screening, so both therapist and patient basically end up fumbling in the dark for a cure. There is also the problem that many physiological causes of ED cannot be identified.

Family doctors, particularly in government-funded medicine, are often reluctant to do such screening because they do not have the budget, and they are not educated about the importance of such tests. They may not understand the tests, their metrics and how to recognise sub-clinical readings (Shoshany et al., 2017).

Laboratory reports are always just an estimate and average and may not be a true reading of dysfunction within that patient. Sometimes when a lab says a reading is normal, a sexologist can see it is less than optimal in that patient.

For most men, psychological erectile function lies at the heart of the male identity. Erections can be considered a measure of male worthiness, fertility, and a man's place in the male pecking order. Like all species, the effective breeder is perceived as the alpha male, particularly in younger men.

Aydin (1997) found hypnosis in the treatment of erectile dysfunction to be superior to acupuncture. We can see how these occasional studies show the efficacy for hypnosis, but the problem is there is no body of studies that show its effectiveness in comparison to drug-administered treatments.

Drug companies have millions of dollars to spend on research that promotes their drugs for sexual dysfunction. Hypnosis research, in contrast, has far fewer funds, so we can see how hypnosis as a treatment is often overlooked.

CASE STUDY: JEREMY

Jeremy was 52 years of age, divorced for five years, with three adult offspring. His wife had divorced him to marry a much younger man when his ability to get an erection began to decline.

Whilst he and his ex-wife were cordial because they shared children, he felt emotionally scarred by what he perceived as rejection of the measure of his maleness.

Jeremy: *"I'm seeing someone new. It's early days but she's very nice, and we seem to laugh a lot together. She's a widow and my age. We slept together but I couldn't get it up. She was okay about it and said* she still wanted to keep on seeing me, but I felt I let myself down."

Tracie: "That's an interesting statement. Tell me, if it had been her who was having some sexual difficulties, would you have rejected her?" (meta challenge, asking him to move to second position.)

Jeremy: "No, she's nice. And I don't judge her just on sexual performance. Tricky – I see what you're doing."

Tracie: "You're right. I asked you to leave self-pity and move to the big picture (direct challenge to render his self-deprecation pointless). Isn't it interesting how such a small shift refocuses things into a different light? (reframing). So, how we can help you?"

Jeremy: "I want to be able to have an erection during sex with her without taking Viagra, which sometimes works and sometimes doesn't."

Tracie: "Well (implied directive), I'm going to order a blood test and some biofunctional tests for you, but also… we're going to point your mind and body in the right direction (therapeutic alliance, direct suggestion)… is that okay for you?" (eliciting co-operation).

Jeremy: "Sure, anything you can do, Doc. You're the sex therapist."

Tracie: "You know, Jeremy, I'm over 60 and I know my body is slowing down and doesn't work as it did at 30. Just a fact of life. Every day I take supplements and treat myself with much more care. I can do many of the things I did when I was 30, and even *more at times. I just have to be more mindful. In fact, I can do things that some 20-year-olds can't. I'm wondering how you might take more care of yourself?" (bringing him on board as his own self-healer, interrogative suggestion).*

Second session

When the tests came back by the second session, Jeremy's testosterone and DHEA were low, triglycerides and HDL were high as he was overweight by about 40 kilos, which was clearly signs of metabolic syndrome. He had been too embarrassed to talk to his family doctor about the ED.

Tracie: *"I'm wondering how much more you could care for yourself?" (holding him accountable, interrogative suggestion)*

Jeremy: *"I could take the testosterone and DHEA supplements you recommended. I am on the diet you gave me and have already lost 7 kilos. As a builder I do get lots of exercise anyway. Do you think I will be able to come off the metformin?" (diabetes type 2 medication)*

Tracie: *"You're doing really really…really well (fractionation, re-enforcing behaviour, ego strengthening). The type 2 diabetes is probably linked to the weight you put on after your divorce. As you keep losing weight you can probably come off the metformin. You and your family doctor can work out when that might happen." (seeding possibility)*

Jeremy: *"I told the lady I was seeing you, what I was doing, and she was so excited for me, supportive. She said she was with me all the way. When I go to her house, she even does the food you want me to eat. I don't work at the weekends anymore and spend time with her and see the kids."*

Tracie: *"That sounds great. It really feels good to be around people who are positive and caring towards you doesn't it?"* (Reaffirming his sense of wellbeing with the partner he is seeing, restoring a sense of worthiness).

Jeremy's sexual identity hypnotic clusters were that he perceived himself to be diminished sexually by the rejection from his wife prior to and during the divorce. He began to associate sex with a heightened risk of future rejection which made him afraid to form new attachments to new women for fear they would reject him sexually.

Trance intentions

1. Inducing a sense of safety.
2. Encouraging adaptability.
3. Ego strengthening and encouraging a sense of self-efficacy.
4. Regression to earlier times when erections came easily.
5. Recall of sensory memory for having good erections.
6. Future pacing competent erections and excitement around sex.

Alright just sit back in the big chair and just relax away from the world (suggestion for exclusion of external sensory distraction)...

close your eyes...**be comfortable and safe in my office**...and whenever you hear my voice (safety anchor)...life changes all the time just like when you're altering a building (metaphor, indirect suggestion for adaptability)...sometimes you know what is going to happen...and sometimes it's a surprise...**you can adapt to every changing circumstance with ease and comfort** (permissive suggestion for adaptability, adjustment for age)...you have made a really good start in rebalancing your body and your life (ego strengthening)...taking care of yourself and feeling good (re-enforcing behavioural changes from the first session, association with taking care of himself and good feelings)...**you're doing well**...you know buildings have memories too (regression by metaphor)...sometimes you take up a floor (double meaning word 'floor/flaw') and you find a beautiful original structure of mosaic tiles intact underneath (accessing memories of erectile function)...**it can be so surprising what you find below the surface** (indirect suggestion that the unconscious has many resources)...go back to when you were young and sex was really exciting and you had a strong erection...life was full of excitement (recall the sensations for the sex response cycle)...**feel that in your body now and nod your head when you do** (memory recall, sensory recall, ratification of trance experience, he nodded his head)... good very good...**your body remembers**...and isn't that good (interrogative suggestion for erectile sensation)...**and when you come to sex in the future you can start with that good feeling in your body** (post-hypnotic suggestion for initiation of the sex response cycle)...now go back to another time when sex in your mind seemed really exciting and you had a sense of confidence...**map those thoughts and feelings** (stacking sexual confidence)...and now a third time when sex was so so exciting for you...map those thoughts and experiences...**join all those**

three experiences together (stacking and fractionation)…and each time you think about sex you sense all three experiences in the present time…**excitement**…**strength**…**good erections**… and such a nice lady you tell me you've met so (word salad deepening trance)…how much you like her (association of the new partner with sexual initiation)…so exciting to make love together (silent suggestion)…it's good to be you…**it's good to have strong erections** (direct suggestion for erections, global suggestion)…**It's good to make love and how exciting** (future pacing the replacement of anxiety with the initiation of the SRC)

The first session was about getting Jeremy healthy, losing the metabolic syndrome, high blood pressure and moving to a wholefood plant-based diet to increase testosterone and reduce vascular occlusions and subcutaneous oestrogen. A plant-based diet is linked to lower risk of erectile dysfunction (Carto, 2022).

Excess adipose tissue produces oestrogen which suppress testosterone, reduces sexual function, produces gynaecomastia and suppresses the SRC. Reverting to a healthy weight helps reverse this process, increasing the sex response cycle.

The second session was about ego strengthening, tracing back the physical and emotional memory for good erections, with post-hypnotic suggestions for erectile function each time he had sex.

It is important to remember with Jeremy that he had a good sex life until the marriage started to go wrong. He became depressed, withdrawn, put on weight and lost his sexual confidence. Using the state recall regression of when he was younger and had a strong erection allowed him to shift his state from erectile dysfunction to erectile function (see Appendix A, item 7).

If a client is unfit, all the hypnosis is the world will not restore erectile function until the client gets control of their health. It is important to work on fixing the physical as well as the psychological problems.

I saw Jeremy once a month for eight months during which time he lost 40 kilos, and came off diabetes and blood pressure medications. His relationship with the new woman deepened, and he gained erectile function during sex. He commented it was not as fast and furious as it was when he was young, but it was marvellous to be able to make love to his partner.

CASE STUDY: VICTOR

Victor registered on the autism spectrum or on the neurodiverse spectrum, as we now say, but he called himself autistic, and had a job in IT as a programmer and designer of video games. At 23 years old he had bought an apartment, lived alone, and had never had a girlfriend. He found it difficult to talk to women, did not know what to say, and could only tolerate a certain number of interactions with other people.

Here it is important not to see his autism as being a pathology from the medical model perspective, but supporting his difference from the neurodiverse psychosocial perspective. We are attempting to support him, not fix him.

I collected him from the waiting area at the clinic where he was playing games on his telephone and wearing dark glasses. In the clinic he asked for the lights to be turned down as he found them too bright. Autistic people can be hypersensitive to light and sound, and many also don't like to be touched (Schulz & Stevenson, 2019). What is notable is that many tend to have repetitive behaviours that start in childhood, and they can become disturbed when routines are broken, leading to difficulties in relationships.

Bryant (2013) posited that the neuropeptide oxytocin increases hypnotisability and increases reactivity to suggestion when the oxytocin receptor gene is more receptive. People on the autism spectrum have also been found to have variances of the oxytocin receptor gene, making them less social (Harrison, 2015).

People diagnosed with Asperger's Syndrome (milder form of autism) also can become angry and reject contact when they are overwhelmed. When someone on the spectrum who is high functioning comes into the clinic, it is impossible to tell if they have Asperger's or not, because we see them for such a short time.

People on the autistic spectrum are often treated for ADHD traits and prescribed amphetamine-type medications (Davis & Kollins, 2012). It is easier to observe ADHD traits because there is a constant loss of focus and often memory. Psychiatric medications used for ADHD can and frequently do cause erectile dysfunction so they can be contraindicated.

In exposing neurodiverse people to hypnosis, we must vary our techniques. They are unlikely to understand or process implied directives and indirect suggestions but may reject constant direct suggestions that become overwhelming for them.

Victor reported having a good erection during masturbation, which was about three times a week. He had recently had his first sexual encounter with a woman, where he was unable to gain an erection and engage in intercourse.

Victor: *"I'm very private. You won't tell anyone, will you?"*

Tracie: *"I'm not legally allowed to disclose information about anyone that I am seeing, unless you have murdered someone. Have you?"*

Victor: "No, not me. I don't mix with many people."

Tracie: "You said your erection was fine during
          masturbation, but you couldn't get an erection
          during your first sexual encounter. I'm wondering
          if that is a syntax error in your programming
          and that you didn't alter your coding to consider
          physical contact with someone else."

Victor: "Okay, what are you going to do with hypnosis to
          fix it?"

Tracie: "Oh I can't hypnotise you (law of reverse effect).
          Your firewall is too high for receptivity to accept
          suggestions in hypnosis from me."

Victor: "What do you mean?"

Tracie: "Well, you tell me you're on the spectrum, you don't
          see many people, and are hypersensitive to light
          and sound. All those things are needed for me to
          hypnotise you."

He looked confused and annoyed.

Tracie: "I'll tell you what I can do (bargaining and creating
          curiosity). I could teach you to code your brain and
          change your unconscious and conscious reactions
          during sex. You're obviously good at coding. Would
          that be okay? (lowering resistance by giving him the
          illusion of control).

Victor: "Okay, let's do that."

His sexual clusters were heavily influenced by his autistic fear of
contact with other people, and being out of his private space in

new circumstances. These things are constants for many people on the spectrum. It takes very intense behavioural therapy to change if they can at all. Therefore, the course of therapy was to give him tools to use himself under his own control. I call it the Incompetent Therapist technique (see Appendix A, item 8).

Trance intentions

1. Put the client in control of his trance experience to reduce resistance.
2. Affirm he is physically competent to have an erection (expert opinion).
3. Allowing him to believe he chooses which suggestions he pays attention to, creating a bind that he pays attention to some.
4. Ego strengthening.
5. Creating auto-suggestion.

Start by closing your eyes so the light does not bother you (using his model of the world)…listen to my voice so you can composite (uncommon words deepen trance) an erection manual for yourself…**be in charge and do it in your own way and direction** (the illusion of choice)…anything that's useful you can keep…and anything that's junk code you can delete (bind to listen to suggestions he wants but listening to all suggestions to determine the difference)…of course biologically we are learning that even junk code has a purpose (reversing logic so that all suggestions can be useful)…**start by listening to every word I say and copying the code** (bringing his focus onto suggestions)…your penis is attached to your brain (truism)…when your mind has the right code your penis does what you want it to (truism)…so put this code in your mind (silent suggestion)…**my penis works just fine** (self-affirmation)…I'm sexually attracted to some women (global suggestion)…I like them…**I'm a young man and healthy** (depathologisation suggestion permitting him to be capable of the SRC)…some women like me…some women find me sexually attractive (ego strengthening)…**I like sex…sex is good…sex is enjoyable** (law of association)…sex is a pleasant experience (silent suggestion)…I'm safe having sex with the appropriate woman (widening his scope of experience whilst giving him a sense of security)…I can spend time with that woman in my own way (compensating for his neurodivergence)…**I can talk to her…it's safe** (broadening his world view)…during a sexual encounter I get a strong erection (psycho-imaginary present tense experience and future pacing)…**during intercourse I maintain a strong erection** (direct global suggestion)…it's good for me to have a strong erection and enjoy sex (association between the two).

Notice the suggestions did not dwell on how he felt. To keep talking about feelings with people on the autism spectrum is fruitless as they often cannot process that internal kinaesthetic information.

> Tracie: *"Now I want you to use this recording three times a day. I want you to write down all the good code you want to keep, and I want you to say it to yourself repeatedly…code it in your brain and neural pathways by habit."*

Whilst many people on the autism spectrum can go into trance successfully, there is always the danger of them rejecting other people's suggestions. They don't, however, typically reject their own suggestions. In fact, they repeat thoughts again and again, creating self-fulfilling prophecies, more than the average person (Cooper, 2022).

This is where we use their tendency to act out repetitive thoughts and behaviours to help them achieve their goals for themselves. For them, there is safety in repetition and familiarity.

I also taught Victor the daily raising of sexual energy exercise, which not only raises general energy and sexual energy but also sexual confidence (see Appendix A, item 9).

I caught up with Victor by Zoom one month later. He had seen the same woman a second time, sex had been good, and he had maintained a good erection. He had told her he did not want a relationship, but the sex was good with her, so they decided to be sex mates occasionally.

CASE STUDY: HARRY

Harry was a very nervous, healthy young man of 19 who was an apprentice plumber. He came from a heteronormative, Catholic, immigrant middle eastern background, with several brothers and sisters who were all being paired off for marriage. He himself was engaged.

Harry: *"We're not allowed to have sex before marriage. My parents are very strict. My fiancée wouldn't allow it."*

Tracie: *"In some cultures that is the way it is, and you are obviously very connected to your family and culture."*

Harry: *"Are you sure everything I tell you is secret, and you can't tell my family? I don't want this getting back to my family. No one knows I'm here."*

Tracie: "Just you and me Harry. I'm like the priest – I can't tell anyone." (creating safety)

Harry: "I don't hurt people and I go to church once a week. I have sex with men. That's it. I've said it. I've never told anyone else before. And I'm definitely not gay. I don't have anything against them, but I don't want to be a gay man."

Tracie: "Well thank you Harry for trusting me with that information. I assure you it will remain confidential. I'm going to confess to you, I'm a little confused why you have come to see me. Tell me in your own words, what do you want from therapy?" (allowing him to tell his story).

Harry: "I've had sex with men since I was 16. I hook up off the Grinder app, using a second phone I have in my car that no one knows about. It was good to begin with and I always had a good hard-on. I always fuck them and come inside them. Of course, I use a condom."

Tracie: "Safe sex is very wise in hook-ups."

Harry: "Next year I get married. The nearer I get to the wedding, the softer my dick's getting. Just over the past few months I can't fuck any guys anymore."

Tracie: "Interesting...and why do you think that might be? And will you stop having sex with men when you get married? You do know it's safe to tell me these things...don't you?" (Triple question, transderivational search, trance induction)

Harry: "I suppose I'm afraid someone will find out the nearer it gets to the wedding I've never talked about it in confession." (grammatically confused trance logic response)

Tracie: "And will you stop having sex with men when you get married?"

Harry: "Sex with my wife might be boring. I want to keep my options open."

Tracie: "I'm guessing she doesn't know. What do you think marriage is?"

Harry: "You get married, have kids, buy a house and love each other."

Tracie: "What would you think if she had secret sex with lots of other people and you found out?" (holding up the mirror)

Harry: "Angry. I might even want a divorce."

Harry's sexual clusters had two main trances. First he was living the expected life of his cultural male narrative of getting married and having children. His libido, however, was directed to having secret sex with men. Both trances conflicted with each other. He associated having sex with men as being unacceptable to his culture, therefore he could not form any attachment to them, which resulted in casual sex only. He did not seek sex with women other than his fiancée and perceived sex with women as being possibly boring. He could not accept that he might be gay and might have been erotically stimulated by what he saw as casual, dangerous sex.

Trance intentions

1. Giving him a second position perspective.
2. Future pacing the realisation of the consequences of his actions.
3. Fractionation deepening of the trance experience by bringing him in and out of eyes closed trance and artificial somnambulism.

Close your eyes...safe in my office...go inside...and I want you to go forward to 10 years' time...put yourself inside your fiancée's body...**see what she sees...hear what she hears... feel what she feels** (future pacing second position)...you've just found out your husband has been having sex with lots of men behind your back...he did not tell you before you got married or during the marriage...**how does that feel...sit with those feelings...processes those feelings** (allowing him to experience her reality)...take your time to understand the impact...lots of time inside your mind (time distortion)...just sit with it and process it...in a moment I'm going to get you to come back to the room...**fully in your own body with what you have learnt**...eyes open and looking at me (reorientation to self and the present)

Tracie: *"Tell me, Harry, what are your experiences as Harry's wife?" (maintaining artificial somnambulism, deepening trance by maintaining the second position)*

Harry: *"Panic. Terrible panic. Ground opened up. Couldn't find a place to stand on. I'm drowning." (notice he is still in trance relating to the second position)*

Trance intentions

1. Giving options other than his present course of events.
2. Inciting psychodynamic conflict resolution.
3. Using the superego to resolve the conflict.
4. Creating parts alignment.
5. Suggesting there are good options and decisions.
6. Restoration of erectile function.

Close your eyes again…I can't tell you where to point your dick (using the client's language frame)…or who to have sex with and enjoy it (giving him permission to have sex with whoever is right for him)…but you said you didn't hurt people (holding him to account)…**so don't hurt anyone** (direct suggestion)… **be kind by being honest** (inducing the superego control)… **be good by being honest with your eyes closed** (trance ratification, eliciting the superego)…it's clear to see you're not ready for marriage (Vi, reflecting back what he has been telling me)…there are conflicting parts inside you (truism)…**you may be ready for marriage in the future** (leaving his options open)…but you indicate physically that it's not now (his actions tell us this)…there is a part of you that wants sex with men… and a part of you that wants marriage to a woman (drawing out the conflicting parts)…**you can hear that at the moment they seem to be opposing each other** (Ai)…to have a happy marriage all parts need to be aligned…all going in one direction…like a universal bolt fitting a universal nut…**all parts of the same system to create harmony and happiness…feeling good** (suggestion for alignment for resolving his Ki incongruency)… that makes happiness…**over the next month you can figure it out** (permissive suggestion for conflict resolution)…you can take your time…think things through carefully…**go**

forward for your best options (indirect suggestion to change direction)…where everyone's long-term happiness has the best chance…**you can make the decision that is good and right** (asking the superego to take over parts negotiation)…**good decisions that you can be happy with**…open your eyes awake and smiling at me.

> Tracie: *"Tell me honestly…what kind of man would you be married to your fiancée and still having secret sex with men?"*
>
> Harry: *"I'd be a nasty man. I don't want to be that."*
>
> Tracie: *"Listen carefully. You're only 19 years of age. You don't have to get married now because the rest of your family are. Don't do something that you may regret for the rest of your life or will hurt someone else (appealing to his values). You can really work out who and what you are and what you want, in time, to have good erections."*

This is initiating time delay conflict resolution (see Appendix A, item 10). The reason I used this was to take the pressure off Harry as he felt cornered to make immediate decisions about his sex life.

One month later he had broken off the engagement, assuring his future bride that it was down to him, and that he was not ready to get married yet, so it would be unfair to her to continue the engagement.

He was continuing to have sex with men and having no problem with an erection, still telling me he was not gay.

> Tracie: *"As I told you in the first session it's none of my business where you put your dick. All I say to you*

is be safe, don't hurt yourself or anyone else. You'll
work everything out in your own time, and the
time is when it's right for you." (taking the pressure
off him to conform to a label)

Sometimes opposing desires in the unconscious mind can go to war with each other and cause conflict, interfering with the sex response cycle. The person may be in a situation where they are unable to resolve the conflict consciously – they might not even understand those conflicts – and a therapist needs to give them a nudge to de-escalate the war.

Zhang (2020) reviewed how brief psychodynamic therapy, combined with medications such as Viagra, can have a positive effect on erectile restoration. I find, however, that in many cases, direct and permissive suggestion, in eyes closed trance and artificial somnambulism, for a psychodynamic shift enables the client to solve their own conflict, in or out of consciousness, without medication.

CASE STUDY: HAVIER

Havier was a 65-year-old South American import/export merchant, dressed in a tailored black suit, with a red cravat, and red shoes with a slightly raised heel to make him look taller. He spoke broken English. In his culture his masculinity is one of the central identities of being a male. It is important here not to confuse misogyny with masculinity and that we are mindful of paying attention to a client's cultural gender roles and working within their framework.

For the majority of men, their sex performance is connected to masculinity. Stanaland (2023) discusses how, when a male feels threatened, he can experience a fragile masculinity that leads to an attempt to restore masculinity. The loss of erectile function can also lead to a perceived threat to men's sense of self, which can create fragile masculinity.

In today's world, masculinity is frequently seen as aggressive, dominant behaviour. From a sexologist's perspective I believe a man's sense of masculinity is a central and necessary driving force for the initiation of the sexual response cycle. Not all men, but most.

Havier: "I like the ladies. I've always liked the ladies. They beautiful. I like to dance with the ladies and make love to them. I never marry, but I'm good uncle to my nieces and nephews. I love my family too."

Tracie: "Yes...it's good to have a good life...how can we help you today?"

Havier: "I have problem. I'm not as young as before. My gentleman parts not so strong. I see doctor in my country and he give testosterone injection and I get Cialis from farmacia. Sometimes it work and sometimes it not. My friend said hypnosis can help."

Tracie: "Yes it can help when the problem is psychological (priming). It can also help to put you in the right kind of mind to help the body work well. How long has the problem been happening?"

Havier: "It started when I am 55. First, I have Viagra but it give me terrible headaches. Then I try Cialis and it was good for some time. After the doctor gave me testosterone, much better but not as good as when I was young. I get afraid it won't work sometimes and then it don't. I don't want to be afraid. I want to make love."

Schardein (2022) found that when the supplementation of testosterone was prescribed alongside phosphodiesterase-5 inhibitors in cases of ageing hypogonadism, erectile function improved. As I have mentioned before, anxiety increases cortisol and blocks testosterone. Also the nocebo effect can be activated.

Tracie: *"You know, Havier…you can remember (creating artificial somnambulism)…have you heard of Casanova? (he nodded his head) (invoking internal association to good lovemaking)…the ladies liked him very much (fractionation)…**he did a lot more than intercourse** (indirect suggestion for sufficient foreplay and sex play)…**ladies like that as you know** (recall suggestion for skills, acknowledging his lovemaking skills)…I'm sure when you make love to a lady…you can make them happy without intercourse (silent suggestion)…**you are such an experienced lover** (ego strengthening)…it's good to have happy ladies…and good to have happy gentleman…**and good to make love…isn't it?"** (interrogative suggestion)*

Havier: *"It's good." (literal responses ratify the trance state)*

Havier had no doubts about his masculinity and had a history of many lovers but had struggled with the advancing of age and declining erections. He strongly associated sex with pleasure and wanted to enjoy it as long as possible in his life. For him sex and intercourse were associated with romancing and lovemaking, as he had never used the word 'sex'.

His sexual clusters were around erections equal his validity as a man. He was a pleasure seeker and needed a psychological and ego boost to initiate and maintain erections.

Trance intentions

1. To restore his sense of confidence during lovemaking.
2. To enable him to have good erections during intercourse.
3. Maintenance of the erection during intercourse.
4. Use mind mechanics to reconstruct his erectile confidence.

Alright close your eyes and be safe in my office (safety anchor)… look up inside your mind…**see a picture of you making love to a lady** (Vi+ imagery and future pacing success)…it's good very good and you're having a good time (initiating serotonin)… she's having a good time (initiating oxytocin)…**you're excited and happy** (stage 1 SRC, excitement increases blood flow to the penis, happiness increases serotonin, endorphins and decreases cortisol, allowing testosterone to improve phosphodiesterase-5 inhibitors' effect on erections)…it's a special time…**it's a lovemaking time** (focus of attention)…you're both enjoying love making…**your penis is full of blood** (post-hypnotic suggestion)…just as you like when lovemaking…inside your mind you say "I have a strong penis" (Ai+)…**your penis is hard and the erection lasts** (direct suggestion, bombardment suggestions, Ki+)…you are strong and a gentleman lovemaker… you like giving your lady pleasure…**you like having a good erection and giving your lady pleasure** (re-enforcement parallel suggestion)…you carry that good picture of you inside your mind (Vi+)…and your voice inside you saying "I have a strong penis" (Ai+)…**it feels good and you are a confident lovemaker** (Ki+)…you remember this every day…the picture… the voice…and the feeling when you come to lovemaking… you're **confident and have good erections when it comes to lovemaking**

The trance was recorded for him to use at home daily.

I have written before about the mind mechanics I use in hypnosis (O'Keefe, 2000):

- Initiating the positive visual internal imagery (Vi+) first.
- Add the positive auditory internal (Ai+) in the client's own voice.
- On top of that initiating internal good kinaesthetic, positive feelings (Ki+).

The three together are strong and activate psychological and emotional shifts in the unconscious that filter through to the conscious mind.

Notice with Havier I generally use the direct suggestion approach as his English was limited and he already stated the problem and informed me of what precise solution he wanted. Although he was experiencing anxiety around his erectile performance, he was dealing with the biological failure of ageing and there was no evident psychodynamic conflict. Therefore I used age-related performance adaption approach (see Appendix A, item 11).

I was due to see Havier a month later, but he telephoned after three weeks to cancel the appointment because everything was working well for him. I asked him to continue to use the recording for the next month as a special time for him each day, and to stay on the testosterone and Cialis under his physician's instructions.

Hypnosis is not a panacea for amelioration of sexual problems. Whilst it can help and even initiate biological function and change, when deteriorating physical function is age-related, it can assist function, but not at times rectify physical deterioration.

Havier stated quite plainly at the beginning that testosterone supplementation along with phosphodiesterase-5 inhibitors worked for him at times. He also said that his fear of erectile failure was his problem: "I get afraid it won't work sometimes and then it don't. I don't want to be afraid."

We as therapists must listen to every single word our client utters. Intentionally or not, they will tell you and display the problem and even the solution.

8 Premature Ejaculation

All males' sexual experiences are different, and the emergence of premature ejaculation (PE) is either a primary (from first sexual experiences onwards) or secondary condition (occurs later in life).

The question of whether this condition is biological or psychological is specific to the individual client or maybe a combination of both. Males are generally too embarrassed to talk about the condition and often do not engage in relationships for the fear of disclosure.

The definition of what PE is varies wildly. There are suggestions it may be associated with hormonal imbalance, infection, neurological hypersensitivity or insufficiency, anxiety, depression, or trauma.

Cia (2014) reported that chronic bacterial prostatitis (CBP) seems to be common in men with secondary PE. The author particularly identifies chlamydia trachomatis infection as being the common pathogen that causes swelling of the prostate or urethra. However, this does not account for primary PE, although immunologically, with infection, we need to acquiese to how little we actually know.

Since PE is multifactorial, it is wise to have biological investigation as part of therapy, even for psychogenic causes. We can never rule out or omit biological investigation.

Masters and Johnson described PE as "the inability of the male to control ejaculation sufficiently to satisfy his female partner in more than 50% of coital episodes provided that she is not anorgasmic" (Crowdis, 2023).

This is a crude and naive perspective that links female sexual satisfaction solely with coitus performance. It is a gross misunderstanding of female sexuality. It also assumes that men normally and automatically have total control of ejaculation.

Strasburg (1990) described PE as "little voluntary control over ejaculation and ejaculates within two minutes or less after intromission in at least 50% of coital attempts."

In fact, some men are able to enter into intercourse after ejaculation occurs, not just at the initial arousal stage or directly before coitus.

Crowdis reports that occurrence of PE can be anything from 30% to 75% depending on the study. It can also be associated with erectile failure, but not in all cases.

I have found some men have sufficient erectile function, and experience an extended plateau stage during masturbation, but fail to have ejaculatory control when it comes to coitus.

The Symonds' (2007) diagnostic tool may be useful in assessing PE. Patients, however, are presenting with complaining symptoms, so I find it too traumatising for them to apply a diagnostic tool. They tend to tell me the problem themselves. They are fully aware of what is happening already.

In considering premature ejaculation in men that occurs within one to two minutes, it is also necessary to treat the person physically as well as for psychosomatic symptoms.

Anxiety during PE is a major component, which may be due to high tissue copper/low zinc, low B vitamins, low vitamin D, hypothyroidism, hyperthyroidism, Graves' disease, diabetes mellitus, metabolic syndrome, heavy metal poisoning, high cortisol due to adrenal or pituitary tumours, pituitary insufficiency, high cortisol and catecholamines due to stress or PTSD, infection in the prostate and urethra, pudendal and other nerves, insufficiency, hypersensitivity or physical trauma, recreational drug and alcohol use, iatrogenic drugs' side effects, disease, testosterone insufficiency, high oestrogen, low sex drive and MTHFR gene variants.

Whilst anxiety, low self-esteem, depression, trauma and mental illness can frequently be found in cases of PE, to presume they are the cause without screening for an underlying physical irregularity is negligent. Whilst many researchers say they cannot find the cause of PE, this bears the assumption that it is one singular disorder, which it is not.

Premature ejaculation describes the symptom, not the cause, so a full investigation of possible causes needs to be carried out. Here we run into patient compliance and them turning up for and completing the tests we order. Sometimes they do not as they deprioritise their importance within their life and treatment framework. So careful explanation at the beginning of treatment is necessary to educate the client on what we need them to be screened for and why.

Psychosomatic causes of PE lend themselves well to remediation with hypnotherapy, but it is not in itself a panacea for all cases. Particularly, as for many men, PE occurs alongside erectile dysfunction (ED).

Here I present cases of males with secondary PE. They have experienced previous ejaculatory control, so they could not be classified as primary PE.

CASE STUDY: OLIVER

This 45-year-old man was a solicitor, never married and had dedicated most of his life to his career.

Tracie: "So, how can we help you today, Oliver?"

Oliver: "I don't know if you can. I've always had the problem, so I don't date women because it's too embarrassing. I saw a program on hypnosis and since you're also a sexologist as well as a hypnotherapist, I thought I'd give it a go."

Tracie: "Well, that's good. I help people with a lot of different sexual issues every week so you can feel perfectly free to tell me what you need. I'm here to help." (creating safety and seeding the idea that he could be helped)

Oliver: "I've always had premature ejaculation, so I have avoided sex and relationships. It's all too messy for me."

Tracie: "I notice from your history you run marathons and go to the gym quite a lot. You're a vegetarian and your diet seems quite good. You say work is not stressful because it's your firm and you have got it well organised. You live in a very nice part of town, have friends and are financially in a good place. Tell me, do you urinate a lot at night and have you had your prostate checked?" (it is important to build client confidence up before intervention and not focus solely on pathology).

Oliver: "No, I sleep well, and my doctor says my prostate's fine. Yes, the rest of my life is just fine. I'm the guy that lots of men want to be. If only they knew the whole story."

Tracie: "Tell me, Oliver, do you masturbate and how often?"

Oliver: *"About twice a week now. I used to do it every day when I was younger. I still use paper porn. I don't want any electronic footprint of my private life."*

Tracie: *"And how long do you last before you ejaculate during masturbation?"*

Oliver: *"That's no problem. I can go for 20 minutes."*

Tracie: *"Mmm, that's really interesting. Have you tried any remedy so far?"*

Oliver: *"Years ago I did try taking my penis out when I was about to come, squeezing it underneath the end, front and back, and waiting. It stopped me coming but I also lost my erection."*

Since he has no problem with ejaculatory control when masturbating, it becomes clear that Oliver's problem is psychogenic. He has also not mentioned why he thinks the PE is happening.

At times it is necessary to regress the client to see if there is any early traumatic sexual experience that may be the root of the original cause of PE (see Appendix A, item 12).

Trance intentions

1. Using his organisational skills to send him into trance.
2. Establish the underlying sense that he is successful in so many ways.
3. Regression to locate any early sexual trauma.
4. Putting that trauma into perspective by metaphor.
5. Beginning to move him on from the trauma.

I want you to just sit in that chair and close your eyes now…I know you're a very organised person…**organise your body to**

relax as I talk to your unconscious mind and you go into a deep trance (causal link, association of me talking to him and him going into trance, occupying his critical mind)…you tell me you're in a good position in life and that's a good thing… and that life is going well for you…**you know how to make things happen** (suggestion for problem solving)…I want you to go back to your first sexual encounter inside in your mind now (initiating regression)…where are you (presupposition he is already regressed)

Oliver: *"I'm in our garden shed." (regression is marked by the person using present tense language)*

Tracie: **"Be aware of your surroundings**…*how old are you…if you're with anyone…tell me who that is…what age are you and who are you with?"* *(bombardment questions to deepen trance)*

Oliver: *"I'm 17 with Lucy from my class at school. It's a hot day. We've taken all our clothes off and are lying on a blanket on the floor in our shed."*

Tracie: *"Be aware of what's happening in the moment…are you having intercourse…***tell me the details** *(during regression you must tell the client to tell you what is happening otherwise they remain focused solely within)*

Olivier: *"We're both virgins. We've planned it for a week. Bunked off school for the afternoon. I'm excited and just put my penis inside her. My dad's banging on the door trying to get in. I locked the door from the inside as I've taken the key. I'm panicking so I come straight away."*

Tracie: "What happens now?"

Oliver: "We're rushing to put our clothes on. My dad's mad.
          He's looking through the window, shouting at me
          that I'm a little pervert. Sent Lucy home. Told her
          dad. She can't look at me for the rest of the year. I'm
          so embarrassed."

Tracie: "That's a long time ago (time shifting, reorientating
          to the present)...coming all the way back to the
          room safe...back to the present time in your body
          (reassociation)...you're a successful and well
          respected man...**eyes open and looking at me** (I
          am not asking him to come out of trance, simple
          to open his eyes and orientate to the present so he
          remains in artificial somnambulism)

Tracie: "You know, Oliver, our first sexual experiences are
          often a fumble. I know myself the third guy I slept
          with was a disaster. I had very little experience
          and he wanted to do it in the straddle position.
          I fell over, banged my head, and passed out. He
          never called me again. I can laugh about it now,
          looking back, but at the time I was so embarrassed."
          (creating empathy through metaphor)

Oliver: "Looking back today I suppose it was bit of a farce."

I taught him the Pelvic Circle Exercise for PE (see Appendix
A, item 13) which includes the pelvic floor Kegel exercises,
the difference between a tense or relaxed PC (pubococcygeus)
muscle, holding in the anus, and relaxing the anus.
Ejaculation happens when these muscles, and particularly the

bulbocavernosus muscle, are engaged, through innervation of the pudendal nerve, during ejaculation and urination. When these muscles are disengaged, ejaculation cannot happen.

Slow, deep nasal breathing

Added to that I taught Oliver the slow, silent, deep nasal breathing that increases nitric oxide, which is associated with better ejaculatory control for extended intercourse (see Appendix A, item 14). Otunctemur (2014) found that nitric oxide levels were statistically lower in men with PE. When we breathe into our chests through our nose, it increases nitric oxide. When we breathe through our mouths, it engages the abdominal muscles more, thereby engaging the PC muscles.

I teach silent nose breathing is because noisy nose breathing in anxious people could cross over into panic breathing, hyperventilation, and annoy a sex partner. Also focusing the breathing slowly through the nose, whilst it gives us more oxygen, produces calm, extending the plateau stage of the SRC.

> Tracie: *"Sex is like riding a bike. We wobble all over the place to begin with, then we get our skills and learn to ride it. If we fall off, we can get back on the bike and get better at it."*

So I'm going to teach you slow, long, silent deep nasal breathing... look at me and follow what I'm doing (modelling)…close your mouth (creating muscle memory)…very slowly breathe in deep through your nose silently as long as you can…then breathe out very slowly and silently as long as you can…keep your breathing in your nose and chest…**continue to repeat this breathing pattern focusing on the out breath**…at the same time relax your anus…PC muscle…and the area where I taught you where the Kegels happen…**relaxing all three areas as you breathe with nasal silent breath very slowly**…relax your body and slow intercourse down…even stopping inside your partner for a time."

It was clear Oliver lacked sexual confidence in his present-day performance. When he thought about or engaged in sex he associated intercourse with panic, having to hurry, and getting caught. His sexual identity cluster was about him being found out and embarrassed. He had developed a phobia around extended intercourse.

Trance intentions

1. To give him a sense that he is in control of his own body and timing.
2. That sex is a private matter between consenting adults.
3. Associating fun and pleasure with sex to cancel the fear response.
4. Teaching him to slow intercourse down.
5. Psycho-imaginary experiential learning.

Close your eyes and go back deep inside…be aware how you grew up into a strong man (bringing time orientation to the present)…**became successful…are an upstanding man**… (indirect suggestion for an erection)…time changes everything (truism and indirect suggestion for change)…acknowledging you are a man in charge of your own life now…**you are free to date anyone you wish** (the power of choice over his father's will)…when you want…how you want…**enjoying that pleasure in your own time** (suggestion for him having the power over ejaculatory timing)…all the pleasure in taking

your time (bind in that pleasure equals taking his time)...
slowing things down during intercourse (post-hypnotic suggestion to reduce anxiety)...taking all the time you need inside your mind and body (cancelling the panic response)... enjoying having intercourse slowly (directed suggestion to slow intercourse down)...**at times you might even stop with your penis inside your lover and wait for some moments**...using the slow silent deep nasal breath...relaxing your PC...anus... kegels and all the other muscles in your pelvis...carrying on when you are ready continue...you can carry on in your own time (silent suggestion, giving him control of his timing during intercourse)...**you and your lover are in control** (this excludes the expectation of external interference)...and deciding between your bodies when it's time to ejaculate...**intercourse**... **fun** ...**and pleasure**...**all in one** (depotentiation of fear and the panic response)...slowing everything down....all in your own time...**all the time you need** (time distortion)...like riding a bicycle you get there when the time is right...(feeding into the metaphor about learning to ride a bike, experiential learning)

He used the recording I made for him twice a day for six weeks. I also advised him on intercourse positions to overcome PE (see Appendix A, item 15). Ejaculation is also linked to the urinary muscles being engaged. When men are about to ejaculate during intercourse, they thrust with their hips. Some positions improve this situation.

INTERCOURSE POSITIONS FOR PE (TEACH TO THE CLIENT)

1. Do not thrust your hips during the plateau period until you are ready to ejaculate.

2. Use the one knee up position, continually bringing the partner towards you as you keep your back straight.
3. Use the supine position as you lay on your back and the partner is on top of you, bearing down on you.
4. Use the position where you are on your knees, sitting on your feet and the partner is bearing down onto you.
5. Use the side-to-side position and push with your straight back, not thrusting with your hips.
6. Use the doggy position but draw the partner onto you, keeping your back straight without pushing with your hips.

Six weeks later Oliver had started an affair with a single woman who was also in the law profession. They had had sex once and he was pleased and surprised how well it had gone.

Crowdis maintained one of the causes of PE is an early bad experience that gave rise to trauma being associated with sex and particularly ejaculatory performance.

In treating Oliver, I did not retraumatise him in regression by continually going back to the original incident. One regression to find the source was sufficient for clinical knowledge. The aim was to reframe his relationship with intercourse as now being associated with pleasure and fun and suggesting he had the power over its timing. His unconscious mind did the rest for him.

However, it can never be said that PE is purely psychologically based, as such reductionism ignores the mind/body interaction. Thoughts and emotions are initiated by hormonal activation. Part of our major job as hypnotists is to suggest replacing fear with pleasant experiences as all men with psychogenic PE experience the fear of failure.

CASE STUDY: MOHAMMED

Mohammed was a 40-year-old practising Muslim living in Australia in an affluent middle-class area. He ran a successful IT company that took up a lot of his time, taking him away from his family, leaving his wife to raise their three children, all under six years of age.

He experienced no notable medical conditions, exercised, had normal blood pressure but tended to get stressed, particularly around business. His weekly schedule was erratic, leaving himself and the family confused about what was their family and couples time.

Sex between him and his wife was functional, in the missionary position and unadventurous. They occasionally fitted it in when they had time, but he often did not look forward to it and ejaculated early.

Both he and his wife were virgins when they married, and he reported their first sexual encounter was not memorable and in the dark. While early masturbation had been satisfactory, he had always experienced PE around intercourse because he was unsure what to do.

Tracie: *"Tell me, Mohammed, what car do you own?"*

Mohammed: *"It's a big Range Rover 4x4 because I have a family and we have to carry lots of things around with us. My wife drives a Toyota."*

Tracie: *"Does each of them have their own manual?"*

Mohammed: *"Yes, both in the glove compartments."*

Tracie: *"And do you own any sex manuals?"*

Mohammed: *"Eeeer, no."*

Tracie: *"Funny that isn't it? You own two cars with manuals. As an IT guy you probably own hundreds of books and manuals on IT systems. If the plumbing goes wrong in your house, you call in a professional plumber who has a lot of manuals on plumbing. You employ 24 people in your company, so you employ an accountant to do your tax returns who has lots of manuals and books on tax law. Do you see the irony here of not having a sex manual?"*

Mohammed: *"I never really thought about it like that. My family don't talk about sex. Reproduction was covered at school. I come from a religious background where the Iman does not address it. I don't hang out with guys who brag about sex."*

Tracie: *"You know, for all of us, the unknown is fearful to begin with, no matter what it's about. We don't know how to manoeuvre something unless we are educated about it or have been given instructions. Imagine how frustrating and humiliating it would be never having seen a car before, having no manual or driving lessons, and being expected to get in and drive it the very first time."*

Mohammed: *"I see. I get your point."*

Time-poor Mohammed was not paying attention to his relationships with his wife and his family. In Islam the family is meant to be a source of peace and tranquility, but his family lived in organised chaos due to his work schedule. He was focused on business, like many men, but was sacrificing taking care of his marriage. He had little knowledge of sex, so approached intercourse with fear.

He associated intercourse with fear of failure, thereby not deepening his attachment to his wife. His sexual clusters were about his duty to procreate but he was deeply confused about how to fulfill the pleasures of sex.

Trance intentions

1. Establishing a locational trance anchor.
2. Trance ratification through catalepsy.
3. Initiating his problem-solving skills.
4. Associating sex with enjoyment.
5. Using the religious superego to regulate his life.
6. Positioning his wife as sexually attractive.
7. Separating lovemaking from the rest of his life.
8. Initiating sex education.
9. Positioning intercourse as something sweet and pleasurable.
10. Deepening the relationship with his wife.
11. Slowing intercourse down.
12. Mind mechanics to focus on being a competent lover.

What I want you to do is just make yourself very comfortable in that…the one you are sitting in…**the one where people go into hypnosis** (confusion technique, locational association with the trance state)…chair where your whole body is supported (associated relaxation)…you don't even have to keep your eyes open…**just let them rest closed as you go into a trance** (causal link)… that's good…very good…very good indeed (trance ratification, ego strengthening)…just like that… even deeper inside (fractionation)…**seeing yourself totally relaxed**…glued to the chair…**immobile…you couldn't get**

up if you wanted (direct suggestion, trance challenge, trance ratification)...**could you** (catalepsy, interrogative suggestion, trance ratification, does not require a verbal response)....**as I talk to your mind**...just a deep conversation (trance deepener)...I know you're a very clever man...you're a problem solver...**when there is a problem you either find or invent a solution** (establishing competency)...you see yourself taking your time and thinking about it (Vi+, indirect suggestion to reassess his life)...now sex is a very natural and enjoyable experience (silent suggestion)...a gift from Allah (enlisting his religious superego)...particularly when you're in love... **like being in love with your beautiful wife** (association with wife and good sex)...like the great blessings of Allah...such a blessing in marriage to have good sex relations (working within his model of the world)...to be savoured and enjoyed at leisure (teaching him timing)...taking your time and being fully present...**exclusive time for lovemaking** (time organisation, focused attention suggestion)...as you learn more about sex... more about...**taking your time and being in the moment**... pleasuring your wife first (introducing foreplay)...**thinking about intercourse as dessert**...like baklawa...when you've had the main course...just time for you and your wife to make sweet love (deepening his perception of the connection between them)...**growing enjoying together**...slowing things down (direct suggestion)...the more you learn the more you are in time with nature (indirect bind for satisfactory ejaculatory control)...a confident sexual man (confidence building)...see yourself now inside your mind...**a confident sexual lover taking his time**...it looks (Vi+)...sounds (Ai+)... and feels good (Ki+, mind mechanics)...everyone's journey is different (depathologisation)...some people learn to ride a bicycle at five and some people at 50...it's your time to enjoy leisurely lovemaking in your own time…**slowing things down and being present**

The modern world is a paradox of rewards and losses. As life becomes more complex it can steal time and attention from relationships. In order to survive, pay mortgages and bills, feed and educate children and keep up with society, much is stolen from our personal lives, including time and attention for lovemaking.

Mohammed presented as a problem solver, with a problem, who needed guidance to resolve the problem, not for someone else to take over the problem. The problems he presented with were lack of knowledge, time, and attention around sex, so they needed to be the areas we worked on.

He had already told me his masturbation history allowed him to maintain the plateau period, so he had no real erectile problems. He appeared naive about sex with a lack of knowledge, time, and experience. He needed to be in the present and have focused attention during intercourse (see Appendix A, item 16).

In relationships both partners can also be rushing sex and not paying attention to high-level lovemaking. If you are working with couples, a focus exercise can help them work together and be present during sex. It's useful to get them to do the couples focusing exercise (see Appendix A, item 17).

He listened once a day to the recording that I made. His homework was to buy four high-quality sex manuals, read them in the couple's bedroom, and keep them locked away in the bedside table when not reading them. He was asked to put a lock on the bedroom door so when they were having sex, the children could not walk in.

I saw him four times. He changed his work schedule to have the same defined days with his family every week, including two nights when he and his wife talked about sex before going to sleep. Over the four sessions, the two nights per week turned into lovemaking nights and they began to explore sex together where he became more confident as a lover and his PE problems disappeared.

Leung (2019) found that a lack of sex education elevates sexual dysfunction. Scientific sex education, particularly in adolescence, leads to a higher level of sexual competence and satisfaction.

When it comes to adult men with poor sex education and sexual dysfunction, as hypnotists and sex therapists, our job is to teach about sex, through suggestion and tasking to initiate the client's sexual curiosity and regular attendance to sex.

CASE STUDY: TONY

Tony, who was a 32-year-old plumber with his own business, had a good sex life until his divorce. He reported his wife started dating another man whilst they were married, and he found out by accident when he passed a hotel they were going into.

The two years prior to the divorce were stressful for him. His wife told him she thought they had got married too young and she was no longer in love with him. There were two children, his son 12 and daughter, aged seven.

His wife employed an aggressive divorce lawyer, wanted the house, maintenance and for him to leave the family home. She declared plans early in the divorce to move her lover in when he had left.

Tony talked about how he was devastated by the divorce, only saw his children every other weekend and had to collect them from and drop them off outside his old home.

Tony: "I just feel like a criminal and that I must've done something terrible. I'm a straight-up bloke, worked hard, gave my family everything they needed, didn't cheat with anyone, tried to be the best husband I could be, and I was still just not good enough. I'm gutted."

Tracie: "I can see and hear you are in a lot of pain about what happened. It's clearly been very difficult for you (authenticating his story and distress). And of course, Tony, such a situation would have been difficult for any man."

Tony: "That's an understatement. I've tried dating and sleeping with a few women since, but as soon as I'm excited, I come. I tried using the anaesthetic spray Dr Numb on my penis to make it less sensitive, but then I couldn't feel anything at all. It's humiliating and the anti-depressants my GP gave me didn't help and made me feel fuzzy, so I stopped them."

The problem with physicians prescribing certain anti-depressants to delay PE is that the side effects can initiate an increase of ED. Hypnosis is, as we have seen from research, a proven better option for psychosomatic cases.

Tracie: "So, what can we do for you in therapy? What do you want to achieve?"

Tony: "Well doc…I want to be able to have a relationship again without coming early. I feel stuck and can't move on with my life."

Tracie: "Well, Tony, you can know…I've seen a lot of men who have recovered from similar situations and *had a good sex life (My friend John technique)...I know when you're in the middle of it, you feel like you're the only one...but you can recover."*

It was important for Tony to know he was not alone and that other men had similar experiences. Repeatedly using the word 'well' initiates healing by interspersal suggestion.

We made his shopping list of outcomes from therapy and one of the biggest issues for him was learning to trust again. His divorce was traumatic, and sex generally requires trust and a sense of safety. Whilst he could get aroused due to his biological libido, continuing along the plateau stage of sex required a greater sense of commitment to sex and feelings of safety.

For that commitment to happen, there must be a strong sense of trust with the women he is involved with. For him, his sexual clusters were that commitment ran the risk of being hurt and rejected again. He was not psychologically and emotionally ready to take that risk, so premature ejaculation seemed his best option to keep himself safe. He constantly regressed to the trauma of his divorce and associated other women with what his wife did.

Tracie: *"Can I teach you something Tony...something you might find useful?"*

Tony: *"I wish you would."*

Trance intentions

1. To teach him to be self-trusting.
2. Arm catalepsy.
3. Metaphor for non-leaking pipes.

4. Create glove anaesthesia and locational sensory transference with the ability to use to desensitise his penis during intercourse.
5. To be able to have sexual sensations in his penis whilst reducing its sensations that lead to ejaculation.
6. To give him control over when he regains full sensations in his penis to ejaculate.
7. To teach him to use auto-hypnosis at will.

Okay lean back in that armchair...be safe in my office and when you hear my voice...**trust you to take care of you** (transferring the responsibility for him to create trust in himself)...the care you take creates your own trust in you (suggestion re-enforcement)...**I'm taking your left hand and placing it in mid air where your unconscious can hold it** (cataleptic hand)...look at that hand...focus on that hand... your unconscious can hold that hand there in mid air (trance ratification)...you know a lot about plumbing (truism)... sometimes to stop a pipe leaking you freeze it (indirect suggestion for extended stage 2 of the SRC, true statement)...**I want you to remember the feeling of anaesthesia you got from Dr Numb in that hand** (direct suggestion for recall of a sense of numbness)...like you have had it in a bucket of ice...10 is the highest feeling and 1 is no feeling at all...**reduce the feeling in that hand to 5 now and nod your head when you have done that** (sensory control suggestion, I nodded my head up and down, then he nodded his head up and down, visual unconscious leading, ideomotor response)...good... very good indeed...**reduce the feeling in that hand to 2 now and nod your head**...(glove anaesthesia, I nodded my head up and down, unconscious leading, he nodded his head)...I'm putting your right hand in the air where your unconscious can hold it (trance deepening)…that's right you got it…(ego strengthening)…**transfer the lack of feeling to the right hand from the hand that's left and let that hand come back to normal and rest on your lap** (anaesthesia transference, sensory manipulation, locational focal shift)…nod your head when you have done that (he nodded his head, he is already trained to nod his head when I ask, Pavlovian response)… that's very good again (fractionation of competence of auto-hypnoanaesthesia)…now you know how to reduce and restore feeling in your body…**transfer the lack of feeling to the left foot and let the hand that's right come back to normal and rest on your lap** (training him in locational anaesthesia)…nod your head when you have done that (he nodded)…**that's very good again**…now transfer it to the right foot and nod your head (he nodded)…your left foot coming back to normal… and nod your head (he nodded)…you can move the reduced feeling to any part of your body…**move it to your penis now and nod your head when you have done that** (he nodded)… right foot coming back to normal…you're learning to reduce the feelings in your penis whilst still having the pleasure of your penis's sensations (silent suggestion)…**you can reduce or increase the feeling in your penis with your mind at any time** (intra- and post-hypnotic suggestion)…you can do this during intercourse trusting in your body and self (permissive hidden suggestion because as it is not tonally emphasised it slips into the unconscious unnoticed)…any time you need… **you have control of the feelings in your penis** (transfer of focus of control to the client)…and when you want… **you can reduce the feelings in your penis** (re-enforcement suggestion)…and when you want you can get full feeling back into your penis to ejaculate…you're plumbing (metaphor for building on his existing skills)…**you can do this during sex**

to delay ejaculation (post-hypnotic suggestion)…until the time is right for you…getting full feeling back at ejaculation

In medical hypnosis we focus the attention to create hypnoanaesthesia during surgery and other procedures (Facco, 2016). In fact, it has been used for thousands of years, particularly before chemical anaesthesia became popular at the end of the 19th century.

Some men delay ejaculation by using skin surface numbing anaesthetic sprays on their penis, so in sex practices, the principle of penile reduced sensitivity has validity.

PE is largely a matter of hyper-sensitivity of the penis but those feelings take place in the mind. By teaching Tony to reduce those sensations when needed, it allowed him a longer plateau period during intercourse (see Appendix A, item 18).

His major problem was separation-induced trauma due to the divorce. He kept reliving that trauma inside his mind as he approached intercourse (see Appendix A, item 19)

I saw Tony for six months, once a month, and he entered a new relationship with a woman. The rest of the work was teaching him to create trust and honesty within himself and the relationship. Sexual ejaculatory competence was restored for him as he also learnt to trust himself again. We also worked on restoring his general and sexual confidence.

CASE STUDY: TOMMY

Tommy was 24 and highly sexually advanced for his age. As a homeless street boy, he started, having regular sex with older men for money when he was 13. He had previously been abandoned by his mother to a range of government homes, but ran away from all of them.

He had been part of a community of street teenagers who looked out for each other, although they slept rough. He went into his first shared house with gay people when he was 17 and was considered handsome and attractive.

There he slept with a bisexual woman who was the first female he had sex with. They both started working for an escort agency individually but were also hired out as a couple. They were not involved, because she had a butch girlfriend, and he hung out in gay men's bars.

During his teenage years he had been heavily involved in the sado-masochism (S&M), leather, and rubber scene, spending time in dungeons, and at multiple sex parties, and for a period of time had a different sex partner every night. Tommy worked as a well-known rent boy (his words), which was how he paid to get through art college for three years.

His artworks began to be exhibited, acclaimed, sold and were highly sought after in his early twenties, which allowed him to live on his own and no longer be involved in the sex industry. Some connections he made with clients as an escort helped him establish himself as an artist. He had mimicked exquisite manners from his wealthy clients. But the more successful he became, the more he took drugs.

> Tommy: *"Something changed. I can't really say when. As a sex worker I used to be able to do sex for hours. Then I used to go out and have sex because it was available. The thing is, I don't need to do sex for money anymore. As a teenager people wanted me for my body. They still want it, but there is this whole new thing going on that people want to hang out with me because I've become a well-known artist."*

Tracie: "And how is that for you?"

Tommy: "I don't know. I worked for it, but it seems a bit
          surreal. I'm feeling sort of like any moment people
          will wake up and say I'm faking the art. They're
          going to wake and realise I'm just a rent boy."

Tracie: "Interesting but rather black and white."

Tommy: "Why?" (he looked perplexed and afraid at the
          same time).

Tracie: "Well, it's like you're restricting yourself to work
          in one medium. You know, monochrome or only
          ever in oils. That you're only one dimensional. Now
          I'm not an artist, but if I remember my classics...
          Shakespeare's players were largely sex workers...
          and Caravaggio spent as much time banging the
          local boys as he did painting canvases...Leonardo
          Da Vinci also liked a nice boy's buttocks...the
          Vatican used to have a trade in selling sex slaves...
          why would being a sex worker be any less legitimate
          than selling paintings...why would your art be less
          than other art...doesn't it negate blind judging
          of art when you don't know who the artist is?"
          (bombardment questions, interrogative induction).

Tommy: "I get all that, but I love my art and I sort of get
          afraid it will all be taken away from me. So, when
          I try sex now, I'm full of fear and I come in a few
          seconds. It's really fucked my sex life up."

Tracie: "And the drugs...it's interesting that trance you keep
          playing inside your mind like an old record stuck
          in a groove...don't ride your motorbike...get in a

car...or on an aeroplane...don't cross a road in case you are run over...don't speak to people unless they attack you (law of reverse effect)...where's the 'don't give-a-fuck' attitude you had when you lived on the streets...night after night, sleeping with men who could have murdered you...why have you stopped being Tommy and become a middle-class prude... what's to gain from fame if you've lost who you are and devalue your own history...the history that contributed towards your perspective as an artist."

Tommy: "What can I do? I've bought a house and studio, have cash, and am selling work but in bed I'm really messed up. I've even tried wearing two condoms at once."

Tracie: "I love Picasso's Harlequin series of pictures...I just get them...but during his blue period he had trouble selling any paintings at all...**at that age you seem to have had great success**...it could all go tits up at any moment...this is the impermanency of life...live with it...**this is the edge that creates great art**...or you can just work as a wallpaper designer or in a supermarket...stop asking for guarantees...there are none."

Tommy: "You're not what I expected."

Tracie: "You're not what you expected either...everything changes...if it didn't...you'd be bored shitless and your art would get stale. "Would you like to learn something neat about multiple orgasms?"

Tommy: "Go on then: What you got?" (it was a challenge)

Orgasmic diffusion relocation

You know when you do watercolours...I don't know about oils (allowing resistance)...but in watercolours when you put too much colour on the brush...**it can spread throughout the picture uncontrollably** (provoking him to examine his psyche bleeding)...it just shoots off in other directions...in abstracts like Jackson Pollock's you randomly...**throw paint at the canvas and see where it lands** (metaphor for orgasms in the body)...just imagine with your eyes closed that your... **orgasm was somewhere else other than your penis**...maybe just maybe (suggestion for permissive curiosity)...you have a little orgasm in your left little finger...or the feeling of a climax in both nipples at once...**sex happens in the brain like art** (truism he can relate to)...just something to play with during sex...a concept...an idea...and then when you want to orgasm in your penis you can later...I wonder how you might explore it during masturbation (interrogative suggestion)

Is this a distraction technique? No, it is teaching a man to be able to put his focus somewhere other than his penis (see Appendix A, item 21). Men who experience psychogenic PE are generally overly focused on the sensations in their penis. In contrast, the average man, without PE, is aware of his penis, aware of his partner and activating motions of rocking and thrusting during intercourse.

When someone is recovering from an addiction or disease, sexual function may be damaged, and as the body takes time to recover, so does sexual function in these cases. Teaching them orgasmic diffusion allows them to have some sense of still engaging in a sex life while the body recovers (see Appendix A, item 20).

Giving Tommy an exercise to do alone allows him to rehearse sensory diffusion without the threat of judgments. Since he had an anti-authoritarian personality, me giving him something to explore was more acceptable than telling him what to do. Firing his curiosity lowered resistance.

Tommy was a thrill seeker. He had lived on the edge and had a high level of resilience. Chronic use of drugs had, however, changed the structure of his brain and he now had a low tolerance to stress. His chronic fear of being seen as a fraud of an artist pervaded every part of his life.

His sexual clusters had become part of this existential crisis of being. He associated sex with being found out, so although he wanted sex, it was now thwarted by the fear of exposure.

Trance intentions

1. Parts integration and accepting the whole of himself.
2. Accepting that his whole history contributed to his success.
3. Stop living in fear.
4. Seeing himself as unique
5. Adjustment to a new lifestyle.
6. Teaching him that sex is not just about libido but also about connection.
7. Confidence during sex and life.

Love the whole of you (the central theme for therapy)…sit back in the chair and close your eyes safe in my office (safety anchor)…know I am not here to judge you but simply help you…**help yourself** (separating myself from his perception of society, calling on him to step up)…as you go deeper inside I want you to think of yourself as a mandala (he is primary visual)...**the deeper inside the mandala you go the greater your fascination with the wonder of the structure** (reframing his complexity in a positive light)...you are art as well as form (framing him as what he loves)...you are a series of magical events in time...**like a river you mould to the available land** (indirect suggestion for adaptability)...the journey changes as is natural...each evolution rests upon the foundations of the past (metaphor, valuing his history)...the further the river gets towards the sea the stronger it becomes...and the more forceful the current (associating his journey with getting stronger)... **everything you have been and are contributes towards the blessing of being you now** (teaching him self-validation)...a work of art to be unique (accepting individualism)...if anything was missing from the past you could not have had your talent (interrogative suggestion, transderivational search, trance deepener,)...**so your whole past created your talent** (suggestion for integrations)...to enjoy art you have to be completely present to take it all in (silent suggestion to come out of anxiety as he has to be present to process the statement)... missing nothing and enjoying all...**sex of course is art to be enjoyed in the moment and art is limitless** (bringing him into the present during sex)...you can be mindfully present during sex (mindful sex, cancelling the panic response)...and as art you can take your time to muse...as much time as you need to enjoy the art in front of you (time expansion during sex)....every lover is different and brings something new... **all the different places in your body you can orgasm** (he is forced to examine the concept to prove or disprove it, since he has already done dungeon work he has seen the concept in action)...little ones...big ones...in a bus queue...on the train... **any time...any place...any part of your body**...take your time and savour (silent suggestion)...like a Caravaggio or Hockney or Tommy...**take your time** (repetition suggestion for extended plateau period)...be present...all of you (self-acceptance)...like the mandala...endlessly rich and worthy...no matter who your lover is...just...**be**...again and again...**simply be** (confusion)... **be art together** (direct suggestion that sex equals his beloved art)...as long as you like...**take all the time you need for sex and desire** (addressing libido and desire)...know your worth as art...know you're art...every part of the mandala...**all the time in the world inside your mind**...exploring all the erotic parts of you (suggestion for exploring sensory diffusion)

In metaphors the client can connect to suggestions with lower resistance. Whilst Hammond (2010) is an excellent source for suggestion, hypnotists must customise metaphors specifically for each individual client to lower resistance, create suggestibility and be effective. Here Erickson understood the value of teaching tales above all other hypnotic theorists (Rosen, 2010).

Although he learned orgasmic diffusion, there was no fast cure with Tommy. Whilst he presented with psychosomatic PE, the effects that drugs had had on his body and brain were devastating. For a period of about a year he had taken LSD three or four times a week and five or six ecstasy (MDMA) tablets every day. Whilst that may have released some of his creative inspirations, it had also damaged his cognitive and emotional processes.

Mohamed (2020) found that people involved in substance use disorder suffered high levels of anxiety and depression. The effects were not just short term but can become lifelong alterations to many areas of the brain, creating permanent mood disorders.

I saw Tommy for two years and a large part of the work was reparenting him and getting him to establish a healthy, low-stress lifestyle, learning to feel safe and connecting with people in a more stable and emotionally enriching way. Much of his life had been centered around sex and he needed to learn life and relationships have many dimensions, changing his primary life criteria of needs.

Naturopathically his diet was changed to plant-based and he was on a regime of daily vitamins and self-hypnosis. Rather than accepting commissions for commercial gain, he refocused his art back to original pieces that he put to exhibition and to market.

As his health began to recover, and he learned to step back from sex, connecting with people first, his PE slowly subsided, and he gained his confidence as a lover once again. He had periods of dating a woman who liked him and a young man he was interested in, both of whom he considered great friends. He learned to trust and take risks in relationships in a way he had never done before.

Tommy suffered from imposter syndrome, which gave rise to extreme anxiety connected with sex because of his history as a sex worker (see Appendix A, item 22). Due to his artistic talents and recognition, his life and financial situation had changed dramatically within a couple of years. He had not had time to mentally adjust to his good fortune which he feared would be snatched away from him.

As his personality matured in therapy and he adjusted to accepting his new status, he was able to learn to become more confident during sex again. Sometimes PE is the symptom of a personality failing to adjust to adulthood. Experiencing an erection and ejaculation in puberty is mainly driven by libido, whereas in adulthood desire and self-confidence rank higher in the criteria of needs for a good sex life.

9 Vaginismus

Vaginismus is a major problem for many women that is rarely talked about or discussed. Most women hide it and just do not engage in intercourse. Pithavadian (2023) discusses a lack of public awareness, poor knowledge in health professionals, and a paucity of research on women's experiences in seeking help. Basically, most health professionals have absolutely no training in helping women with this condition. This can lead to women being anxious and feeling ashamed about raising the issue.

Raveendran (2024) reports a clinical prevalence of 5-7% of women who can experience primary (never had intercourse) or secondary (previously had intercourse but now more difficult) vaginismus. It is seen as a difficulty in gaining entrance to the outer third of the vagina and at times the upper regions of the vaginal canal. The merging of the vaginismus and dyspareunia (painful intercourse) classifications has increased confusion around the condition. Reissing (2014) noted all women who experience vaginismus have vaginal pain.

Also, many doctors fail to diagnose the presence of vaginismus because they can, under examination, sometimes with anaesthesia, gain entrance to the vagina. So, they diagnose psychogenic vaginismus, which can, at times, be inaccurate.

It is important to remember that vaginas are all shapes, sizes and depths. They also tilt forwards, backwards, to one side or may be poorly developed (Slaoui, 2020). Painful resistance to vaginal entry can also indicate possible uterine, vaginal vault, bladder, rectal, or small bowel prolapse, fibroids, vaginal, cervical, uterine, pelvic or bowel cancer, and sexually transmitted infections. Some women's uteruses can tilt excessively backwards or forwards but this does not generally cause intercourse problems.

This is why I always insist on women being medically screened before I treat them. I frequently receive telephone calls from women who do not want to undergo such screening and I decline to see them. I will explain to them the need for such thoroughness, but some women dismiss it as irrelevant. Many family doctors also do not consider such exams necessary so a physiological diagnosis may be missed.

In addition, copulation can fail because males have penises that also have different shapes and tilts, which can mean that the couple's genitals are incompatible for intercourse.

The condition in some women can have a psychological cause, but also a fear and rejection of intercourse can occur when physical difficulties are present. This becomes more complex when concurrent mental health problems are present, and in cases where patient compliance is low.

The interaction of physiological and psychological barriers to intercourse needs to be examined on an individual basis. Angın (2020) found in a systemic review that patients were more resistant to treatment when they had a relative who also had vaginismus, or a partner who blamed them for the condition.

CASE STUDY: GLORIA

Gloria suffered from genital lichen planus. This is an inflammatory condition that causes a considerable amount of vulva and vaginal pain (Farhi & Dupin, 2010). The cause and triggers of the condition are generally unknown, but it is believed to be an atopic autoimmune disease and associated with the Hepatitis C virus (Machin, 2010).

Gloria was 46, had one son of 18, by caesarian section, had begun menopause and experienced vaginal atrophy. Vaginal atrophy is reduction in the volume and size of the vagina, often missed in menopausal and post-menopausal women (Carlson & Nguyen, 2024).

She was using topical steroids and was taking prednisolone daily to reduce inflammation. Due to the family history of oestrogen-sensitive breast cancer, she felt she could not take oestradiol which has proved useful in some cases (Bhardwaj, 2019). Whilst less invasive oestrogen cream is more recognised now (Desai, 2023), it was not generally used for this purpose back when I saw Gloria.

Autoimmune disease – when the body mistakenly identifies itself as a foreign invader so attacks it – can be sparked by many causes including genetics, exposure to toxins, allergies and trauma, initiating an inappropriate immune response, and cytokine storm (Pisetsky, 2023).

Even though Gloria still menstruated, she was clearly perimenopausal. Hormone changes occur from 30 years of age and the occurrence of autoimmune diseases become more common in some women.

Mohan (2017) found that oral lichen planus was more common in perimenopausal women than in the general population, particularly related to depression, so we could equate the same increase in the genital condition.

I am going to come back to my frequent statement here that there is no separation between mind and body. When one is diseased, the other becomes diseased. This is particularly poignant in the cases of depression, anxiety and stress in patients with auto-immune diseases (Kalkur et al., 2015).

As hypnotherapists we need to soothe and direct the mind and emotions to help rebalance the body. Also, through relief of trauma, we are able to influence epigenetics, and ramp down cortisol and catecholamines to reduce inappropriate innate and adaptive immune responses. We can see researchers have reported successful outcomes for relief from lichen planus using hypnosis (Cruz, 2018). This should also include hypnosis to help change lifestyle choices.

> Gloria: *"I'm devastated and overwhelmed. My husband's left me. I can't focus on work. I feel rejected and useless. I'm in pain. I'm so unhappy and left to deal with my teenage son who is now depressed. I don't know what to do."*

> Tracie: *"Well Gloria, you are so right. You just told me about the most important piece of information, 'You're overwhelmed', and why would anyone in your situation not be?"* (acknowledging distress)

> Gloria: *"Thank God. At last someone's listening to me."*

> Tracie: *"Let's do an exercise. Here's a clipboard and a pen. Put a line down the middle of it. On the left, put everything that is a problem. On the right, put what you might think are assets or would-be solutions."*

We talked through each item briefly and brought them down to a maximum of five-word statements.

> Tracie: *"Let's look at the negatives. Read them out."*

Gloria:

1. My husband has left me.
2. He is filing for divorce.
3. Work is horrendously busy.
4. I'm overwhelmed.
5. I never have enough time.
6. I'm constantly in pain.
7. No sex for five years.
8. My son is depressed.
9. I feel old.
10. I don't know what to do.

Tracie: "Well let's look at the positives. Read them out."

Gloria:

1. I've got a job.
2. Money in the bank.
3. Somewhere to live.
4. Still alive.
5. Live in a beautiful country.
6. Roof over my head.
7. No one shooting at me.
8. I have food.
9. I'm getting help.
10. I'm a free woman.

This exercise helps people voice their problems out loud and witness their resources. Gloria was clearly consumed by her internal kinaesthetic distress which was distracting her from and creating a negative hallucination for her resources Ki-. By changing her assessment to auditory (Ae+) and witnessing her resources out loud and seeing them written (Ve+), she is breaking state and beginning to cancel that negative hallucination.

Gloria was clearly not coping with her life and the pressures she believed she was under. This was compounded by the rejection from her husband because she was not available for sex. Her sexual clusters were about 'sex equals pain' which had become a continuous trance of her not engaging in intercourse even if her marriage depended on that happening. She associated her genitals with the complete failure of her womanhood.

Trance intentions

1. Establishing artificial somnambulism.
2. Chunking problems down.
3. Presupposition that the problems can be solved.
4. Initiating systemic solutions.
5. Regression for resource mining.
6. Affect bridge to feeling good about herself.
7. Identifying existing caring skills.
8. Initiating self-care.

Tracie: "I'd say that's a pretty good start (validating therapy)…the problems can be broken down into small pieces to help you solve them (shrinking her perception of the problems)…**one thing at a time** (intra-hypnotic suggestion, chunking down)…not all today…but just (preparatory conjunctive)… one thing at a time…**and everything becomes manageable** (direct suggestion, future pacing success)…everything is manageable for you (silent re-enforcement suggestion)…when you break a problem down you solve one piece…peace at a time (double meaning)…**piece**…**by peace**…**by piece** (de-escalation of overwhelm)…do you think that will take pressure off you" (interrogative suggestion).

Gloria: *"Guess so." (notice the monosyllabic response as she goes into trance)*

Just close your eyes...be safe and calm as you hear my voice (contingent suggestion)...as a chief librarian (tapping into her identity of being in charge)...**you have and have had systems** (identifying existing resources)...as a mum you had systems in place to care for your child...it's good to be able to use systems again and again to get control (fractionation of existing resources)...you already know how to catalogue... file...and retrieve information...**you're really good at systems already**...let's start with how you learnt to walk (regression, resource mining)...one step after the other...**and you remember how to do those steps**...then you learnt to skip... bouncing along happily (Ki+)...**you remembered how to jump rope**...then you learnt to do your hair as a teenager... looking really pretty (Vi+, Ki+, ego strengthening)...**feeling good about yourself** (Ki+)...you said to yourself when you looked in the mirror I look pretty (Ai+)...and you learnt how to keep your baby safe and take care of him (recalling caring skills)...kissing his knee when he fell down...**being very very loving**...so you know all these things...you have those caring resources...**all ready** (suggestion for activating change, call to action)...it's time to remember...**take one step at a time**... having systems for dealing with life's challenges...working through life's difficulties one thing at a time (re-enforcement suggestion)...**feel good about yourself** (Ki+)...being very loving to yourself every (initiating self-healing)...every... every...every single day (global suggestion, future pacing)... **and more some self-care** (suggestion for exceeding perceived limitations)

I put Gloria on a wholefood plant-based diet which increases microbiome balance, reducing inflammation in autoimmune diseases (Tomova et al., 2019; Alwarith et al., 2019). What was also necessary was to create a food diary and do an elimination diet to see if any specific plant-based foods created inflammation. We also removed all grains as some people with allergies and autoimmune diseases are allergic to grains.

A herbal prescription was used, containing Rehmannia (Rehmannia glutinosa: anti-inflammatory), Hemidesmus (Hemidesmus indicus: reducing immune activity), Passion flower (Melissa officinalis: calmative), Rhodiola (Rhodiola rosea: adaptogenic for eliminating anxiety, depression and fatigue).

Added were multi-vitamins, B complex 3 x a week, vitamin E 400iu 2 x daily, vitamin D3 5000iu 2 x a week, a daily probiotic (taken away from herbs), quercetin daily, NAD (nicotinamide mononucleotide) 250mg daily, Vitamin C (liposomal) 3000mg 2 x a day, zinc 25mgs daily, magnesium at night 350mgs, and only chamomile tea (no caffeine or alcohol).

The earlier script was used for hypnosis twice a day on a recording. The biggest need was for Gloria to eliminate being overwhelmed and make everything manageable for her.

Three months later she had reduced stress and trauma. Withdrawing someone from steroids is a huge task as withdrawal can be worse than the disorder being treated by them. The side effects of withdrawing can be horrific, even in some cases the entire shedding of the skin (Margolin, 2007).

Trance intentions

1. Getting her to recognise her success and resources.
2. Dissociation from marital trauma.
3. Re-enforcing self-care behaviour.

4. Accepting her single status.
5. Re-enforcing the habit of chunking.
6. Installing boundaries and governors to reduce overwhelm.
7. Re-association to her body.
8. Hypnotic dreaming to counteract hyper-analytical thinking.
9. Lowering the out-of-control autoimmune response.
10. Changing her relationship with her genitals.

Okay so you have been doing well…you have changed your eating to healthy…**taking more care of yourself** (validating the client's work, re-enforcing the action)…now is time to step back from the drama of your separation (dissociation from trauma)…spend more time taking care of you (activating the survival mechanism, expanding her self-care)…**a lot of time taking care of yourself** (post-hypnotic suggestion)…you have raised your son and he is 18 and going off to university (triple ratification of competence)…you're getting used to being on your own (acclimatisation to new life)…**you're taking one thing at a time**…you have three months' paid leave coming up just for you…it's okay to have time (permission to have time for self)…attention…and self-care…**time just for exclusively eyes closed and going deep inside** (incorrect grammar, word salad, trance deepener)…over the next three months… no internet…no work (installing governors)…just being at your sister's holiday home by the sea (removing her from her stressful environment)…**lots of time…space…attention to taking care of your health** (direct suggestion, time expansion reducing life pressures)…peaceful life…relaxed…comfortable (silent suggestions for convalescence)…just in nature…talk to your body...hello body everything is okay (reassociation to the body)...and you can balance your... **body...mind...emotions** (intra-hypnotic suggestion)...creating peace and comfort within (ramping down the immune system)...your skin and pelvic regions can be bathed in a beautiful soothing colour (Vi+)...and feeling (Ki+ & Ke+)...**so comfortable and calm** (reducing cortisol and increasing serotonin and endorphins)... just like when you would sing a lullaby to your baby (bridging resources)...quiet peaceful and dreamy (disengaging hyper-analytical thinking)...**all your skin can be comfortable and peaceful** (intra-hypnotic and post-hypnotic suggestion)... **focus that peace and comfort in your genital area in your dreaming now** (suggestion for hypnotic dreaming, lapse of 5 minutes for hypnotic dreaming)...and you feel good...you feel at one with nature...**you feel at one with yourself** (somatic reintegration)...you feel free...you're in control of your life... **really loving your body** (esoteric generalised commands bypass critical conscious filters)....I love you...say that to your body...I love you...**say that to your genitals I love you**...your body is happy...your mind is happy...your skin is happy...your genitals are comfortable...**and happy**

Inducing endorphins is crucial in pain management as they are our natural painkillers, possessing morphine-like effects (Sprouse-Blum, 2010). We have known for a long time that B-endorphins reduce serum cortisol, stress, oxidative stress and pain in virtually any circumstance (Myint et al., 2017).

Patterson and Mendoza (2024) show us the extensive use of hypnosis in pain relief. Erickson's less direct and more metaphoric, interspersal hypnotic techniques were also effective in reframing pain (Erickson, 1966).

Gloria used the recording twice a day whilst on sabbatical. After two months her lichen planus was gone. After three months she could get three fingers or a dilator inside her vagina comfortably with lubrication. When she came back to the city, with her high-pressure job and the imminent divorce, the condition returned. She began to understand that it was agitated and activated by stress.

Song (2018), in a Swedish study, showed that those exposed to high levels of stress and trauma were more likely to develop autoimmune diseases, regardless of the source of the stress. We know that stress affects the brain/gut axis due to destruction of the balance in the microbiome between commensal bacteria and non-commensal bacteria (Moloney, 2014). This further disturbs homeostasis in the central nervous, immune and endocrine systems. Since the skin is the largest organ, disturbance of the microbiome also disturbs the balance of protective bacteria on the surface of the skin, and can cause dermal dysbiosis.

After two years the divorce was finalised, Gloria moved interstate to a small town by the sea, living a low-stress life, focusing on her health, and the condition went away again. After six months she started a sexual relationship with a local man who she became fond of, but reported she made it clear to him that she never wanted to get married again.

Whilst this disorder is often positioned as a psychiatric disorder associated with anxiety and depression, I think it is dangerous to presume there is no underlying physiological etiology that is exacerbated by stress (Maseroli, 2018).

We can see in Gloria's case that the reduction of stress and change of lifestyle reinitiated homeostasis, gave relief from the lichen planus and allowed her to restart her sex life and intercourse once again (see Appendix A, item 23).

CASE STUDY: PENNY

Penny was 26, married for two years, but was never able to have intercourse because her husband could not gain entry to the upper regions of her vagina.

Penny: *"My husband is the most wonderful man and has been very patient. I had a gynaecologist examine me under anaesthetic and he says there's nothing wrong with me, but my husband can only just get into the very beginning of my vagina."*

Tracie: *"That must have been very frustrating for the both of you. How can we help you today?"*

Penny: *"I'm an infant teacher and love children. Obviously, we want some kids. We do everything but intercourse. I need to get over the vaginismus. The gynaecologist said it must be psychological."*

Trance intentions

1. Therapeutic alliance.
2. Safety anchor.
3. Muscular relaxation, initiating the parasympathetic neurological system.
4. Bring her attention to self-exploration of her vagina.
5. Suggestion for daily vaginal dilation.

Usually if it is psychological it's because someone is tensing up at the beginning of intercourse...let's try to change things...**sit back and be comfortable in that big armchair safe in my office** (contingent suggestion)...think of a lovely relaxing colour as you close your eyes (bind)...tell me what that colour is (wait for response)...yes orange is a lovely colour and of peace...just fill

your body with that colour of peace now (direct suggestion)…
piece by peace in your own time as your body completely relaxes…I want you to start having sex with yourself often (giving her control)…once a day spend 15 minutes' private time using lubrication and slowly putting your finger inside your vagina…slowly and gently…**progressively spreading your finger as you widen your vagina**…put a ball of relaxing orange light all the way throughout your vagina inside your mind and body (universal relaxation)…**comfortable progressive exploration of your vagina**

Penny used the recording once a day before she did the exercise. She successfully managed entry into the beginning of the vagina but still experienced the same problems further up the vaginal canal. Since most vaginas range from one middle finger to one and a half middle fingers in depth, most women can manage to touch their cervix.

We then substituted her fingers for a series of progressively larger silicone sex toys. Unfortunately, surgeons and pelvic physiotherapists recommend glass or plastic dilators. The problem with these is that they can increase pain because they are not flexible like a penis. I much prefer patients to use silicone, flexible sex toys. A new recording was made for Penny to use each day in the same style, but with the suggestion to progress with the sex toys.

Added to that was a clitoral stimulator such as a magic wand or masturbation at the same time, then transferring that activity to doing it with her spouse to increase endorphins and oxytocin. Some women can use a sex partner, friend or sex surrogate to get comfortable with their vagina opening with another person. Adding clitoral stimulation also increases natural vaginal lubrication, reduces cortisol and increases serotonin.

The easiest and most comfortable position for vaginal insertion in vaginismus is the missionary position with a pillow underneath the hip. The straight missionary, rear entry, or on top position can leave the woman with less control as they give deep access to the vagina.

Chermansky (2016) discussed how dysfunctional pelvic floor muscles cause retention of urinary flow. This is a greatly under-researched area, and muscular contortion can also block intercourse. Earlier in this book, I talked about how under-developed vaginas can lead to a shallow pouch, unable to facilitate intercourse. Also, cases of vaginal agenesis can lead to almost a total absence of vaginal depth and structure.

Two months later there was the same lack of progress. When I reviewed the case, I noted the gynaecologist had gained entrance to the full vagina under anaesthesia, told the patient there was nothing wrong and that the vaginismus was psychological. I was beginning to think this was an incorrect diagnosis.

I have worked for many years with trans and intersex women who have undergone vaginoplasty, vaginal realignment or correction. They must use dilation to train the neovagina to stay open. The hypnotic relaxation technique is successful in these cases and with many women with vaginismus.

Due to lack of progress, I was beginning to suspect that Penny had an upper vaginal obstruction. I sent her to Australia's most experienced sex realignment surgeon who found that the musculature at the top of the vagina had a tendency to become contorted, blocking entry. On her second visit he performed vaginal Botox injections.

I saw Penny two months later and she had had successful intercourse with her husband several times. In this case my work turned out to be a supporting role to help her get to the root of the problem and find a solution (see Appendix A, item

24). As intercourse became a regular occurrence, the top part of the vagina stretched, and intercourse was possible.

Melnik et al. (2012) carried out a systemic review of studies for treating vaginismus. The problem here was that part of the research was based on the Cochrane Depression, Anxiety and Neurosis Group's Specialised Register. All too frequently, outdated, misogynistic, Freudian concepts of female sexual dysfunction are overly associated with neurosis when in fact there may be a physiological cause.

It was necessary, however, to inform Penny that the top part of her vagina may revert at times due to lack of sex or dilation, particularly during menopausal vaginal atrophy, or it may change after childbirth when the vagina stretches. For the time being, however, she was very happy with the results.

CASE STUDY: ILLENA

Illena was 32, in the army, and had appeared to go into early menopause at 30. No clinician could tell her why, but they suspected it had something to do with the stress of her working in a war zone for two tours.

Her oestrogen, progesterone and FSH were low, and LH, SBGH, cortisol, DHEA, TSH and inflammatory markers were high. In menopause we expect to see FSH elevated. There were no clear physiological signs of infection. She had no hot sweats. These markers were a clear sign of adrenal stress and dysregulation of the hypothalamic pituitary adrenal axis (HPA-Axis).

Sex had been intermittent in her life because she focused on her career first, thinking she would have a family later.

Illena: *"I was 17 when I enlisted, thought I'd retire at 43 and then have children. It's all been such a shock, and I haven't had sex since my periods stopped.*

I tried it with this guy in the field a year ago, but my vagina has shrunk. It's like I put it on a hot wash, and it came out smaller. It was too painful to have intercourse and do sex. He couldn't get it in."

Tracie: "It appears you're possibly in menopause and the vagina can seem as if it's smaller, particularly as you might not have the natural lubrication you used to have. But that would be an unusual diagnosis at 30 years of age so let's explore it further. Tell me, was it very stressful being in war zones?" (giving her space for catharsis)

Illena: "Very. I had to be vigilant and aware all the time. Sleep with one eye open. It's not just the enemy you've got to watch out for – it's your own guys misbehaving too."

Tracie: "Are you signing up for another tour?"

Illena: "No, no and no. I've done my duty. I'm taking three months' leave and transferring to a desk job in logistics at home. I need to focus on me for a time."

Tracie: "So how can we help you today?"

Illena: "I'm now afraid to try sex again. If you point a gun at me, I can handle that. I know 50 ways to deal with disarming you. But I'm now afraid to have sex because my vagina has shrunk."

Tracie: "Do you have any flashbacks, sleepless nights, nightmares or signs of PTSD?"

Illena: "No. I'm so tightly coiled and I've never let go of control."

Despite Illena being in the army and trained in combat, that would not exclude her from the effects of PTSD.

Musheyev (2022) reported on a 33-year-old woman who exhibited hypopituitarism, hypothyroidism, PTSD, amenorrhea, and panhypopituitarism. Some people with PTSD do not show outward signs as they internalise stress somatically, which affects their physiology and particularly the HPA axis.

Shufelt (2017) described some women who experienced PTSD functional hypothalamic hormonal disruption. They can seem, for the most part, asymptomatic, and were referred to as the 'walking well'. Bonazza et al. (2023) tell us this psychological change may lead to underlying depression and amenorrhea, which would naturally lead to vaginal atrophy and dryness.

Illena had been in a combat situation for two tours in a high state of alert. It had disrupted her natural sexual evolution because she focused primarily on her career. She initially appeared to have started early menopause and experienced vaginal atrophy. Her sexual clusters were around shock that she could no longer have children and that she could not engage in intercourse.

Trance intentions

1. Creating secure multiple safety anchors.
2. Orienting her body to the present time.
3. Regression to identify the drivers of the hypervigilance.
4. Validating the need for hypervigilance in a war zone.
5. Placing and recontexualising hypervigilance as a past need.
6. Reorientating her to the present.
7. Tapping into her survival mechanism to change fast, adaptive behaviour.
8. Direct commands to stand down and relax. Soldiers respond to direct commands.

9. Balloon imagery for vaginal expansion.
10. Training in using progressively-sized sex toys to restore vaginal flexibility.
11. Reassociating sex with good feelings.
12. Reassociating her to her sexual body.

Close your eyes and be safe in that chair…you're back home in your country which is also very safe because you're in my office (double locational anchors)…**when you hear my voice you can feel safe** (contingent suggestion, triple safety anchor)…you said to me 'I'm so tightly coiled and never let go of control'…that's an interesting statement (transderivational search to confirm the statement, trance deepener)…and when you were in the field it may have been a good statement (acknowledging the validity of the statement, placing it in past timeframe)…**and here we are now…today…in my safe office in the present**…go back to your time of being in the field inside your mind (regression)…tell me what is the statement doing for you when you're in the field?

Illena: *"It's keeping me alive."*

And that was a really good thing at that time (reorientating her back to the present, time shift)…but you know soldier that you must be aware of your surroundings at all times…**when your surroundings change you change and fast** (utilising her military training)…your life has changed…your surroundings have changed…**you are safe so stand down and relax soldier**… this is your mission now to relax…let go…do fun things…hang out with friends…and play for a while safe at home

There is always a danger when working with military or ex-military personnel who have seen action that when they return home from active duty, they then experience explosive decompression and full-blown PTSD.

Hacker Hughes (2008) clearly identifies the need to use controlled psychological decompression in reorientating post-combat soldiers back to normal life. The problem in researching this area is there are no clear guidelines or agreed methodology, due to cross-cultural, time and motivation difference. A therapist needs to feel their way on an individual patient basis, constantly observing the client's reaction to treatment.

This was a script I put on a recording that Illena used twice a day. I prescribed a herbal mixture of Valeriana officinalis (balancing the body system), Vitex agnus-castus (female reproductive regulator), Passiflora incarnata (calmative) and Glycyrrhiza glabra (adrenal regulator), daily probiotic (taken away from the herbs), plus daily B complex, Vitamin C 1000mgs, Zinc 25mgs, and magnesium 325mgs at night.

I also taught her the pelvic floor circle exercise for vaginismus to learn to relax those pelvic floor and vaginal muscles (see Appendix A, item 25). To relax those muscles requires a person to come out of beta and high beta brain wave activity, activate the vagus nerve and parasympathetic nervous system, reducing cortisol, and creating endorphins and serotonin. This gives greater access to the vaginal vault.

I saw Illena once a month for four months to reorientate her to a desk job at home in the army, at which time her menses returned. The return of the menses could not have been predicted and the treatment was a case of trying and seeing what happened.

In the fifth session:

Tracie: "So you've got your periods back."

205

Illena: "I didn't expect that. I guess I was much more
          stressed than I thought I was."

Dimoulas (2007), in studying female naval training recruits, found that 88% reported experiencing multiple symptoms of dissociation during peak training stress.

Tracie: "Well, in combat zones, people dissociate from
          their bodies as a form of self-defensive mental and
          emotional protection. Of course, that will now
          mean that your vagina will become more flexible
          and supple again."

Illena: "That's a relief."

Close your eyes and go inside…see your vagina inside your mind…**see it like a balloon that naturally stretches a great deal** (Vi+)…vaginas are very flexible because that's how babies get out (confirmation of its ability to stretch)…**you can be gentle with it just like you would a ballon** (permissive suggestion)…you stretch the balloon before you inflate it… **your vagina becomes more flexible as you relax and insert a nice soft sex toy inside daily** (post-hypnotic suggestion, contingent suggestion)…gently does it…take your time…lots of lubrication…you're in control at your own pace (gathering resistance)…**increasing the size of the sex toy as time goes by**… and when you come to sex you're happily enjoying your flexible vagina feeling good (Ki+, association between intercourse and positive kinaesthetic experience)…being in your full female sexual energy (reassociation to her sexual body)

Several months later Illena contacted me and told me she had started a relationship and intercourse was going well. It became clear that Illena experienced stress-related amenorrhea which led to vaginal atrophy. Resolving the stress was the key to restoring her menstruation and normalisation of her vaginal tissue, enabling her to have sex (see Appendix A, item 26).

CASE STUDY: HADIZA

Hadiza was visiting Australia from England on her sabbatical year between school and university. She was of African parents.

Hadiza: *"My boyfriend split up with me on the telephone this week. He's not in our church and my mother never wanted me to see him in the first place."*

Tracie: *"How can we help you today?"*

Hadiza: *"He tried to have sex with me, but couldn't get it in. He said I was too tight."*

Tracie: *"What do you think?"*

Hadiza: *"I think I should never have let him try but he pressured me. Then my GP said everything was normal so it must have been me to blame."*

Tracie: *"When do you think you will be ready for sex?"*

Hadiza: *"My parents are very strict and traditional from their country so they told me I shouldn't have sex until I'm married. But I grew up in England and I just want to be ordinary."*

Tracie: *"What's ordinary to you?"*

Hadiza: *"Well, trying sex with someone before I'm married to see if we are suited. Even to have sex without getting married, but I need to be more selective*

> *about the boys I date. I think I might like to try sex*
> *while I'm here in Australia."*

Tracie: "Why?"

Hadiza: *"Nearly all my friends have done it, or they are*
          in relationships. And I can try sex here in private
          without my parents interfering."

Here was a young woman feeling pressured to have sex by her ex-boyfriend and comparing herself to her friends who had sex. She believed she did not match up to her boyfriend's expectations, and experienced peer pressure from other women her age, and her parents. Her sex clusters were associated with her being in the position of not being able to please everyone, so she failed herself.

Trance intentions

1. Therapeutic alliance.
2. Self-autonomy.
3. Recontextualising sex as a good experience.
4. Changing sexual behaviour governors to sexual possibilities.
5. Elevating sex from the necessity of marriage to the heightened pleasure of free choice.
6. Promoting communication during sex.
7. Giving her control over the speed at which intercourse takes place.
8. Erickson's pseudo-orientation in time.
9. Learning the fun art of sex.
10. Taking her through the SRC. Psycho-imaginary experiential learning.

I would like you to trust me (eliciting therapeutic co-operation)…my intentions are to help you but not tell you what you must do (dissociating myself from those who told her what to do)…**only you can decide when it's right for you to have sex** (putting the decision in her hands)…of course for everyone it's different (liberating her from others' expectations)…and that's a good thing…**you'll know when it's right for you as your mind and body will tell you** (initiating intuition)…it's an individual choice that you have the right to make for yourself (positioning any choice she makes as right for her)…sex can be wonderful and…**a good experience…pleasurable…fun** (re-enforcing positive perspectives on sex)…it can even be a spiritual experience of ecstasy just as nature intended…it's such a natural experience when you take the time and communicate well with your partner…**each of you saying what's right for you** (giving her a voice)…close your eyes and relax inside your mind (taking her out of flight/fight/freeze)…relax in your body too because it's nice…slowing things down can make it right for you…**going at your own pace** (post-hypnotic suggestion)… you choose the time…place…pace…circumstances…and partner (silent suggestions)…just imagine inside your mind the future perfect way to have intercourse for the first time…**how do you look up inside your mind** (Vi+)…**how do you sound** (Ai+)…**how do you feel** (Ki+, triple question interrogative trance deepener, two minute elapses as she processes)…with that knowledge you can choose the person that's right for you… **when you know it's right you can relax your body and relax your vagina**…having a good time…bring the experience back with you to the room as you open your eyes and smile at me (association between the experience and good feelings)

Tracie: "*Hi…how was that for you?*"

Hadiza: *"It felt good. I took my time and was in control of my own body."*

Tracie: *"Sounds like a feminist manifesto to me. Great. It's what we all want as women. What we are all entitled to as women. To be able to control our own bodies and sometimes enjoying losing control to ecstasy."*

The United Nations (Raday et al., 2017) discussed in a position paper women's rights to autonomy over their own body. Less than half the world's women have that right and sexual freedom. Control over their bodies comes in the form of tradition, religion, legal constriction, misogyny, women upholding misogyny, and negative social views on sex.

Hadiza stated what her parents, religion and last boyfriend expected from her around sex. No one had asked her what she wanted before, so when it came to sex, she shut down out of fear of lack of bodily autonomy that translated into vaginismus.

Close your eyes again and go inside…be excited about sex (initiating stage 1 SRC)…I don't know how that will happen…and maybe you don't know how that will go well yet (presupposition it will happen)…**you will know what you know when you know how you know** (confusion, trance deepener)…in a way that's right for you…of course we are all learning about sex all the time (validation of progressive sex education and learning)… sex is different with different people…at different times…**we are all learning and experimenting and that's fun** (eliciting serotonin around the thought of sex)…and you can enjoy the journey of exploring your yoni and your clitoris…nipples…lips and each erogenous part of your body (stage 2 SRC)…and as the fun of exploring in a safe and relaxed way (silent suggestion for safe sex)…**you can build your sexual energy**…and when it peaks…what parts of your body will that sexual ecstasy explode from…your clitoris…vagina…or the whole body (stage 3, SRC)…**and your body just melts afterward into your lover's arms** (Stage 4, SRC)

First sexual experiences can often be clumsy, particularly if we have no or little sex education. They can carry with them a level of anxiety and fear of the unknown, which causes our body to tense up when it needs to relax. Sex education, learning and exploration leads to greater sexual satisfaction at the primary loss of virginity and subsequent sexual experiences (see Appendix A, item 27)

Hadiza listened to a recording of this content each day and read the *Complete Kama Sutra: The First Unabridged Modern Translation of the Classic Indian Text* (Vatsyayana, 2012).

Hadiza came to see me on her way back through Sydney to London. She had an affair with her diving instructor whilst up on the Great Barrier Reef. It lasted three weeks and she reported he was a very caring and experienced lover.

Tracie: *"So what made the difference?"*

Hadiza: *"That it was all my choice. And I could explore sex as little or as much as I wanted. Also learning that sex is so much more than just intercourse. Although the intercourse was very good, I mean really good, I will probably never see him again. And I now see sex as a form of connection to someone that has an ecstatic spiritual element. I now have a beautiful yoni, not just a vagina."*

10 Becoming orgasmic

Orgasm is one of the great ecstatic human experiences, but it is hugely misunderstood. On one side of the spectrum is suppression of sexuality that can mystify and suppress the experience, through the nocebo effect. On the other side of the spectrum is pornography, and unrealistic expectations of the earth moving beneath us, frequently setting us up to never be enough with our orgasms.

SO, WHAT IS AN ORGASM?

Well, that depends on your body, mindset, emotional state, experiences, cultural interpretation and expectations. Saffron (2016), from a mechanistic perspective, describes it as a neurophenomenology of sexual trance and climax, which would co-ordinate with stage three of the SRC, but this is very male centric.

Some females begin to orgasm in childhood and puberty, others may have a very low sex drive and no personal or cultural frameworks to perceive being orgasmic. Most males begin to orgasm during the dream state at puberty, often producing night emissions.

The problem here is that Saffron equates it to the ultimate goal of reproduction, ejaculation, manipulation of the genitals and a reproductive seizure. It is limited to a heteronormative point of view that belies the understanding of multiple orgasms and whole-body orgasms. He is correct, however, that it is the result of a trance-like altered state of focused attention, no matter how brief or how long.

Female ejaculation is thought to be the expulsion from the urethra of fluid from the Skene's gland before and during orgasm. It is commonly known as gushing or squirting. Research shows, however, that female ejaculation and squirting are different. Squirting is a sudden expulsion of liquid containing urine that partially comes from the bladder (Rodriguez, 2021).

Anorgasmia is the inability to achieve orgasm. Various treatments, such as transcutaneous temperature-controlled radio frequency (TTCRF) have been proposed with varying success (Alinsod, 2017). But these do not take a psychophysiological approach and are reductionist.

The ecstasy of an orgasm happens in the brain as a perception of genital and whole-body experiences. The parallel evidence we have for this is a sensation of pain, which regardless of the state of the body, we can manipulate with hypnosis and suggestion, which changes the perception of pain (Hilgard, 1983).

Wise (2017) reported when monitoring brain activity in women who self-stimulated and partner-stimulated that, "Extensive cortical, subcortical, and brainstem regions reach peak levels of activity at orgasm." The brain activity reduces considerably post-orgasm.

Holstege et al. (2003), using positron emission tomography, found measurable increases in regional cerebral blood flow (rCBF) during ejaculation. He stated, "Primary activation was found in the mesodiencephalic transition zone, including the ventral tegmental area, which is involved in a wide variety of rewarding behaviors. Parallels are drawn between ejaculation and a heroin rush."

ANORGASMIA

Starc (2019) tells us about the use of hypnosis in female anorgasmia where orgasm was achieved by masturbatory stimulus with the person's partner. The problematic issue with much research is that it continually refers to dysfunction. As therapists, we should avoid such language with clients because it cements them into that self-perception of failure. It is far better to use an approach of learning about how to make orgasms happen.

Bridges (1985) associated failure to orgasm in women with an unwillingness to relinquish control during coitus. Whilst that is true for some women who deprioritise orgasms, it is also a Freudian perspective that tends to ignore primary biological failure or lack of knowledge around sexual experiences.

Jenkins (2015) found that complete anorgasmia in men is far less frequent, and they are more likely to present with retarded ejaculation. This concurs with what I have found in my own practice. It is likely to be linked with lower levels of testosterone in men, though it can occur when testosterone levels are high. This suggests that sex binding hormones may be failing. I have also found it happening with men who experience MTHFR gene variations.

There is an incalculable combination of physical, mental, emotional, educational, ethnographic, social, and interpersonal dynamics that collide to produce anorgasmia. Therefore, we must test, observe, analyse and treat every case uniquely and differently.

For us as hypnotists and sex therapists, we cannot manually stimulate clients, even if we know how to physically teach them to move towards orgasms. That would be crossing ethical boundaries and leave us open to malpractice accusations. We can, at times, however, use and work with the client's partner and sex surrogates.

We do have the ability to use suggestion, help the client create erotic imagery, and to train them to be orgasmic. This of course is from a knowledgeable sex therapist's skill set. Unless the cause is a lack of psychosexual development or psychodynamic conflict, hypnosis alone is insufficient treatment. Since this is a multifaceted experience, the research in this area is piecemeal and anecdotal at best, and hypnosis generally forms a supportive role in sex therapy.

In each of the following cases I will show you some aspects of the way I work with clients who present with anorgasmia. There are many more, but these cases may give you some insight.

CASE STUDY: KYLIE

At 28 Kylie was in a relationship with a man who was becoming disinterested in her because she did not orgasm during intercourse with him.

Kylie: *"He's a nice guy, would make a great dad, but he's disappointed I don't come when he's inside me."*

Tracie: *"Let me get this right. He finds fault in you because you're not orgasming when he's having intercourse with you. He sounds pretty insecure to me. What do you want for yourself from therapy?"*

Kylie: *"Well, I've never orgasmed. I don't know if I can. What do you think? Do you think you could help me orgasm?"*

Kylie is like many women who have not been encouraged to explore their own orgasmic adventures. Most women are discouraged and shamed whilst men are encouraged to explore their sex adventures. Her sexual clusters were around feeling there was something wrong with her because she was being told she does not meet the boyfriend's sexual expectations.

She now associates intercourse with her being inadequate. It is important in these circumstances to explore all possible contributory factors to the anorgasmia and help people to discover their first orgasm (see Appendix A, item 28).

Trance intentions

1. Changing her perspective of what an orgasm may be to make it achievable by recontextualising.
2. Recalling past pleasurable experiences.
3. Recalling past pleasurable life orgasms.
4. Teaching her control over her body.

Sure...you can expand your idea of what an orgasm can be... it's a little seizure of pleasure...the French call it 'la petite mort' which means (sex education via metaphor)...**the little death of pleasurable tension**...that's all...it's simple...you've already had lots of pleasurable orgasms in your life (conversion of her self-perception of failure to success)...for instance...**the excitement (Ki+) and satisfaction you got when you saw (Vi+) you had good money in the bank** (kinaesthetic affect bridge to initiate SRC)...you can remember that feeling of relief...that feeling of joy...**that long shudder of pleasure you had throughout your body** (Ke+, regression to mine for past seizure experiences)... when you tasted your favourite ice cream (Gi+)...**that great feeling of pleasure** (reinitiating endogenous enkephalins and endorphins: the body's natural opioid experiences)....when you're on holiday and hear friends laughing (Ai+)...the smell of your favourite flower (Oi+)...**this even happens when you think about those things inside your mind** (transderivational search, intra-hypnotic suggestion, future pacing pleasure)... they are life orgasms...they are relatives of a sex orgasm...and of course there are many different kinds of sex orgasm you can enjoy (presupposition she will have different orgasms)... **and you will get that really good feeling as you spend time pleasuring your body** (post-hypnotic suggestion)

Here I am rehearsing her for the stage 3 of the SRC.

She looked confused, which makes her susceptible to suggestion.

Kylie: *"Isn't a big sex orgasm different from that?"*

Tracie: *"Do you want little orgasms and big orgasms?"*

Kylie: *"Well, yes."*

Tracie: *"Are you sure?" (nodding my head up and down)*

Kylie: *"Yes" (establishing a yes set)*

Tracie: *"Don't want to change your mind?" (shaking my head from side to side)*

Kylie: *"No."*

Tracie: *"Absolutely sure you want these?"*

Kylie: *"Yes." (locking the gate)*

There are many different kinds of sex orgasms (de-escalation of the polarity of orgasm and non-orgasm)...and they are only different like money in the bank is different from ice cream or being on holiday (rational comparatives)...**they all make you feel good** (validating different orgasms)...of course having an orgasm is something you practise...**and then get better and practise and better** (conditional suggestion, reducing the anxiety around whether she climaxes or not)...**having great sex does not necessarily mean you need to have the big orgasm** (allowing resistance)...you can have all sorts of orgasms where...when...and in a way that is right for you (self-determination)...**I will teach you beginning today**...a really good thing is to have control over your body...orgasms are a mechanical, chemical, neurological, emotional and even spiritual experience (information overload trance deepener)... you can first learn the circle exercise...**well...it's really three exercises joined together** (overload):

The circle exercise (as taught to client) (see Appendix A, item 29)

The seat – Sit in the chair and literally pull the exterior of your anus in as much as you can. Keep your mouth open as you inhale.

Kegel exercise – Lie on your back with your legs bent halfway up, and feet on the floor and suck your vagina up inside you like you have a vacuum cleaner inside (or if male, the space behind the scrotum). You can even do this practising with a vaginal barbell (particularly the Betty Dodson design). This engages your pelvic floor muscles that run behind your vulva and increases blood flow to the genitals. It stimulates the urethral nerves and sponge where you find your G spot. It also causes inhalation.

PC (pubococcygeus) muscle exercise – This muscle runs underneath your body from your genitals to your anus, attached to the top of the front pelvis, with the insertion at the coccyx. Try this when you are sitting on the toilet peeing, suddenly stop the flow and then start it again. Feel the perineum engaging. Try to push the muscle down and notice how the urinary flow increases. Then relax and notice the difference. Now practise it without urinating. When you push down, it also causes you to breathe out.

These are pelvic floor exercises. Start doing them in a circle, sucking in the anus, then drawing in the kegels, then pushing down the PC (bearing down). Continue the circle as you practise this rhythm for 10 minutes. You can do it lying on your back, thrusting your hips up and down at the same time as you masturbate. Do this at least once a day for 10 minutes or longer. It stimulates the feeling in your clitoris and urethral sponge (via the urethral nerve). When you find yourself moving towards high excitement and orgasm, focus mainly on the PC exercise and work it by pushing the PC down.

Golmakani (2015) used a randomised control trial administering pelvic floor exercises to primiparous (bearing a first child) women for eight weeks. The experimental group saw significant improvement in sexual self-efficacy, but there were no improvements in the control group.

Pastore (2014) reported a trial of giving pelvic floor muscle exercises to men with lifelong premature ejaculation, over 12 weeks. He reported an 82.5% success rate of gaining ejaculatory control.

There are many different kinds and systems of pelvic floor exercises. This training is given within the context of also strengthening the abdominals, gluteal, adductors, latissimus dorsi and spinus erectus muscles through exercise.

Muscles must work in co-ordination to create pelvic floor balance, providing good sexual function and genital stimulation. When some muscles are too loose or too tight, it causes sexual problems. This is particularly noticeable in post-partum women, who, during pregnancy and birth, have over-stretched muscles that become flaccid, and can also cause urinary incontinence.

This looseness of the pelvic muscles is also prevalent in modern adults in developed countries who lead sedentary lives and have poor muscle tone, or in ageing individuals.

There is a caution here, however, as women's bodies are different from men's, particularly more mature women or those with osteoporosis. Lunges and squats can put too much pressure on older bodies. Stretches, aerobics, and resistance exercise are far more effective.

I tend to break these sessions down to between three to several sessions, so the person is not overwhelmed and abandons therapy. It is a lot of information to take in if you have not had a life that involved erotic stimulation before. I also back everything up with written information and videos so the client has resources to use at home.

Hypnosis was used to help Kylie implement these changes, including listening to recordings I made for her each day. She was taught to raise her sexual energy through sexual energy breathing and to alternately tighten those pelvic floor muscles as she emulated intercourse. This process was to get faster to take her to climax during masturbation or sex with a partner.

Sit comfortably back in my office and close your eyes… you have been learning that small pleasures can be enlarged…**a pleasant sensation in your clitoris gets magnified**…which feels good (Ki+)…you enjoy those sensations…an exciting feeling in your vagina and clitoris is pleasing…**that you can times by 10 inside your mind**…(fractionation)…you can feel good in your breasts…which can be really nice when you just let go… **experiencing that again and again**…when you masturbate you can rub your clitoris with your hand…massage the area above your pubic region with the other…**and thrust with your pelvis faster and faster**…as you get more excited…the faster you get the faster your breathing gets….**the pleasure keeps on increasing until it explodes into relief and bliss** (fractionation)

Here I am also teaching her to find her G spot (Gräfenberg Spot) at the urethra sponge, getting her partner to press his fingers on her midriff whilst she is masturbating and using a sex toy. The urethral sponge surrounds the urethra and the clitoral nerve. During arousal it becomes engorged with blood and compresses the urethra to prevent urination.

The urethral sponge contains many nerve endings that can become highly sensitive during arousal which increases sexual pleasure. It can also be stimulated during rear entry intercourse because the penis or sex toy presses against the front wall of the vagina that presses on the sponge.

Therapy was also about her taking control of herself and ownership of her body and not just allowing her vagina to be another way for her boyfriend to masturbate. This empowerment was to allow her to determine when and how she would orgasm.

Most women give up on orgasm far too early. It takes practice and dedication to creating those orgasm trances. It is important to encourage our clients to stay with it as they practise getting better and better at creating those orgasmic seizures.

Kylie was also tasked to work from the Barbara Carrellas (2007) book *Urban Tantra*. Along with further therapy and coaching, she achieved orgasm within two months.

CASE STUDY: JUSTIN

Justin was a local government civil servant. At 35 he had worked his way up the career ladder, been married for 10 years and had two children.

Justin: *"I can come okay after about 30 minutes, but I don't orgasm. My wife gets enough sex because I can last, but she's disappointed I don't get excited, even when I'm coming. She jokes it's like having sex with a civil servant."*

Tracie: *"I'm just wondering what you think an orgasm is?"*

Justin: *"Well, my wife says it's like jumping out of a window with no parachute and landing safely in heaven."*

Tracie: *"And what do you think it is?"*

Justin: *"I guess you get all excited and out of control."*

Tracie: *"What I notice is you hold your breath, and you are quite a shallow breather. How do you breathe when you come?"*

Justin: *"The same really. I think I breathe the same all the time."*

Everything about Justin pointed toward a form of autism: restricted breathing, sensory restricted monitoring, the flat (unexpressive, emotional blunting) face when talking, and chronic and persistent perfunctory behaviours. He was undiagnosed and highly functioning with no excessive behaviours. It was important here not to give him a pathological behavioural label that could damage his quality of life.

Tracie: "So, what do you want from coming along here today?"

Justin: "I want to perform sexually like other men, so my wife is happy."

Justin functioned well in all areas of his life due to his persistent perfunctory nature. His marriage seemed to be going well. His monotone emotional state continued into his sex life where, whilst he performed intercourse adequately, he was not altering his state in moving towards ejaculation. His sexual clusters were around believing he might be missing out on what he referred to as normal people's experience of orgasm. Cognitively he associated intercourse and sex with performance and not necessarily getting excited.

Trance intentions

1. Ego strengthening.
2. Associating ejaculation with success, achievement and happiness.
3. Changing breathing patterns towards orgasms.
4. Conscious awareness of breathing patterns.
5. Teaching him to be aware of when in his body he is coming to the end of the plateau stage of the SRC.
6. Learning to gather and direct his sexual energy.

Tracie: "Interesting (pause, engagement)...you tell me your wife gets enough sex because you can last during intercourse (transderivational search)... **that's really good** (ego strengthening)...you tell me you can ejaculate and indeed have two children... **which I'm sure you and your wife are happy**

223

*and feel good about (initiating endorphin and serotonin)…orgasm of course is an individual experience (reduction of comparatives with other people)…your individual experience just for you (presupposition one will take place)…**just right for you** (inferred satisfaction)…did you know orgasm is connected to your breathing patterns (interrogative association)…I know you're a smart and analytical sort of person so let's…**examine those breathing experiences now** (analytical challenge)*

Chakra locational breathing identification exercise

Taking Justin into the esoteric concept of the chakras disables his analytical critical inferences.

Close your eyes and monitor your body as you locate where you are breathing from, and what part of your body is moving. I am going to help you locate your main chakras:

1. Breathe in from underneath your undercarriage between your scrotum and your anus. This is your base first chakra (the Root Chakra (Muladhara).

2. Then move your breathing in up to just around your midriff, just above your genitals. Your second chakra, the sex chakra (the Sacral Chakra (Svadhishthana). At this lower level, the breathing is quite slow.

3. Move your breathing in up to your mid abdominals above your belly button and below the ribs. This is your third chakra (the Solar Plexus Chakra (Manipura). This

is where you sense your emotions because 95% of your serotonin is created in your gut. As you move up your chakras, you are accumulating and gathering sexual energy.

4. Move your breathing in up to your heart space and lungs. This is your fourth chakra (the Heart Chakra (Anahata). This is the centre of your connection to your wife and your good feelings and love towards her.

5. Move your breathing in up to your throat. This is your fifth chakra (the Throat Chakra (Vishuddha). This is your centre for communication where you tell your wife how beautiful she is as you make love to her.

6. Move your breathing in up to your forehead between your eyes. This is your sixth chakra (the Third Eye Chakra (Ajna). This is where your intuition lives and where you see yourself as a sexual, passionate man.

7. Move your breathing in up to above the crown of your head (the Crown Chakra (Sahasrara). This is like a control centre that balances your body and your sexual energy and can explode out of you when you ejaculate and orgasm.

Open your eyes and look at me (still artificially somnambulistic)…becoming aware of your breathing and the amount of oxygen going around your body (silent suggestion)… **you can fully appreciate oxygen is the breath of your life** (intra- and post-hypnotic suggestion)…the more oxygen you have the more excited you become with more sexual energy (plateau stage of SRC)…it's a really simple analysis (appealing to his analytical ego to ingest the concept)…**as you control your breathing you control your level of excitement**… your breathing gets faster coming up your body…the higher you move up the chakras the more sexual energy you gather (contingent suggestion, fractionation)…as you keep gathering the excitement up to your crown at some point you just let it go out through the crown of your head…**it feels great and you just let go and relax whether you have come or not** (resolution stage 3 of SRC or non-ejaculation orgasm)…of course you can have an orgasm in any part of the body…**which will be really interesting for you to experiment with** (post-hypnotic suggestion).

Casula (2022) reviews the use of metaphor in psychotherapy and its ability to bypass conscious critical thinking and resistance. In hypnotherapy we have a history of this theory from Franz Mesmer to Milton Erickson. It is unimportant whether Justin believes in chakras or not as what I did was provide him with a framework within which to learn to monitor and relate to his body and its biological rhythms. It gave him a system he could use because he was a systemic person who was goal-orientated.

It is important to remember that Justin had no complaints about the desire or plateau stage of the SRC. I also did not focus on his feelings or any conflict. He was task orientated. I gave him a mechanical awareness exercise which he could follow analytically.

Only at the end did I give a suggestion for "letting go" and "feeling great". So, we are creating a sexual seizure trance. It was important not to panic him by increasing oxygen without it being associated with performance rewards and the release of the sexual energy he had gathered, framed as an orgasm.

I put the instructions on a 10-minute recording that he used every day. He was to practise the process during sex and share what he was doing with his wife.

Along with that, I did other state-shifting work with him, teaching him to change states fast around joy, sadness, excitement, and acceleration of feelings. This included mind, body language and facial expression changes because neurology is hard-wired, and people with limited emotional ranges need to be taught these states which they normally do not do naturally (see Appendix A, item 30).

With practice Justin was able to experience what he thought was an orgasm within three months, which was a large release of energy. The important factor was he thought it was an orgasm.

Men can also learn to experience multiple orgasms using edging which is holding back near to an orgasm and experiencing orgasms in other parts of the body, rather than the genitals at ejaculation (see Appendix A, item 31).

Final session six months later:

Justin: *"Yes. I looked up 'la petite mort' as you asked me to. When it comes to sex, it means the little death and sort of loss of consciousness. The bit at the end of sex when you come or climax. I get it now."*

Tracie: *"It's good to have a full life, isn't it?"* (sealing therapy)

CASE STUDY: CAROL

Carol: *"Believe it or not, I'm 38 and I only started masturbating one year ago. I've learnt to orgasm, but it takes me nearly an hour with different sex toys and vibrators."*

Tracie: *"A big congratulations for connecting deeper with your sexuality. What can we help you with today?"*

Carol: "I can't orgasm with my husband. He gets tired and it puts me off. I want to be able to reach orgasm more quickly."

Tracie: "What do you think an orgasm is?"

Carol: "It's me losing it and shouting 'Yes'. The fireworks moment at the end of the show. It seems I'm a noisy one. I'm loosening up a lot and no longer care about being so controlled."

Carol was an upper-class housewife. She was brought up to marry into high society and behaved in a controlled way. Sex had been something she did to keep her husband happy. At 37 her body revolted against her repressed upbringing, giving her the first orgasm on her own. Although she could orgasm more quickly in private, her sexual clusters were still around pleasing her husband when they had sex. For most of her adult life sex had been associated with being a good wife.

Trance intentions

1. Associating fun with experimenting with orgasm.
2. Expanding her orgasm repertoire.
3. Positive hallucinations of orgasms.

What's really fun to learn (reducing anxiety)...**there are many different kinds of orgasms that can happen during sex**... or even not during sex (expanding sex skills)...playing with multiple orgasms is really great (implied directive)...**there are little mini orgasms...long orgasms...OMG orgasms**...and of course...**multiple orgasms that keep repeating** (information overload, recontextualising orgasms, causing trance induction)...close your eyes and dream...just imagine...a really wonderful dream of you having…**many different kinds of orgasms** (engaging sensory positive hallucinations)…as you're dreaming those… **mini**…**long**…**OMG**…**and multiple orgasms**…(she was left in hypnotic dreaming for five minutes, reducing conscious resistance)

If the client is already on the road to their goals, we do not need to push the boulder up the hill. Simply supplying them with more options allows the client to expand their experience.

The rest of the session was spent teaching Carol breathing and tantric sexual chakras work. It was also putting what she learnt on a recording, and she was given back-up written material to practise daily and follow at home.

Session two was four weeks later.

Tracie: *"Let's continue with the learning today. Have you ever looked at someone and just thought, 'Oh My God he's hot', and got a shudder going through your body?"*

Carol: *"Yes. Tom Cruise, naked, in the a film* The Right Moves. *He's cocky and hot. It's a turn on."*

Trance intentions

1. Locational fantasy erotic stimuli.
2. Fractionation of that stimuli.
3. Teaching her back-to-back orgasm.
4. Recontextualising what an orgasm may be.
5. Teaching her how to create multiple orgasms.

Close your eyes and just re-run that scene of Tom Cruise naked in your mind and…**get that shudder again** (affect bridge)… nod your head when you've done it and got the shudder (she nods her head)…**wow quick you know that scene really well**

don't you (interrogative suggestion, intra-hypnotic suggestion, the speed bypasses conscious interference and resistance)...in a moment I want you to run it again but times that shudder by 10...and nod your head when you have done that (fractionation, she nods her head smiling)...and run it again and times the shudder by 100 and nod your head (she squirms in the chair and nods her head, nudging suggestion)...**good very good enjoying yourself** (validating the work)....this time I want you to transfer that shudder to your genitals...clitoris...vagina...or both while you (silent suggestions, creating anticipation)...**run the scene again now** (the illusion of choice because whatever option she chooses she enters the plateau stage of the SRC)... nod your head when you've done (she nods her head)...was that good for you (louder voice)...or not (softer voice, tonal direction, she replied yes)...**really really good feelings**...now I want you to run the scene again and again as many times as you can really fast...back to back really fast...**and I want you to get those shudders in your genitals each time you re-run the scene** (after 30 seconds)...open your eyes and look at me (artificial somnambulism)

Tracie: *"So how was that for you?"*

Carol: *"Fuck! Mind the language. Is that legal?"*

Yes...we are doing hypnosis and sex therapy...**and you seem to be having a good time**...people get precious about what they think an orgasm is and that's setting themselves up for failure...you are not one of those people (direct suggestion)... you can wonder about enjoying many different kinds of orgasm (searching for referential index, trance deepener, indirect suggestion)...**remember in your mind...body...and genitals** (intra-hypnotic suggestion)...an orgasm can be...**mini**...

OMG…**long**…**or multiple**…every orgasm is a sex seizure that is…**thrilling and ends in a sense of pleasure and sometimes release**…now some women orgasm in their clitoris during masturbation…and some in their vagina…and some during intercourse when the man's or partner's body is rubbing against them stimulating the clitoris during intercourse…or even during intercourse when the clitoris is also being manually stimulated…you can orgasm just thinking about a really hot person (expanding sexual experience)…**there are so many ways to orgasm and you can choose what gives you pleasure at different times** (generalised suggestion, direct suggestion)… of course practice is the key…close your eyes…every day you can try different kinds of ways of orgasming…**you can enjoy the excitement** (stage 1)…**a period of sex** (stage 2)…**and the orgasm** (stage 3)…whatever feels good as it happens (silent suggestion)…**afterwards you're feeling good** (stage 4)… during sex you can gather your sexual energy up through your chakras…be aware of your breathing…**keep pushing your PC muscles down during the multiple orgasms**…and pump them and breathe out to help another one happen…and even when you have an orgasm you carry on for another if you want

In perimenopausal and postmenopausal women, it is important to use lubrication to restore sexual fluidity. Not water-based because it dries out. Try plant-based and of course hypoallergenic. It needs to be viscous and remain viscous. Some younger women also need lubrication.

The G spot is more sensitive during a fuller bladder. When the urethral sponge is inflated, it tends to make the G spot hypersensitive. When teaching women to orgasm, a pre-sex fuller bladder can increase sensitivity.

I gave Carol an exercise for her and her husband to do:

FINDING THE G SPOT

1. Get your husband to give you cunnilingus.
2. He puts his middle finger up inside your vagina with the palm of his hand facing forward.
3. He presses forward up inside your vagina with that middle finger.
4. At the same time with the other hand, he presses down on your midriff just above your pubic area as he continues cunnilingus.
5. His hands pulsate towards each other with the rhythm of you thrusting your hips. He needs to pay attention to your rhythms as you get more excited towards orgasm.

The delusion that sex comes totally naturally is just that. We need to learn the art of sex, just as we need to learn the art of walking or carrying three plates at once. A large part of our work as a sex therapist is to rehearse the client in the art of sex.

Two months later Carol had expanded her sex and orgasm repertoire. She was enjoying the different kinds of orgasms. In the final session she commented, "If only the carpenter, who is building some wardrobes for us, knew what I was thinking about and what was happening in my knickers. My husband is quite confused by what's happened now I'm orgasming a lot, but he's certainly not complaining."

Gérard (2021) published the results of an online survey of 419 sexually diverse women, aged 18 to 69, who identified as multi-orgasmic. They were assessing sociodemographic backgrounds, context and characteristics of a recent typical multi-orgasmic experience. The data found that such characteristic experiences were not the same for everyone.

What is important for a sex therapist to remember is that we know in the Tantric, Kundalini and Taoist traditions the ability to reach multiple orgasms has been taught for thousands of years and is not a matter of some women and men getting lucky (see Appendix A, item 32).

CASE STUDY: JAMILE

This young man of 23 was brought up in the Middle East in a strict Muslim family. Any mention of anyone being gay was dangerous, put the family in danger, and carried the risk of being imprisoned or killed.

Jamile: *"I knew from an early age I liked men. I didn't really understand it because there was no information. It was clear that I couldn't tell anyone. My family and everyone I knew said it was bad and the religious police hurt people like that."*

Tracie: *"That must have been difficult and frightening for you as a teenager."*

Jamile: *"I was very good at English studies, watched American films and decided I wanted to study to become an engineer in another country. My family didn't want me to go to America, so I came to an Australian university. I'm never going back to my country of birth. When I went to the Gay and Lesbian Mardi Gras here, I couldn't believe it, there were gay police."*

Tracie: *"Well, how can we help you today?*

Jamile:	"I'm embarrassed to talk about sex. I've had a boyfriend for two months, we slept together four times, but I can't come."
Tracie:	"Do you masturbate, and do you come and have an orgasm?"
Jamile:	"Yes, it's no problem. I'm just too embarrassed to come in front of him. If my family find out, they will stop my allowance and disown me. I will be forced to go back to my country and be hurt."
Tracie:	"I see...that's a difficult situation for anyone...what do you think the solution is?"
Jamile:	"I don't know. That's why I came to you."
Tracie:	"How many more years before you finish your degree and change from a student visa to a work visa?"
Jamile:	"Two years but I have a boyfriend now."
Tracie:	"Are you okay to be guided by me?"
Jamile:	"Yes, if you can help me."

Jamile would be in danger in his country of birth. His life had been about trying to live in another country, which he managed as a student. His sex clusters were centered around the fear of being found out and forced to move back to his country of origin. Whilst his libido drove him towards sex, it was always in a state of fear.

Trance intentions

1. To ensure him a private, safe place to consider his dilemma.

2. To separate the conflicts so each became manageable.
3. To propose and consider an engineered solution.
4. To suggest the safe options of staying in the closet for the moment.
5. Regression to uncover the drivers for the anorgasmia.
6. Suggesting there are mental engineering solutions.
7. Conflict negotiation for him being able to ejaculate but have an orgasm in other parts of his body instead.

Okay I want you to know first of all that I tell no one about your visits to me...in fact that would be illegal for me to do that (safety was important to him and his number one driver)... **you can know you are safe here with your eyes closed now** (contingent suggestion, locational safety anchor)...it seems there are two problems you face (separating the problems to make them more manageable)...one your family can't find out about you being gay at this moment in time...two your mind still thinks it's back in the country you came from...**both have an engineering solution** (presumption there are solutions)... for safety you will only see your boyfriend privately and not in public (post-hypnotic suggestion)...no posting on social media (hypnotic governors)...and you begin to engineer your mind more in a Western way of thinking about being gay (cultural adjustment)...**these are the pillars to hold up your bridge to the work through the next two years to hold up the bridge so it doesn't fall down**...go back to the last time you slept with your boyfriend...you're having sex...tell me what are you thinking about?

Jamile: *"I'm so ashamed. What if someone finds out? What if my family finds out? It's wrong. I'm a bad person. I like him to fuck me, but I just can't come."*

Now as an engineer you have to use the right tools for the right job…you may use a theodolite to survey the ground…you may use a computer to make your calculation…**the right tools for the right job** (metaphor for appropriate skill sets)…you have to use the right steel concrete rock wood glass cable support beams roofing and contractors (cognitive overload, trance deepener)…the right tools for the right job…for sex…**you can have the right thoughts for sex to be good** (modal operator of possibility)…carefully engineering those thoughts… **the thoughts that are right for the culture you live in now** (locational re-adjustment)

Some immigrants live the same life they did in their original country, just in a different location. Johnsson (2015) found that immigrants' major reason for failing to adapt to a new culture was directly linked to the levels of stress in moving.

Whilst Jamile faced little discrimination for being gay in a major city in Australia, his source of income was derived from the homophobic culture and family he came from. This was a daily stressor that prevented him from fully identifying as a gay man, so he faced constant psychodynamic conflicts around sex.

The only safe option for him was to stay in the closet until he could finish his degree and become financially independent. Normally as a sex therapist, I would want a client to adopt their identity as soon as possible, but many people's lives are far more complex. By supporting Jamile staying in the closet for the time being, it relieved some of his stress because a professional had advised him to do that.

The second conflict was his internalised homophobia, due to two decades of religious programming, preventing him from climaxing during sex with a man. Both conflicts were interrelated and co-dependent.

Jamile I'm wondering if we might engineer a solution (engaging his interest)…a workaround for just the next two years (conditional bargaining)…**allowing you to ejaculate during sex** (post-hypnotic suggestion)…because as you know it feels good to ejaculate and orgasm (truism)…let's try this (participation invitation, therapeutic alliance)…**for the next two years when you ejaculate during sex you feel an orgasm in other parts of your body instead of your penis** (disintegration)…go forward in your mind (future pace)… the next time you have sex with your boyfriend you can have an orgasm in all the other parts of your body apart from your penis…**you allow yourself to ejaculate**…the orgasm which can be very intense…**it can happen everywhere else in your body but not in your penis** (we are retaining the codependent conflict but changing the way it works)

Dąbrowski (1964) wrote about positive disintegration theory of personality development, noting that it must be created and shaped by the individual to reflect their own unique character. Jamile partly needed the stress of his life to force him to create a change of his values and beliefs as he adjusted to a new life.

He had told me that the difficulties in his childhood had motivated him to study English and leave his country of origin. When we serve the client everything ready-made on a plate, we can infantilise them and disempower them.

When working with clients we must be careful not to project all our values onto the client. Such massive sudden change can cause a collapse of coping skills and psychotic decompression in some people who are highly vulnerable. Heffer (2017) states that an alarming number of university students experience depression, anxiety and suicidation due to the stress of too great a cultural change and are unable to cope mentally and emotionally. The workaround worked for Jamile, allowing him to ejaculate during sex but not have an orgasm in his penis.

Like clockwork, after he had got his degree, job, working visa and was now financially independent, and had been through five other sex partners, he came back to see me.

We worked on eliminating his internalised homophobia and embracing himself as a gay man. I also helped him bring his orgasm back to his penis at stage 3 of the SRC, whilst at the same time having whole body orgasms. This allowed him to resolve his two conflicts and be publicly known in Australia as a gay man.

He intended to never go back to his country of origin or mention his sexuality when communicating with his family.

Tracie: *"Your duty Jamile is to live the blessed life that Allah gave you the best that you can. To respect and love the gift of life. Your family are entitled to their lives in their world and you to yours. As-salamu alaykum."*

Orgasm is a deeply personal experience and dependent on so many aspects of the person's physical, mental, emotional and social topography. In Jamile's case, whilst he still wanted to experience orgasm, it had to be within the context of his current personal and cultural situation (see Appendix, item 33).

I do not accept the majority of people who telephone me with anorgasmia if it becomes clear they are not prepared to invest the time, money, or effort in making the change. They often deprioritise the importance of an orgasm in their lives to the point that they are not prepared to make the protracted effort, but just want someone else to fix it with hypnosis.

I explain to them it is a process and they will need to go through different steps of sex therapy to achieve their goal. Hypnosis is a vehicle that can help the process go faster and more comfortably.

11 Unwanted Sexual Behaviours

I am calling this section, 'unwanted sexual behaviours'. I wanted to avoid the word 'paraphilia' (to like something additional or alongside normal sex) because of its pathological connotations (American Psychiatric Association, 2022).

The foundations of this kind of pathologisation and the fight against it reaches back to Ellis & Symonds (1896); Gebhard et al. (1965) and many more. We can see in Unwin (1934) how he opens his enquiry into culture and sex by describing different groups of people as 'civilised and uncivilised'. Many of these researchers may not have intended their studies to be ammunition for commercialised psychiatry and psychology to market a supposed normality and abnormality, but that is what often happened.

The pathologisation of sexual behaviour has also been used as a political tool throughout the ages, and used by politicians and religious groups to push their own agendas, divide people and control public narratives. We can see from Foucault's discourse that he equates politics to mean power (1991). Politics, religion, medicine and pharmaceuticals are all industries that seek power over human sexuality by naming and shaming for profit.

The same is happening again in sex therapy today with many university-educated sex therapists trying to turn sex into solely a reductionist science, devoid of the art of therapy, or the art of sex.

Indeed, in ancient Greece, where same-sex relationships were commonplace, there were no words like 'homosexual' or 'lesbian', as all such relationships were generally considered part of everyday life.

There is no 'normal' with sex, as everyone's experience and developed taste accumulates individually. Paraphilia in the legal sense has often been used to condemn different groups of people.

It is also important to remember that every generation and cultural group creates its own sexual preferences due to the individual's and group's exposure to influences.

It is not that I never use the word 'paraphilia' in court reports, only that it must be the individual who claims its common usage and owns the word if they feel their attachments are highly pathological and detrimental.

The idea that sexuality develops exclusively at puberty is a myth. Like many other attachments, sexuality is influenced as soon as cognition, values, beliefs, emotions, and behavioural routines begin. Its beginning in formative years tends to happen outside conscious awareness. In some cases, it is also influenced by physiological aspects.

Whilst primary sexual attachments establish during formative years and escalate at puberty, other attachments can also form during any period of life, adding to or extinguishing previous attachments.

Here I want to emphasis that what I do with clients is not correct them to become 'normal' but assist them to make the alterations they want and need to live the best lives they can. As a sexologist, this will, of course, include guiding them in all cases where they seek help.

I have had thousands of telephone calls from spouses and relatives of potential clients asking me to correct the sexual behaviour of the person they are telephoning about. My answer is always the same: "Unless you're the official carer or guardian of the person, the person must telephone me themselves." Even when they are the official carer, I still want to talk to the person on the telephone in advance to screen whether they would be suitably compliant for hypnosis and wish to change their behaviour.

CASE STUDY: SEBASTIAN

Dorothy, Sebastian's mother, telephoned me to ask if I could help as she was his official carer. He was 24, had an IQ of around 65, was verbal, lived at home with his parents, was on no medications, and had never worked due to his intellectual disability. The family addressed him as Seb.

On going out into public recently, he had started to exhibit sexual advances to unknown women. Three months earlier the family had attended a festival and whilst in a crowd Seb had placed his hand on an 18-year-old woman's backside. She was very upset, and the police were called.

Seb's family explained he was disabled and apologised profusely, but the young woman's family insisted on pressing charges. When the matter went to court, the magistrate found that he was not guilty due to diminished responsibility, but still made a court order that he attend corrective therapy.

In working with intellectually challenged people there is a strong need to frame the therapy as a carrot, not a stick. Such people often have lower cognitive ability to control their emotions. It is important to focus on the positive experience of coming to my office and keep the sessions short.

I asked that the day Seb was brought to my office it was treated as a family outing into town, and he was promised ice cream after they had visited me. His mother had told me on the telephone that he loved ice cream.

Seb's family were traumatised by what happened and said that they had ceased to go on family outings. Since the incident Seb had also not gone to the daycare centre he usually attended during the week.

Much of the history-taking was done by telephone and email in advance of the session. There was no history of violence or aggressive behaviour. At the beginning of the session Seb's mother was present and handed me some documents, then waited in the waiting room whilst Seb and I worked together.

Tracie: *"Well, hello Seb. How very nice to meet you. Have you been having a good day in town?"*

Seb: *"Yeah we went Opera House see pigeons."*

Tracie: *"Why, that's great. Did you do anything else?"*

Seb: *"Shoes. I got new trainers…smart!"*

Tracie: *"Lucky you. It's fun to have good trainers, isn't it?"*

Seb: *"Yeah, smart."*

Tracie: *"Your mum told me you got into trouble at a festival when you touched a lady's bottom."*

Seb: *"Yeah she was nice but got angry."*

Tracie: *"Well…you know Seb…**you can't touch people without asking them first**…don't you?" (direct suggestion within an interrogative suggestion)*

Seb: *"Yeah, but she was pretty."*

Tracie: *"You know that touching her without asking hurts her."*

Seb: "I didn't want to hurt her, just touch."

Tracie: **"If you touch someone without asking, that hurts them**...do you understand that?" *(initiating cognitive understanding)*

Seb: "Yeah, I ask first".

Tracie: **"I want you to ask your mum or dad first**...if it's okay to ask the person if you can touch them...you can do that...can't you?"

Seb: 'What if mum and dad not there?"

Tracie: **"You wait and ask them later or ask a carer... okay?"**

Seb: "Yeah, okay."

Tracie: **"You don't want to get in trouble with the policeman**...again...do you?"

Seb: "No way."

Tracie: **"You don't want to hurt or frighten anyone**...do you?"

Seb: "Not hurt anyone."

Tracie: **"You want girls and boys to feel safe**...don't you?"

Seb: "Yes, everybody safe. I kind."

Tracie: **"And you'll be kind doing that**...very kind to everyone."

Seb: **"Be kind to everyone**...and get ice cream at home every day."

Tracie:	*"Can we play a game…the be nice game…**you want to play before ice-cream?**" (interrogative suggestion)*
Seb:	*"We play now."*

Algahtani (2017) discusses the combined use of constructivism and behaviourism in teaching people who are intellectually challenged, rather than exclusively using one or the other. My professional experience as a hypnotherapist and psychotherapist is that parents and carers who lean towards respective behaviourism generally produce better automatic behaviours. That must, however, have very positive experiential associations with the behaviourism for the client.

It is important to remember in hypnosis with people with intellectual challenges that they will take everything you say as literal. The Committee to Evaluate the Supplemental Security Income Disability Program for Children with Mental Disorders et al. (2015) found that there can be reduced ability in cognitive processes, problem solving, reasoning, judgement and abstract thinking. Therefore, I observe that direct suggestion will encounter less resistance because there may be less processing through the frontal lobes.

Seb was a young, intellectually challenged man whose libido was still normal for his age. He was, however, not clear about the boundaries around acceptable sexual behaviour. His sexual clusters were finding women attractive and wanting to touch them, driven by libido, having less impulse control than the average person, and not intellectually understanding the rules around sexual engagement.

Trance intentions

1. To instill stronger boundaries around sexual advances.
2. To install behaviour governors.
3. To allow him to have sexual thoughts and behaviours.
4. To associate kindness with good sexual boundaries.
5. To give him a sense of pride in his good sexual behaviour.
6. To get him to use the parents and carers as filters to check what was safe sexually.

Alright mum knows you're safe (the dependent attachment to his mother validates the statement – validation by association)…we're having a good time (framing constructive therapy)…**close your eyes and sleep a little** (inducing trance but not too deep)…**you will be safe and very comfortable in that chair** (direct suggestion)…so comfortable…you like being comfortable (framing constructivism)…I want you to… **remember to be kind** (post-hypnotic suggestion)…remember to be kind all the time (behaviour governor as we have already established that using carers as sexual behaviour filters equals kindness)…kind to girls and boys (universal suggestion)… **kind to everyone that's good** (re-enforcement suggestion)… you always ask mum dad or a carer before you touch someone (direct suggestion, first governor, the instructions must be complete and precise for him to understand and process)… keep them safe too (moral imperative as he has already said he is kind)…**keep everyone safe and happy** (suggestion for global behaviour)…you will remember never to touch anyone before you ask them (installing second governor)…never touch anyone before you ask…**mum…dad…or a carer the day before you ask the person if you can touch them** (direct suggestion for behavioural filters using a time delay)…mum and dad know best…and every day mum and dad will ask you if you have been kind (expectations for behavioural regulators)…**and when you have been kind you can have ice cream** (Pavlovian response)… good people can have ice cream every day…when you are good and kind you can have an ice cream (triple re-enforcement)… keep everyone safe…**I know you are good Seb**…you know you are kind (linked behaviours)…**you will remember to be good… kind…and respectful to other people** (re-enforcing behavioural boundaries)…and then you get an ice cream (Pavlovian response)…**you get rewards for kind behaviours**…people like you when you are kind (conditional reward)… it's good to be liked…**means ice cream** (behavioural incentivisation)

In the initial conversational trance, I used some interrogative suggestions that hid direct suggestions. However, in deep trance, notice I did not use any interrogative suggestions as that may have pulled him out of trance for clarification.

Also, I did not go over his past incident, charge, or traumatising court hearing as that would simply have been too re-traumatising for him. It was, in my opinion, a mistake for the police to allow the proceedings to go that far, knowing his intellectual challenges.

Because of his limited attention and cognitive processes, it was important to keep the trance short. The family were instructed that he listen to the recording 3 x a day in a quiet place, sitting in a chair. The daycare centre staff also got instructions that he was to listen to the recording at lunchtime under their supervision.

I saw Seb two weeks and then three months later and he was doing fine. The family were going on social outings again and he had returned to the daycare centre five days week. I also had to write a report for the court.

246

Every day his parents asked if he had been good and kind and when he answered 'yes', he would get ice cream. The ice cream was made at home by Seb and his parents from frozen bananas and fruit with three flavour options and no additives or sugar: flavours being strawberry, raspberry or vanilla.

Working with people with intellectual challenges requires suggestions to be literal, direct, and repetitive. It's pure behaviouralism. There is also a need to include instructions for boundaries and governors (limitations on behaviours), as positive instructions alone do not clarify acceptable behaviours. Indirect suggestions can leave the client unsure of what they need to do and do not work due to limited cognition, although metaphor can work at times if the story is consciously memorable.

Considering the element of sex drive in the equation, establishing boundaries around behaviour and sexual activity needed to be the primary aim of therapy. Installing behavioural governors must always be associated with positive rewards (see Appendix A, item 34).

I am firmly of the opinion that people of limited cognition are entitled to sex, but for everyone's safety, there needs, at times, to be supervision because they often are unable to identify the dangers of inappropriate interpersonal contact.

CASE STUDY: FATHER FRANCIS

This was a 28-year-old priest from South America who was in a panic when he telephoned me. I could hardly hear him because he spoke so softly and I had to ask him to speak up several times.

When he arrived at my office, he was not dressed in his cassock, but in ordinary civilian clothes to try to blend in while visiting in London. His father had been English so he spoke perfect international English.

He told me he had terrible troubles around having impure thoughts about women and masturbating. As he told me, he averted his eyes and seemed highly embarrassed and believed what he was doing was a mortal sin, a gross betrayal of his vows and that he would go to hell.

It is common to see people who may be highly educated in certain fields of life but have such poor knowledge around sex, such as Father Francis. They can have all their logical and rational cognitions distorted by extreme religious beliefs.

He wanted hypnotherapy to stop him having what he called "impure thoughts and actions". In other words, he wanted to stop fantasising about women sexually and to cease masturbation. I have spent many years considering different religious perspectives of controlling sexual libido, following the principle of 'saving the seed and focusing the mind'.

Whilst I had an appreciation of his religious perspective, I also saw a danger here as a sexologist. There is a huge history of religions subduing sexual libido, particularly in the Catholic church. This transmutes into suppressed sexual desire, sometimes emerging as sexual abuse, which has recently thrown the Catholic church in particular into turmoil throughout the world (Bruni and Burke, 2002).

We can see that hundreds of priests over the past several hundred years have spawned secret love children. There is also a rich history of sexually frustrated nuns who have been immensely cruel to children and other women (Justice for Magdalenes Research, n.d.).

There are those who have a low sex drive, but suppressing a healthy young man's sex drive and covering it in guilt and shame creates neurosis and is unnatural (Carroll, 2010).

Tracie: "If I were a Catholic and needed confession, should I trust you in confession?"

Francis: "Yes."

Tracie: "Well, I'm not a Catholic, but I am a sex therapist, so will you trust me?"

Francis: "Okay."

Tracie: "Let me ask you: In your religion it says God made man in his own image. Is that correct?"

Francis: "Yes, it does – in Genesis."

Tracie: "So it follows God must have genitals and those genitals are sensate and perfectly acceptable. So, God must see that having genitals and using them cannot be a sin but a celebration of God."

Francis: "Where are you going with this?"

Tracie: "Well, if a single man came to confession and told you he thought about women and masturbated, would you tell him he had sinned?"

Francis: "No."

Tracie: "I know for a fact, because I have read the King James bible, that it doesn't say that masturbation is a sin. You're a Christian and Jesus, according to the bible, said if your right hand causes you to sin, cut off your right hand and throw it away. But you have told me man is made in God's image, that masturbation is not a sin, and that you have not had sex with anyone."

Francis: "But the papal guidance says different."

249

Tracie: *"Mmm…**interesting**…and here we come to the*
folly of man…thinking they know more than God…
*because it was…**God that gave you functioning***
***genitals**…not man."*

I sent him away on a mission to the London Catholic Library
to investigate the origins of celibacy in the Catholic priesthood.

On his return he told me he had found texts that explained
priests got married before the 11th century. The problem for
Rome was that the properties the clergy were being given by
the church were then inherited by their children on their death,
so, the church was losing that property. For economic reasons,
it initiated a policy of chastity for all priests.

Here was a man conflicted in his beliefs, knowledge, values
and actions. The institution that he works for, the Catholic
church, used controlling, abusive behaviour to make him feel
guilty about being a man and having sexual thoughts and
urges. He associated sex with being a sinner himself but not his
parishioners. His sexual clusters were that if he did not follow
the Vatican's edicts, he was an impure sinner.

Trance intentions

1. To allow him to expand his knowledge of chastity.
2. To position the church as the source of that knowledge.
3. To validate his mission as a priest.
4. Reframe him as a good man inside his mind.
5. To take the church out of his internal conversation.
6. To allow him to resolve the issues with God himself.

Alright Francis just close your eyes and go inside…you can
understand your dedication to the church and their missions

(transderivational search to validate the statement, trance induction)...**noble the cause of your mission to be a good man and priest with genitals** (paradoxical intent, using the problem as the solution)...I'm reminded of Jesus's conversation with Pontius Pilot..."Render therefore unto Caesar the things which are Caesar's; and unto God the things that are God's"... your orders come from Rome...**your genitals are from God** (ultimately God is his boss)...you are a man of this earthly realm...you have the same body as other men...**God gave you sexual urges and pleasures**...you find women beautiful and sexually attractive and they are children of God (leverage, God always trumps the church)...your earthly vows don't allow you to have relationships...**think where does that leave you** (interrogative, transderivational search, trance deepener)... perhaps you have to honour God and the church separately in your own way (initiating parts negotiation)...well God gave you your genitals and...**you want to honour God above all else and what he gave you...don't you** (impossible for a priest to refute)...the church gave you orders not to have relationships...it seems you're respecting both of those...**what you do by yourself in private is between you and God**... what you do in public is between you and Rome...if you were sexually obsessed you would not be a priest...**so it seems you have found a compromise already**...it's clear from your research that God didn't give you orders not to masturbate or have sexual thoughts...but also Rome wants you to be its emissary...perhaps...just perhaps...**you can find a personal compromise**...of course I don't know how you will do that because I am not you (indirect suggestion for him finding his own solution)...and in this moment you might not fully know how you will do that (implied directive he will find the solution later)...but I know as you pray on it you will find a way (prayer

251

is his medium of communication with himself)…**creating your agreement between you and your God**…and the answer will come to you in your prayers (post-hypnotic suggestion)

In such a client with religious inner conflict, a therapist should never suppress the person's inner dialogue. There were so many thoughts and feelings that Francis was experiencing, and the only peaceful solution would be the one he worked out for himself (see Appendix A, item 35).

To try and suppress his sexual urge would be medically unethical because it would be interfering with the body's natural mechanism. As a therapist, I would be placing myself as the third dictatorial entity in his life, which would have increased the inner conflict.

Hunter (2005) talks about how parts negotiation aids resolving inner conflict and initiates unconscious learning. Sometimes as a therapist all one really needs to do is give the client information so the unconscious can execute that process of resolution.

Taking the church out of the equation (which was the contentious party) and suggesting he resolved the conflict directly with God allowed him to follow his faith.

Some months later when he was back in South America, we had a telephone conversation and he told me he had worked out a solution. I didn't ask him what his solution was. It was none of my business. He came to find a resolution and simply told me he had found one.

CASE STUDY: MARY

Mary was a 48-year-old lesbian, as she described herself. She had only had one brief sexual encounter with a woman many years ago, which involved no relationship. She had never had any sexual contact with men.

She was also a committed Christian and saw that identity as a large part of who she believed she was. There was much confusion around her religious beliefs and her sexual identity.

When she said 'lesbian' she stuttered and shuffled in the chair. She looked me straight in the eyes when saying the word 'Christian'. It was clear she repressed her sexuality.

Tracie: *"Tell me, how we can help you today, Mary?"*

Mary: *"Well, you are my second choice. I looked for a Christian therapist but was afraid what I said might get back to the church. Since you are a sex therapist, I decided to give you a try."*

Tracie: *"Well…we'll try to help you and…what do you need help with?"*

Mary: *"I'm embarrassed to tell you and need to be sure everything is confidential."*

Tracie: *"Well, your family doctor referred you to me, but I am by law unable to share any information from the session with anyone without your permission. That's unless your life, or someone else's life is in danger."*

Mary: *"No, it's not that. What it is…Oh I don't know how to put it. I can only masturbate in the shower."*

Tracie: *"Well, many people masturbate in the shower, it's quite common, or of course in the bath."*

Mary: *"You don't understand. I can only come when the shower head is pointed towards my clitoris."*

Tracie: "Hot or warm water is very stimulating to the genitals as it opens the blood vessels, so your clitoris becomes engorged and more sensitive. When it's enlarged, there is more pressure on the nerves, so you get increased messages of pleasure going to your brain."

Mary: "But it's not normal."

Tracie: "I'm not sure what normal is. I sit in my office each year listening to hundreds of reports of people's sex lives. They are all different. That's the only normal: that everyone's experience of sex is different."

Mary: "It can't be normal. I've heard of no one doing it."

Tracie: "You don't exactly hang out with women talking openly and freely about sex and their genitals. So, your knowledge on the subject could be open to some further education. What is it you want to achieve in therapy?"

Mary: "I want to have sex normally."

Tracie: "I'm confused...you've told me you don't have sex with women. You've never had sex with men and don't want to. So is masturbation your kind of sex?"

Mary: "Having sex with women is a sin in my church. Even me thinking about having sex with women is a sin. So, I started masturbating in the shower when I was young to wash my sins away."

Tracie: "You must be exhausted with that heavy load of shame you are feeling."

Mary: "And I cut. I often cut after the shower, on my arms. No one knows. I always wear long sleeves. Even my GP doesn't know. No one's ever seen my arms since I was 13."

Tracie: "Thank you so much Mary for trusting me with all this information, your thoughts, feelings, frustrations, and pain. I will do my very best to help you, but I want you to agree to do everything I say."

Mary: "Everything?"

Tracie: "Well, yes...**everything**...otherwise you're wasting your time and money."

Mary: "I'll try."

Trance intentions

1. Eliciting commitment to change.
2. Accepting she deserves more in life.
3. Normalising lesbianism.
4. Promoting the concept that she is not an outsider and there is a place in the world for her.
5. Calling in her superego to be kind to herself.
6. Using her moral Christian imperatives to initiate self-acceptance.

No good...'I'll try'...gives you another way to sabotage yourself...**and I say my clients deserve much better** (validating her, creating therapeutic alliance, she can't dispute me protecting my client)...which you can learn to say all so well (modal operator of possibility for self-esteem)...you see I've been around lesbians since I was 12 years old...many of my friends are lesbians...I've lived in lesbian culture for most of my adult life...**I've loved lesbians**...very nice people...from all different faiths...I've been married to two men...**I'm now married to a lesbian** (again she is unable to dispute my statement)... wonderful woman and love of my life...kind soul passionate about animal welfare...you grew up being told lesbians were sinful (truism)...you were afraid of being a lesbian (truism)... **lesbian are just human beings** (suggestion for adjusting her value system)...people identifying as lesbians (which includes her)...**deserve respect...love...kindness** (leading)...close your eyes and go inside safe and fully accepted in my office (contingent suggestion, by closing her eyes she concedes to being fully accepted)...**imagine a world were God is a woman** (initiating feminism)...like you she is worthy...she is fully valid...**like you she's beautiful just the way she is**...it's okay for you to imagine a world where you fit in with kind people (moral imperative, her religion requires her to be kind, adjusting her superego)... it's okay for you to be one of those kinds of people (forming an alliance with people who are kind to lesbians)...**acceptance of course begins with yourself** (a double bind, in that she has to be kind which requires her to be kind to herself)...as you have faith...whatever faith that may be...it's important in your faith to be accepting of all equally Jesus's words not mine (leverage)... you can always choose your faith...but that faith can be about being accepting too...**people of faith can be accepting and loving** (permission to accept herself)...sometimes people say things because they live in fear...sometimes they get caught up in a web of not knowing...**you can say things that allow you to live in love and acceptance** (permissive suggestion)... you can say accepting and loving things to others (principle of reciprocity)...and it begins with you saying loving accepting things to yourself...**saying accepting kind things to yourself** (re-enforcement suggestion)...isn't that nice...isn't it being moral...isn't it being a good person (triple question creating cognitive re-adjustment)...it's good to be a good person... **and you can be an accepting person all the time having faith** (global suggestion)

The first-time I saw Mary was about desensitising her to the word 'lesbian' and reasoning with her sense of goodness. Saying the word 'lesbian' several times, at the beginning of the eyes closed trance state allowed her to process that identity without the amygdala interfering and sending her into internalised homophobic panic and shame. Accepting that identity was the way for her to connect with her whole self.

Repetitive use of the words 'lesbian' and 'acceptance' was a form of exposure therapy to reduce her anxiety around identifying as a lesbian. Marks (1979) discussed how controlled, progressive, constant exposure, as a form of behavioural therapy, to a fearful stimulant, can reduce and eventually eliminate the fear response.

Mary was clearly not connected to her body and sexual identity except for her sexual activity in the shower. She had experienced the early childhood and teenage trauma of being brainwashed into believing lesbians were bad, therefore she associated herself with being bad. Low (2011) found how early childhood trauma can lead to self-harming behaviours in women. Gold (2011) explored how childhood physical abuse, internalised homophobia, and experiential avoidance leads to psychological problems in gay men and lesbians.

As soon as Mary climaxed and left the shower, her internalised homophobia kicked back into play. Boyer (2022) examines how trauma, particularly early trauma, can initiate dissociation and this would include physical and mental dissociation. Mary's early learnings in her community were that being lesbian is wrong, dangerous, bad and evil. This initiated her early internalised homophobia and self-hate, and she became dominated by two opposing personalities.

Sobanski & Wagner (2017) report that besides the hippocampus, thalamus, hypothalamus, periaqueductal gray region, and locus coeruleus, the amygdala is the main site in initiating the panic reaction. So, it is clear that all learned homophobia and internalised homophobia is a panic response. Working in trance, however, taking the brain waves down to alpha and theta, reduces the ability of the amygdala to initiate the fear response when exposed to a fearful stimulus.

The second part of the first session was about reframing and relearning that lesbians can be good, loving people. Therefore, by proxy, she could be a good, loving person as a lesbian.

> Tracie: *"Here are the details of a women's social group. It's run by an ex-nun, she's very nice. I want you to go twice over the next two weeks. Use the recording we made today twice a day in private."*

I saw Mary two weeks later.

> Tracie: *"How were your women's groups?"*

> Mary: *"They seemed nice. Not what I expected. They're lesbians, well not all of them but a lot seemed to be. And some of them had small children and babies."*

> Tracie: *'They didn't burn you at the stake, force you to join a coven or drag you into sin then?"*

> Mary: *"No – and I did my recordings as you said."*

Mary's sexual clusters were around her escaping into the shower to satisfy her libido, then punishing herself by cutting and destroying her body. The cutting had also allowed her to maintain that trance for many years because she had been punished. It was a coping mechanism. Her problem was the coping mechanism was now failing.

Trance intentions

1. Initiation of artificial somnambulism, thereby controlling the fight or flight response.
2. Defining self-identity.
3. Reassociation to her body by the process of ownership.
4. Self-validation.
5. Acceptance of human differences.

Be safe here again (re-initiating the safety anchor)...I want you to work on ownership with yourself today please (confusion to send her deeper into trance as she had little understanding about self-ownership)...think about your birth certificate and how it has your name on it...think about your passport and driving licence (legal identifiers)...**you are identified as a valid individual** (initiating independence)...your tax number... the ownership document for your car...**all identify you as an individual** (bombardment suggestions)...your school certificate...your electricity bill...the name on your credit card... **all identify you as being a bona fide person in your own right** (separating her from old moral imperatives of being part of an organised religion)...did you know no one has exactly the same shape head...or the same shape feet...or even exactly the same eyes...**everyone is just different all just naturally different** (dissolving generalisation about right and wrong people)...not mother and daughter...not father and son...not even identical twins are the same...**so you are a special individual... unique...recognised as valid as yourself a valid individual...** every part of you is valid and special (parts integration)... you are of course not like anyone else...and anyone else is not like you (simile suggestion)...**we are all different and valid...** whatever you believed in it made you as different as the rest of us are (silent suggestion for not berating her previous self)... **by nature you are you**...they are your feet...ankles...legs... hips...tummy...back...arms...hands...shoulders...head... ears...nose...breasts...clitoris...**all of you is real** (indirect suggestion that being lesbian is real)...all of you is valid and real...**deserving**...real...you own you...feet are beautiful for walking...hands are useful for writing...eyes for seeing...ears for hearing...**body for feeling like a lesbian** (intra-hypnotic suggestion) every part of you is valid and true...**your clitoris is beautiful**...your breasts sensitive...**your sexual desires are valid and true**...breathe...sit...stand...walk...move in your space...**own and validate every part of the woman you are** (post-hypnotic suggestion for claiming her identity)

In hypnotically-induced saddle block and pudendal block anaesthesia, sensitivity and feeling is reduced by suggestion (Erickson J.C., 1994). Back further to Esdaile (2023) in the 19th century, we can see the phenomenal effects of suggestion in anaesthesia in over 300 patients undergoing surgery.

What can happen in sexual repression, and probably did in this case, is that an internalised homophobia created a psychosomatic pudendal nerve block and anaesthesia through unconscious autosuggestion. This affected the sensitivity of the pudenda, hypogastric and pelvic nerves that service the genitals. What she was left with was a sensation in the urinary nerve. She developed a negative hallucination, eliminating perceptions of genital sensitivity.

I saw Mary every month for several months on the condition she stayed in the women's group. After several months she became fond of one of the women, they became an item and she climaxed during sex as she became desensitised to the lesbian experience through a form of exposure therapy (see Appendix A, item 36). The last time I saw her she had not been cutting for three months.

My job was not to tell her where, when and how to climax, just promote fertile ground where she could work it out for herself by reducing and eliminating her internalised homophobia.

CASE STUDY: MELISA

Melisa was in a submissive BDSM (Bondage, domination, sado-masochism) relationship with her husband. At 36 she had been married to him for eight years, had a daughter of five and a son of seven.

The relationship had always been master/slave based and operated dynamically purely on that basis. That was how they met – through a BDSM network. To avoid unwelcome prying eyes, Melisa wore an ankle bracelet with a lock on it, rather than a collar. These items in BDSM culture symbolise being owned by a master or mistress.

Modern BDSM births from the works of the 18th-century French writer the Marquis de Sade (1969), and in modern culture very much promoted by James (2012) in her book *50 Shades of Grey*. Being a sub (submissive) means you fully comply with all your owner's instructions and wishes, without question. In vanilla (ordinary) BDSM, the submissive has a code word that they can use to ask for the proceedings to stop, but in highly bonded S&M relationships there is none.

Melisa's master claimed her as his property as soon as they met. It was what she was looking for at the time. She was fully comfortable with the relationship at that time.

She attended the session during school hours without the knowledge or permission of her master. She had confided in a friend, who helped her make the appointment, that she thought she was in trouble and needed help.

Melisa: *"I've always been submissive. I hardly spoke to anyone at school and had sex with the boys whenever they wanted. I was on the pill from 13, so I didn't get pregnant. Other girls would call me a slut, and I secretly liked it."*

Tracie: *"Thank you for trusting me with that information which is completely confidential between you and myself. I also need to tell you that I will not disclose to anyone at any time that you are seeing me."*

Melisa: *"Thank you. Part of me wants him to catch me for being here and punish me for coming to see you. He's very strong-willed and very successful in business. But I think I am drowning and out of my depth."*

Tracie: *"Can you explain a little more please?"*

Melisa: *"When it was just the two of us, it was my purpose to be his sub, which was before my son was born. We were on the BDSM circuit, and we have a secure, fitted dungeon in our cellar."*

Tracie: *"What changed?"*

Melisa: "We had children. He has been seeing a woman every weekend for the last six months and given me away to other masters at weekends, while the children are at their grandparents. He's a really good dad and provider. I can't leave him. I have no money or way to make a living. He wouldn't let me take the children. I feel it's all out of control and I don't have his attention."

Tracie: "So what options are you left with?"

Melisa: "I can't do it. I can't give him back the chain and lock. Who would I be? I know it's my only option. But I've never been myself before. You've got to help me."

Their relationship was based on him owning her if she wore the chain and lock (Taormino, 2012). He could do anything to her and give her to anyone he wanted for sex and anything else. It was not an abusive, coercive, or illegal relationship, neither did she experience Stockholm syndrome, as Melisa's behaviour was legally voluntary. In such a relationship, she had no voice.

As I started to write this book, the New South Wales Government in Australia began to bring in a bill to criminalise coercive control (Rose, 2022). Whilst it was meant to protect vulnerable women and families from abuse, it sent fear though the BDSM culture as they could go to prison for seven years for their practices. The bill is part of a suite of modern-day morality laws that should be operated with great caution. We can see in the UK that police sometimes use laws that are a thousand years old to prosecute people to elevate their arrest quota.

Melisa had parents who were not interested in her as a child. She associated being controlled with being wanted and valid. Her sexual clusters had always been around belonging to another person, even if that person was a stranger that her master had given her to.

Trance intentions

1. To help her cancel the master/slave relationship.
2. Support her already indicated decision to give her husband back the chain.
3. Save the marriage and structure of the family.
4. Creating the illusion of free choice, not absolute necessity.

Close your eyes and go inside...have a time of peace and comfort for you (personal time safety anchor)...**just for you and you only listening to my words** (bringing her focus to suggestion, giving her space to adjust)...you know you face a choice...you already know what the choice is...**it's your choice and your choice only** (presupposition she has already made her choice)...no one else can make that choice for you... sometimes we are faced with hard choices (acknowledging how hard the choice was for her)...**and can make the right choice** (modal operator of possibility to bypass resistance)... it's a choice you have already thought about...it's a choice you have sought help to make (truisms)...**make the right choice for you** (changing her criteria of needs to put self-preservation first)...I want you to see up inside your mind your children all grown-up and happy (future pacing the success of her decision, initiating her maternal instinct)...they're smiling and well balanced human beings (leverage)...**your children you help build** (re-enforcing the future pacing, ego strengthening)... you helped them become happy...like every parent there are hard choices along the way…it can be challenging…**you know happy parents help children become happy adults** (bind to be a happy parent to protect her children)…sometimes it's time for change…everything ends…**everything changes all the time** (indirect suggestion for change)…perhaps it's time for you to change (permissive suggestion)…your change that's right for you (silent suggestion to take action)…**freedom to make you and your family happy** (appealing to the superego to regulate behaviour)…we all have to take the lead sometimes… sometimes it's the right thing to do…**shed old chains and become someone else now** (direct post-hypnotic suggestion to give back the chain)…is that time now (interrogative suggestion)…learning to make new boundaries around sex and relationships (silent suggestion)…putting limits on what you will allow (initiating boundaries)…**your time is now**…it seems you've made the choice already (presumption the choice is clear)…it seems you know what to do…you indicated what you want to do…**give back the chain and lock** (post-hypnotic suggestion, reflecting her own decision)

Melisa was in two different relationships with the same man. The first and most central to her life so far was as a submissive where she must be obedient all the time. The second was as his wife, a role she had not yet played in her own right. My caution in working with her was to help her opt out of one relationship (master and sub), without damaging, and indeed to fertilise the other (husband and wife).

That night she gave her husband back the chain and lock after the children had gone to bed. She did not ask him to take it off, but she cut it off with plyers.

For a submissive to give back the symbol of bondage is complete severance of their contract. Apparently, he was completely shocked. She stopped doing what he told her to do, neither did she tell him she was seeing a therapist.

Melisa continued in therapy for a year, discovering who she was, who she wanted to be and how to create that. The marriage continued but with no sexual relationship, until he gave up his mistress several months later. They then had to both embark on a journey of how to be husband and wife.

In many ways mine was a supportive approach in this case, allowing the client to adjust the relationship with her husband to a dynamic that now suited her as a mother and wife (see Appendix A, item 37).

12 Sex Addiction

Sex addiction is different from other addictions as it is largely driven by a biological urge. This biological urge accelerates at puberty due to increased sex hormones. We can also see when we give people testosterone, generally their desire for sex rises.

In fact, testosterone therapy as a hormone replacement therapy is used to increase sex drive in men, women, intersex people and trans men. Inversely, we can see that low levels of testosterone, oestrogen and progesterone are linked to hyposexuality (AlAwlaqi, 2017).

Batrinos (2012) tells us how elevated testosterone can give rise to aggressive behaviour in men, which would include aggressive sexual behaviours. We can see that elevated testosterone and oestrogen together seem to increase women's sexual desire (Cappelletti, 2015).

Some people's natural sex hormone levels can be very high and others can be genetically hypersensitive to ordinary levels. As we are discovering more about genetic hypersensitivities, as well as hyposensitivities to sex hormones, we learn that it is not always elevated sex hormones that lead to aggressive sexual behaviour or addiction (Bloom, 2015). In these cases, people either enjoy an active sex life or find the high sex drive distressing, and they can even become disturbed about being overly aggressive.

Alesi (2023) reviewed blocking the effects of androgens with anti-androgen medications such as Flutamide, Spironolactone or Cyproterone. These are used with sex offenders and to treat prostate cancer, polycystic ovary syndrome (PCOS), excess body hair, acne, female pattern baldness, congenital adrenal hyperplasia (CAH), precocious puberty and in intersex and trans women's medicine.

In pregnant women, on the other hand, a rise in oestrogen and progesterone can increase the sex drive, particularly in the second or third trimester. With that, however, can come allergies due to elevated sex hormones (Untersmayr, 2017). What we really don't know yet is the extreme effects of sex hormones on the function and efficiency of the brain.

The voracious need for sex is not, however, solely driven by the biological urge or the need for sexual satisfaction. Indeed, many sex addicts have often commented that they do not enjoy sex but are hopelessly driven to seek sexual encounters and be promiscuous.

There are psychological and emotional drivers involved. Many people measure their self-worth by their level of promiscuity. For them, the more sex they have, the greater, they think this adds to their value as a person.

The problem for some, however, is that they never seem to reach a satisfactory level of self-worth. So, they are trapped in the delusion that success, promiscuity, and a high sex drive will make them happy, but ultimately it makes them dysfunctional as a personality, often leading to anxiety and depression.

In teenage years, when good risk-taking skills are not yet fully formed, the fear of missing out (FOMO) can become a driver in over-sexualisation and promiscuity, particularly in males.

Boys can tend to have sex due to peer pressure in trying to establish their place in the pecking order of the man pack. Girls can tend to have sex for emotional validation of their beauty, desirability and worth as a potential mate.

There is also a large influence of social drivers that promote high sexualisation as being linked in many cultures with success and intellectual freedom. Influences include what is permissible within the social order, how much power men have over women in misogynistic societies, and how promiscuous women are permitted to be.

This is the opposite in groups such as Hasidic Jews, chastity-sworn Christians and in religions including Catholicism, Hinduism, Jainism, and Islam, all of which promote no sex before marriage. Added to this is the spiritual practice of controlling sexual desires as with Catholic priests, nuns and Buddhist monks.

So, mind over matter can reduce the effects of testosterone, oestrogen and progesterone in hypersexualisation, even though levels may be high.

Compulsive sexual behaviour disorder (CSBD) is not listed in DSM 5TR (American Psychiatric Association, 2022). It is, however, listed in the ICD 11 (World Health Organization, 2024) under the Family of International Classifications (WHOFIC), code 6C72. It is not listed under paraphilia.

CSBD is the compulsive, excessive engagement in sexual thoughts, fantasies, and activities, and having sex that extends to beyond the person's physical, mental, emotional and social wellbeing.

I insert a caveat here, in that hypersexuality is not a sex addiction unless it is detrimental to the wellbeing of the person or the persons around them.

CASE STUDY: CLAUDE

This was a high-ranking civil servant, department head and gay man of 43. He had been married with two children until coming out as gay at 29. The divorce had been acrimonious as he had been secretly having affairs with men, whilst still married to his wife.

Since coming out, Claude became firmly attached to the inner-city gay scene, which included bars, clubs, sex on premises venues and chem sex parties. For him, these became a relentless stream of weekly events that rolled one weekend into another, joined together with the use of cocaine, methamphetamine and GHB (gamma hydroxybutyrate), at least four times a week.

The chem sex scene was where men he knew had sex with everyone in their circle, and as soon as someone had scored drugs, everyone else would get invited. If you were part of the in-crowd, you would get a phone call or message and if you were not, you would be left out.

Claude's life revolved around staying in with the in-crowd. Despite having had two heart attacks due to the drugs and being pronounced dead for 10 minutes the second time, he had no concept of himself as being other than part of the drug-taking, sex-focused in-crowd. He was engulfed in that identity.

Tracie: *"So let me get this right, Claude. You say you want to break your addiction to sex, but at the same time you want to stay as part of the friends who make up the chem sex circle."*

Claude: *"That's about it."*

Tracie: *"Fascinating…that level of delusion you have built up for yourself…such an intelligent man who holds down a high-pressure job requiring a clear grasp on reality…yet your social life and sex interactions are the complete opposite where you have little grasp of reality at all…how did you get to be such a Jekyll and Hyde character"* (shock technique)

Claude: *"Ow – is that what you think?"*

Tracie: *"There's not enough magic in the world to turn the story you're telling me into a fairy tale (jolting him out of the delusion)...you wouldn't be sitting in that chair if the story you were living was working for you (transderivational search to verify or dispute my comments, forcing him into trance)...but (15 seconds silence, confusion)...and I do say but...a really big but (fractionating the confusion)...because there really is an alternative option...**you could change that story into a better life** (permissive directive, modal operator of probability)...if that's truly what you have come to see me for...to change your story...stay alive... **become someone different** (direct suggestion)... someone who enjoys sex...deeper meaningful relationships...reunites with your daughters...since you're not yet dead (leverage)...just maybe it's time to live as a happy gay man...**having a meaningful sex life."***

The shock technique is the hypnotic equivalent to ECG in a life-saving situation. It is a confrontational shock technique to motivate the person towards alternative life-saving and enriching options.

People will not leave their delusions because of their perceived cognitive logic, empathy or sympathy. My experience is they will only consider a new viewpoint when they are uncomfortable in their delusions. Since Claude had had two heart attacks and been pronounced dead for 10 minutes, yet continued to take drugs, it was clear logic did not appeal to him.

He was in the chem sex trance, yet also living in a trance of being successful professionally, so he needed a jolt to work out the incongruencies of his life. As we travel through life, living diametrically opposed trances, it cancels out the benefits of our stated intentions. We develop amnesia and negative hallucinations around the damage that battle causes.

By pointing out the destruction of the two opposing stories he is living, it forces Claude to confront the incongruencies of his narratives (apposition of opposition).

Here is a man who associates connection with destructive drug use and co-dependency within a chem sex circle. His sex clusters are around high-risk-taking and life-threatening behaviours around sex and drugs that have no deep and meaningful interpersonal connections.

Trance intentions

1. Reflective self-assessment.
2. Drawing his attention to the incongruencies of his life trances.
3. Provoking solution-focused problem-solving.
4. Integration of opposing trances.
5. Suggestion for a more wholesome and healthy way to live.
6. Hypnotic dreaming.

All I'm doing is holding up the mirror to you and showing you what you told me...nothing more...nothing less...**look into that mirror as you go forward**...close your eyes and look deep deep into that mirror in front of you inside your mind (visual internal reflection)...what do you see (interrogative suggestion to go deeper into trance)...are your different stories competing with each other (interrogative suggestion for confronting the conflict)...**living in harmony with all your stories allows you to be your whole self** (metaphor for stopping drugs and changing friendship circle)...it allows you to be more self-accepting...more self-loving...more self-caring...**health...happiness...deeper friendships...a kind lover** (permissive alternative options)...of course this requires you to change your stories today (it is a medical emergency)...yes...today...here...now...here today now... (time frame for change, call to action)...**live a different sex... friendship...and relationship story**...it requires a high level of self-respect...**you can wonder how you will do that** (interrogative suggestion, strategy challenge)...what do you need to do to work that out...who do you need to become... **what new stories do you need to live every day** (question bombardment, generating options, sending him deeper into trance)...I know you don't want to be at war with yourself... you know you don't want to be at war with yourself (nudging suggestions)...**as a caring lover you take care of many of the other person's needs too**...you keep yourself and the other person safe (forcing him to redefine sexual contact)...physical needs...emotional needs...your lovemaking makes you smile for a long time (future pacing, changing his time frames as they are very short as an addict)...**you are fully present during sex**...every minute is memorable...you take time to make love and be caring...perhaps you can think about that in every part of your mind...**take the time now and rewrite your stories as you sit there** (he is left in hypnotic dreaming for 10 minutes just thinking)

Claude's life patterns were often about running away. He ran away from being gay by getting married to a woman and having children. Then he ran away from his marriage by having affairs. He escaped his marriage by jumping into the middle of the gay scene. He ran away from meaningful relationships by being part of the chem sex scene where no one talked about love, just drugs and sex. He now associated sex with escape.

His sexual clusters were around drugs, plus chem sex parties, and perceiving those as self-validation.

He had to find his own way forward and, for that, he had to reassess and remake his life trances. He was not someone who a therapist could tell him not to do something as this would have raised resistance. I believe that would have failed.

I was not forcing or commanding him to look at his life but inviting him to consider a different story for himself forthwith. Since he was highly successful in his career, he already had high-level problem-solving skills which he could use to create his new story.

Tracie: *"And in your own sweet time you can slowly and comfortably come back to the room and look at me."*

Claude: *"I guess I need to get away. Have some space and time."*

Tracie: *"It's interesting you should say that. I have a client who has just come back from a silent retreat in the mountains. He said it really cleared his head and gave him a different perspective on life (my friend John technique)."*

Claude: *"I like warm, hot tropical beaches like north Queensland or deserted beaches in Thailand."*

Tracie: "Mmm that sounds nice. Perhaps you can write
a journal of your thoughts while you're away and
bring them to the sessions when you return, and we
can talk about them."

Before Claude left for his vacation/sabbatical, I worked with him in four further sessions to stop taking unnecessary substances and become clean and sober. He continued the program whilst he was away.

For his homework on holiday, I asked him to find several Buddhist temples and just sit in them and meditate. One of the major teachings of the Buddha is to be present, not lost in the chaos of the past or future.

Claude went to Thailand for a month but then extended his stay by two weeks. The last two weeks he invited his teenage daughters to join him, and they had family time. He said it was the best two weeks he had had in years.

I saw him three more times and each time he told me about his changes inside and out. I explained to him that people who continually take drugs with him are not respecting or caring for him. They will either change or not in their own time, and it was not his responsibility to make that decision for them.

He severed all links with the chem sex circle and decide to be celibate for a while, until he worked out what he wanted from a lover and relationship (see Appendix A, item 38).

Evers (2020) tells us of the need for mental health help for men practising chem sex and using multiple drugs. Evers reports that 56% of those preferred to be counselled by sexual health workers. Vykhodtcev (2022) reported a study of 65 sex workers in St Petersburg, Russia, of whom 46% took drugs as a psychological defence mechanism. So, it is important to remember that not all chem sex is motivated by hypersexuality alone.

CASE STUDY: JEANIE

Jeanie was 50, divorced, financially independent and retired. She had run a large agency that she had sold for a considerable sum two years previously.

Jeanie: *"I got really stung. I don't know how it happened. I'm such a smart woman and have been successful. I dated a series of younger men and I fell for one."*

Tracie: *"And how can we help you today?"*

Jeanie: *"He's 29, the same age as my son, and the sex was amazing. I'd never had sex like that before, we did everything. I couldn't get enough."*

Tracie: *"You said you got stung?"*

Jeanie: *"He's an escort or gigolo as they call them in Europe. I met him in Italy. I was his customer and he came to my hotel. I kept going back to Italy to have sex with him. He stopped charging me after a while but then I lent him money to start a business which failed, and the money was gone."*

Tracie: *"You stopped paying smaller amounts and instead gave him a lump sum?"*

Jeanie: *"I suppose you could say that. I employed a private detective who told me he had a girlfriend and baby, and bought a house with the money I gave him."*

Tracie: *"What do you think about that?"*

Jeanie: *"Well, I guess I became his mark. To me it was not a lot of money. I understand why he did it, but I still want to see him. It's the sex, you see, it's been out of this world."*

Tracie: *"Well, for that money it would need to be. Was it worth the spend?"*

Jeanie: *"To be honest, yes. I never knew you could have sex like that, all night, and every fantasy you could imagine."*

Tracie: *"And what do you need help with?"*

Jeanie: *"My son is an accountant and is asking where that money went. I think I'm addicted to sex with this young man. Can you help?"*

Jeanie associated her new sexual experiences as part of her rebirth as a person, making up for the years she had denied herself. Her sexual clusters were bound up in extreme risk-taking to achieve sexual adventures she had never known before, where she abandoned and abdicated reason. It was about reclaiming her youth.

Trance intentions

1. Reassertion of her sense of privacy.
2. Metaphor about people losing control.
3. Self-analysis of her personal sexual adventure.
4. Reducing her lapse of judgment to only temporary.
5. Reassessing her sexual contracts.
6. Mapping the changes across all sensory systems.
7. Reducing the obsession.
8. Future pacing her having control over the encounters.

Close your eyes and sit back in the chair in the privacy and safety of this setting…privacy of course is an inalienable human right…**you know you can**…**have a right to privacy** (both direct and indirect suggestion…there are things a mother and son don't need to discuss…a long time ago in my house in the South of France I would have guests to stay…one day a very prim friend from London came to stay…she did not drink but in the middle of the French countryside she got drunk every night… very drunk…she was not used to intoxicants…for two weeks she became a completely different person…but it was at my house so her tango with alcohol remained confidential…if you don't have an experience of something…you might not know how to handle it (parallel metaphoric meaning)…**just sit there thinking about your own journey of sex with this man** (lapse of five minutes whilst she sat in trance)…only you can calculate the cost of your sex intoxication…there were good times…and deception…**how will you go forward differently** (interrogative suggestion to change what she is doing)…what would you change about the agreement…would you see anyone else…are you looking for sex or a relationship…(triple question, trance deepener)…sex is fantastic…friendship is good…relations can be rewarding…**the best time is when you know exactly what you are experiencing and have control**…now I like chocolate ice cream (multiple sensory engagement)…you may ice cream like to or not (word salad provoking cognition)… but you probably would…**not like it all the time** (installing governors)…some things are special because they are new… some things are special because you have them sometimes… some things are special because they're fascinating and fun… some things are special on Tuesday Thursday or Saturday (boredom deepener)…**you can feel good when you have special things on your own terms** (contingent suggestion, reducing the compulsion)…feeling good…open your eyes smiling at me (artificial somnambulism, creating serotonin and endorphins to accelerate change)

Back in 2006 Fong reviewed whether sex addiction could be classified as a standalone psychiatric disorder under impulse control disorders. This, however, has turned out to be a commercialisation of human nature and a form of social control.

In Jeanie's case she did not have a lifelong addiction. If she had bought a sports car that turned out to be stolen and then was repossessed, would she have been considered a person with risky behaviour?

If she were a man in the same situation, would she be considered unbalanced? Remember, she said the money she lost was not a great deal to her and she could afford it.

Tracie: *"You were a wife, mother and businesswoman who serviced a lot of other people. Sex with your husband, according to you, seemed to have been unadventurous. Divorced and lonely, you embarked on an adventure into sex, which you could afford financially. You had a really good time but didn't understand some of the business rules around buying sex from young men (holding up the mirror). Tell me what you will do differently in future?"*

Jeanie: *"I will do my cost/benefit analysis in advance."*

Tracie: *"Do you understand that many of these young men selling sex, that you had contact with, are unlikely to be able to provide a rewarding emotional attachment?"*

Jeanie: *"I do now."*

She decided to still see the young man for sex but on a per hour, contractual basis when she was in Europe a few times a year. She also changed her accountant to someone who was not related to her.

Conde (2021) found cognitive changes and decline in post-menopausal women were more frequent and accelerated than pre-menopausal women, due to a decline in oestrogen and progesterone. The changes are more dramatic in women than in men.

Jeanie told us in her history that she had been successful in business, but during her time with the young man, she had suspended her due diligence when she lent him money. Added to that was the intense high levels of oxytocin she experienced during and after sex, linked to her new sexual discoveries with the young man, all of which reduced her risk assessment skills. Plus she was going through menopause.

Close your eyes...**know sex is beautiful and rewarding** (it is important not to damage her newfound appreciation of sex)...and sex when you want it can be good too...safe sex under controlled circumstances (silent suggestion)...**life of course is much more than just sex** (recontextualising sex as a just part of her whole life to reduce the obsession)...how else might you enjoy contact with people (interrogative command to expand her social life)...who might you see...where might you go...**you can wonder how life might be** (initiating life strategy changes)...have a dream about that now (five minutes elapsed, hypnotic dreaming)...when will you know (interrogative time expansion for creating solutions)...**opening your eyes... smiling...and awake**

I saw Jeanie six weeks later.

Jeanie: "After I saw you last, I had a busy night tossing and turning in bed. When I got up in the morning I signed up for bridge and mahjong courses."

Tracie: "How is it?"

Jeanie: "So much fun and fiercely competitive. I'm having a great time."

Tracie: "Have you seen the young man?"

Jeanie: "Yes, I went to Italy for five days and booked him for the week. The sex was good, but I think he's losing his edge. I told my son I'm going to have my own accountant from now on to get more clarity, no reflection on him."

Tracie: "Do you still think you're addicted to the sex?"

Jeanie: "No, but I think I could get addicted to bridge!" (we laughed)

People can become lost in lust without tethers to their present-day reality when they are unused to high levels of sexual excitement, causing an addiction. For us as therapists we need to help them gain perspective on their new-found experiences and their reality (see Appendix A, item 39).

CASE STUDY: CHRISTOPHER

Christopher: "I can't handle it. It's getting worse and it's driving me crazy. Now at 28 I seem to want sex all the time. I'm horny."

Tracie: "How long has that been happening?"

Christopher: "I've always had a high sex drive and before we had kids my wife was up for it twice a day. Now we've got kids she's not up for it, so I'm meeting women on a dating app. She doesn't know about that."

Tracie: "That's sounds like a difficult situation."

Christopher: "It's not just that. I'm on edge all the time, like I want to jump out of my skin."

Tracie: "I'm going to get you to have a blood test. We want to look at your testosterone and your thyroid."

Christopher had bulging eyes, a high respiration rate, was a shallow breather, fidgeted, and talked fast. These are all signs of Graves' disease, a form of hyperthyroidism.

Christopher: "How long will that take?

Tracie: "We can have the results in a week."

Christopher: "Can you help now?"

Tracie: "Absolutely and I am going to tell you how."

He now associated the availability of sex with women outside his marriage. His sexual clusters were bound up with his biological drive and need for sex that he perceived as being out of control.

I placed both his hands in mid air in front of him, turned upwards, palms open, level with the bottom of the rib cage, creating instant artificial somnambulism.

Trance intentions

1. Cognitive awareness of the dangers of having sex outside the relationship by changing his awareness to visual representations.
2. Helping him listen to his unconscious messages.
3. Allowing him to prioritise the right choices for his family.
4. Installing behaviour boundaries.
5. Sub-modality deprioritisation of sex outside marriage.

Look at those hands (focused attention)...**in the hand that's right** (double meaning)...you can place your wife and family... in the hand that's left you can place the out-of-control sex drive and anxiety (implying it has a less valuable content)...**clear to see easily** (visual hallucination)...tell me what's the family one look like?"

> Christopher: *"I love them. I love my wife. I'm afraid of losing her."*

> Tracie: *"Now look at the contents on the one that's left...the out-of-control sex drive...**what's that look like?**"* (creating cognitive awareness, dissociation from the sex drive, changing his sensory modality from kinaesthetic to visual, breaking state)

> Christopher: *"It looks like it's chasing me, and I can't run fast enough to get away from it. It's going to catch up with me and hurt my family."*

Frequently, the unconscious alerts us to physical, mental, behavioural, and emotional disturbances by producing metaphorical danger. Gieselmann (2019) described how nightmares can be a sign of psychological disturbances. However, I have often found with patients that their stories can be a sign of physical illness. The idea that the psyche is separate from the somatic to me seems bizarre.

Here I am not projecting a meaning on Christopher's unconscious metaphoric revelations, simply observing his present life map as he describes the trances he is living.

The obsession many hypnotists have with trying to elicit ideomotor response as a form of answer, solely through finger signals, is not superior to verbal responses. The unconscious will communicate what it wants to communicate, when it wants to communicate, and our job as hypnotists is to lower resistance to enable that communication.

Close your eyes still seeing the contents of those hands… focus on the family…**build a protective wall around them to keep them safe** (installing boundaries)…nod your head when you have done that (he nodded)…change your focus to the hand where the sex drive is out of control…**I want you to slow that whole picture down** (sub-modalities work)…nod your head when you've done that (he nodded)…interesting how you can change the way you feel (silent suggestion)…**now change that picture to black and white** (sensory reduction)…nod your head when you've done that (he nodded)…when you have done all that tell me about the difference (presupposition there has been a change)

> Christopher: *"Oh my God. It's like I've used an inverter to downgrade the current from 240v to 12v."*

> Tracie: *"Open your eyes and calmly smiling at me (remaining artificially somnambulistic, adding the new, calmer, kinaesthetic sense of control to the*

*calmer visuals imagery)...so how are the contents
of the hand that previously held the out-of-control
sex drive...how would you say...**it looks different**"
(interrogative indirect suggestion for change having
taken place)*

Christopher: "It's quieter."

His original comment was, "I'm on edge all the time, like I want to jump out of my skin." This indicates kinaesthetic distress. I worked with Christopher in the visual psychoimaginary modality to reduce resistance and break the kinaesthetic state. I then introduced suggestions for kinaesthetic promotion of serotonin. He then naturally mapped that new state across himself to the auditory modality saying, "It's quieter."

Trance intentions

1. Hand drop induction.
2. Hand drop deepener.
3. Changing breathing.
4. Submodality work.
5. Time distortion.
6. Creating self-efficacy for having physical control.

I'm going to turn your hands over now...when I press the right one down you will...**close your eyes and go into a deeper trance** (presumption he is already in trance)...that's good you feel comfortable and fine (silent suggestion)...when I press the one that's left down you double that trance (fractionation)... **now deeper deeper deeper** (bombardment fractionation)... good good good comfortable easy and peaceful...**breathe very very slowly just only through your mouth** (this breath kills the sex drive because it reduces oxygen)…when the sex drive becomes noisy…breathe slowly only through your mouth (time-specific post-hypnotic suggestion, re-enforcement suggestion)…**slow everything down inside your mind** (Ki- & Ke-, time distortion)…**change everything to black and white** (Vi-, dissociation)…**reduce the sound** (Ai-, the volume of my voice became lower and my delivery slows down by a half)…it's easy when you need…it's easy when you want…**you have control** (intra-hypnotic suggestion)…reducing your sex drive…when you need…**any place** (post-hypnotic suggestion for multiple locational competency)…**any time** (post-hypnotic suggestion for competency at any time)…any circumstances (post-hypnotic suggestion for competency for any situation)… **you have control**

Christopher used a recording of this trance 3 x a day. When his results came back his TSH was very low. He had further scans and it was clear he had Graves' disease. He did not take beta blockers because he was learning to control his body with hypnosis, but his GP placed him on Neo-Mercazole which is used to reduce the formation of thyroid hormones.

Whilst Graves' disease is an autoimmune disease, adverse reactions can be controlled with hypnosis. We can see that Torem (2007) tells us hypnosis was reported as being highly beneficial in lowering overzealous immune responses. So, I worked with Christopher on better control of his immune response.

His testosterone was high and further investigation confirmed he had high cortisol and an androgen-producing adrenal cancer of the right side (Mușină et al., 2020). Surgery was scheduled for a unilateral adrenalectomy to avoid malignancy. The oncologist decided not to remove the thyroid at this stage due to concurrent adrenalectomy. A double surgical shock could have sent Christopher into an adrenal crash when he may have become hyposexual.

Hypnosis was used to help him through surgery, recovery and adjustment. Several months later his sex drive was manageable.

Here we can see another example of the importance of medical screening in such cases, before we presume the symptoms are completely psychogenic (see Appendix A, item 40).

CASE STUDY: CAMILE AND MARK

This couple were in their early thirties, both worked full-time and had two children aged five and six.

Mark: *"I know you didn't want to come here Camile. I feel like we're arguing all the time because I want sex and you don't."*

Camile: *"I've told you, you're addicted to sex, get over it. It's all in your mind."*

Tracie: *"I'm going to give you both a clipboard. Could you please write down, individually, what you would like the outcome of today to be."*

Five minutes passed.

Tracie: *"Now read your list to each other."*

Mark: *"I want sex once a day. I'm a man. I'm frustrated."*

Camile: *"I want sex once a week because I'm a woman, work full time, have the kids most of the time, and look after the house."*

Tracie: *"What I'm hearing is frustration from both of you (truism)...I can see how both of you work full* *time...**and look after a young family** (indirect suggestion)...you know I see this so much with couples who have young children...so much to do... bills to pay...school runs to do (acknowledging both their pressures)...you don't seem to have a lot of time for each other anymore...**perhaps you can connect more** (permissive modal operator allows for possibilities to be considered, without instructing them to do that, it is a soft, permissive suggestion)...what did you do together before you got married (interrogative suggestion for regression to more romantic times)*

Camile: "We used to go away on holiday to Bali or Europe. I loved our time in Greece."

Mark: "Yes that was good. Everything was slower. There was time for sex."

Here was the age-old story of a couple with mismatched sex drives. He associated sex with daily stress relief. She associated sex with yet another thing to fit into her overwhelming schedule. They had forgotten what drew them together in the first place.

Their joint sex clusters were like two ships passing in the night with no lights on. They were crashing into each other as communication and agreements around sex were poorly worked out. They associated sex with each other with stress.

Trance intentions

1. Regression for resource mining.
2. Reinstating good feelings towards each other.

3. Bringing those good feelings into the present time.
4. Future pacing, creating good feelings towards each other.
5. Implementing the boundary of respectful communication.
6. Promoting interpersonal negotiation.
7. Eliciting reciprocity through planning.
8. Bringing sex back to fun.

It's obvious you're having a really good time on holiday (maintaining regression)...both close your eyes and remember how that feels (regression, kinaesthetic resource mining)...**feels good** (Ki+)...**you look happy** (Vi+)...**saying sweet things to each other** (Ai+, mind mechanics)...oh to be in love (silent suggestion to reinitiate connection and oxytocin)...such a nice way to live...just imagine inside your minds how you both can make that happen today...in the future together (shared responsibility, working as a team)... **incorporating some of those good times into your present life** (direct suggestion)...being respectful to each other (silent suggestion)...considering each other's needs (eliciting co-operation)...**how good can that be** (interrogative suggestion, emotional change)...of course this requires co-operative planning (call to action to work together)...it requires careful scheduling (re-enforcement suggestion)...**compromise on all levels by everyone** (interpersonal negotiation)...of course you have done all this before...**remember**...you were experts at this when you were courting...time on your own (silent suggestion for independence)...**time as a couple having fun with sex**... at appointed times of course...**so everyone gets their space** (double suggestion as time for individuality and time for coupling)...when you have a good schedule time seems to be on your side (contingent suggestion)…**you might try sex twice a week at an appointed times if that's right for you** (inferred solution)…how do you think that might work inside your minds…how would you organise that…**time goes slower with good schedules**…time is on your side…getting someone else to look after the children…**just having fun sex time as a couple just for you two**…in a moment I want you to both come back to the room with positive solutions (time appointed post-hypnotic suggestion)

Vowels (2020) cited better communication as a major tool used by couples with sexual desire disparity to take them towards resolution. The demand of bringing up families can be stressful for all parents who sometimes mistake mis-scheduling for rejection by a partner.

I saw Mark in a second session three weeks afterwards.

> *Tracie:*   "*You know, Mark, you need to come off those steroid motivators you are taking to bulk up your body. They are messing with your body. Sure, at the moment, they have increased your sex drive, but in the last session with your wife, it seems that has caused problems in your marriage and what she considers is your aggressive sexual demands.*"

Normal males' testosterone levels are 300 to 1,000 nanograms per deciliter (ng/dL) or 10 to 35 nanomoles per liter (nmol/L). Mark's blood tests revealed they were 2500.

He was not taking synthetic steroids that are often bought illegally at gyms. What he was taking was labelled as a natural testosterone booster that he bought off the internet which contained Vit D 2000IU, Zinc 20mgs, Bulbine naturelis 200mgs,

Fenugreek 200mgs, Maca root 125mgs, Urtica dioica, 125mgs, Bioperine 10mg. Due to his self-administration, the problem was that there was no blood test before administration. This meant that if he had sufficient testosterone before he took the supplement, he would develop high testosterone.

> Mark: *"You think it's the steroid boosters? I love the sex on them. I took them this time for 12 weeks because I've got two compressed vertebrae in my neck and nerve pain due to lifting heavy weights above my head. Because I had to have time off from the gym, I've lost between 35% to 40% of the strength in my pecs (pectoralis major and minor)."*

Trance intentions

1. Awareness to stop the testosterone-raising supplements.
2. Focusing on his health more naturally.
3. Associating strength with rational behaviour.
4. Eliciting co-operation to work with his wife.
5. Appealing to his superego to regulate his demand for sex.
6. Giving him the option of solo sex when his wife is not available.
7. Suggestions for communication and co-operation.

Look at me now (law of focused attention)…your bloods don't lie (citing science as the validator for the change of his behaviour)…your testosterone is extremely high (truism)… **it's time to focus on your health more naturally** (direct suggestion)…family before vanity…your marriage before vanity…**it's good to be strong and healthy naturally** (implied suggestion to stop supplements)…and as your eyelids get heavier and heavier you find you can't keep them open (presupposition of eyes closing)…and (preparation conjunctive)…**go into a deep trance now** (intra-hypnotic suggestion)…a strong man is one who is strong in character (silent suggestion, linked suggestion going back to the couples session for him to work with his wife)…he works with his family (indirect value re-enforcement suggestion)…**he works with his wife** (implied directive to reduce sexual advances)…happy homes have good co-operation…communication…and care…how will you make that happen every day (interrogative suggestion for taking action and personal responsibility)…**you can know you're a good man** (suggestion to activate those changes immediately)…and sometimes you have sex sessions with yourself if your wife's not available (venting sexual energy)…you can have a good time… **and sometimes you can have sex with your wife** (indirect suggestion to reduce sexual approaches to his wife)…when she is available (conditional suggestion)…perhaps a couple of times a week (flexibility on timing)…organising yourselves well… **you can have a good time together**…remember…remember… everything balanced (silent suggestion)…**everyone happy in your family** (suggestion for superego regulation)…you make that happen by controlling your sexual energy…**listening to your wife about what she finds unacceptable**

Armstrong (2018) tells us that whilst anabolic steroids elevate testosterone and increase libido, cessation of use can lead to reduced testosterone and sex drive, and in some cases ED. Park et al. (2022) shows us that continuous use can also lead to secondary steroid-induced hypogonadism, low testosterone, gynaecomastia and ED, due to feedback suppression of the hypothalamic-pituitary-gonadal axis and reduction in luteinising hormone. This is the same with nutritional and herbal supplements that create high levels of testosterone.

I saw Mark and Camile as a couple for a follow-up three months later. Mark had stopped taking the supplements. They were getting on much better as a couple and had sex twice a week.

When Mark and Camile were courting, they only had sex two or three times a week. Mark's increased demand for sex was driven by his supplement-induced heightened libido.

Hanson (2009) considered how men can feel displaced and disempowered in a woman's life by the arrival of children. This greatly under-researched area, around the displacement of men in industrial and post-industrial families and post-feminism societies, needs to address men's sexual insecurities.

What Mark needed from Camile was attention, and what she needed was space away from having so much responsibility. By creating the space for them as a couple to date and be together, without the demands of the children, they were able to renegotiate their sex lives to both their satisfaction (see Appendix A, item 41).

13 Recovery from Rape and Sexual Assault

It must be clear in a therapist's mind that rape and sexual assault are acts of violence. They are not mistaken, amorous advances, whether they are carried out by adults or children.

Those acts contain intention and conscious choices, so there is always a perpetrator and a victim. The victim can suffer physically, mentally, and emotionally for life unless treated. Some people never recover.

Our family, society, medical and legal systems, however, are often prejudiced against the victim, so most of the assaults are never reported. Even if an accusation is made, establishing burden of proof means the victim must relive the event, which can be equally devastating.

Thomas (2023), in a systematic review of studies, found that self-reported surveys showed current estimates of 27% of men and 32% of women had been sexually assaulted at some time in their lives.

I caution here about men providing rape counselling for women and female-identified people. If a woman has been sexually assaulted by a male, she may be less comfortable discussing these issues with a man. Some female clients may consider this to be 'women's business'.

If a male has been assaulted, he may be more comfortable working with a male therapist. This is not always the case because women may be perceived as more empathic, but the client may consider it 'men's business'.

Here we are also talking about male and female-identified people, although none of us are strictly 100% biologically male or female. Those who are sex and/or gender diverse can also be at a high risk of violence and abuse.

Sexual acts never take place out of context of the person's whole life. Sexual assault creates mental and emotional dysregulation as well as physical trauma. It can result in personality decompression, lack of coping skills, mood disorders, borderline personality disorder, disassociation disorder, damage to the person's ability to operate healthy personal boundaries, attachment disorders, PTSD and, at times, suicidation.

To help the client initiate or reinitiate a healthy sex life, these mental health problems must generally be treated first, but not always. There is also no one single way of working with trauma victims. No one quick fix treats all. There are ways to accelerate treatment, some of which I show here and also in my book *Inspiration for Survive and Prosper: Personal Transformation Out of Crisis* (O'Keefe, 2013).

As a therapist I have thousands of strategies I may use with a client and the combination of those strategies are solely dependent on the individual client, how they present, their needs, and their progress.

Here I shall present on creating a sense of safety for and in the client, helping them read other people's intent, choices of interaction, better communications, cancelling victim guilt, emotional control, operating good boundaries, decisions to disclose or not, psychodynamic resolution of internal conflict, reinitiating self-agency, ego strengthening, and systematic desensitisation to sex.

If there are pre-existing mental health issues, diagnosed or undiagnosed, prior to the assault, this complicates recovery. A great deal of time and care is needed by the therapist to tease out the separate mental health issues and treat them.

Pre-existing mental health issues may also render someone more vulnerable to sexual assault as they may have reduced cognitive processing and risk assessment skills.

The age of the therapist can also be a factor in these dynamics. Older therapists can be seen by the client as less threatening, with more life experience.

In some cases, therapists closer to that person's own age may make the client more comfortable. They have social experiences in common and this is particularly relevant in drop-in and youth centres.

CASE STUDY: JANET

This 27-year-old woman had been referred to me by a former client. She lived on social security benefits in her ageing mother's home. A friend paid for six sessions in advance.

She had been raped twice as a teenager, had shut down socially, and became a recluse at 21. She had never had a relationship or consensual sex.

A man was interested in dating her, but she could only tolerate being around other people for about 10 minutes at a time. She had a phobia of being physically touched in any way. No family or friend could even hug her.

There had been two years of weekly sessions with a psychologist that had not remedied her daily trauma state in any way.

On the telephone:

Tracie: *"I have to be clear with you Janet that in taking you as a client I require you to follow my instructions and do everything that I say. You tell me you've already had an extensive number of sessions with other therapists, and nothing has changed. I want us to focus on solutions for you. Is that okay?"*

Janet had no communication with her mother, even though she was living with her, because the mother experienced major depression and did not communicate. Her father left them when Janet was three years old.

In short, she had no family confidante or role model and no example of a well-behaved, kind man in her life. She did not understand what boundaries were or that she had a right to them. Neither could she read men, so they all appeared potentially threatening to her. She had one female friend.

She had two sisters who also lived at home and the main way of communicating between the siblings was arguing and getting angry with each other.

Janet: *"I get angry very quickly. I can't control it. I blow up because no one respects my point of view, particularly my sisters. I hate it when they bring a boyfriend home."*

She associated sex with potential rape. Her sexual clusters were all around avoidance of physical contact which is why she had never had a consensual relationship.

Session one was about teaching her to create safe spaces where she could go to when things became too heated and uncomfortable.

Trance intentions

1. Creating psychological and emotional safety.
2. Handing over the control for creating that in the client.
3. Teaching her to use that process at any time.

From what you are telling me you seem to have felt unsafe most of the time (acknowledgement)...**be safe here...close your eyes and relax...safe here always** (locational safety anchor)... inside your mind I want you to see a safe place where you can be safe and alone...**see** (Vi+)...**hear** (Ai+)...**and feel that space** (Ki+, mind mechanics)...perhaps your room...the garden... going to the park in daytime...**wherever is right for you to be safe** (freedom to choose)...and nod your head when you have done that (wait for ideomotor response)...when you go to that place physically...and inside your mind...**you create safety** (self-agency)...privacy and safety...**you can make that space safe for you** (modal operator of possibility for self-efficacy)... it's your very own space... peaceful...relaxing...private...safe (silent suggestions)...you don't have to explain it to anyone... **carrying that safe place around with you inside your mind wherever you go** (paradoxical intent, turning dissociation into a resource)...nod your head when you are there (she nodded her head)...if there is a potential argument you just excuse yourself and find your safe place...**you are fully present in that safe space enjoying it and feeling comfortable at any time** (universal safety procedure)

Rothbaum (1992), in a longitudinal study, found 94% of rape victims experienced PTSD immediately after assault, and 47% within three months. But the problem with PTSD is that it is a time bomb and can suddenly be triggered 60 years after the original traumatic event, often by an unrelated trigger.

It was clear that not only was Janet experiencing PTSD from the double rape, but also that she had been raised in a home with a single parent with chronic depression. The parenting had been inadequate in teaching her life skills and resilience. So, part of my job was to reparent her in resourceful ways.

In session two we focused on boundaries and a person's right to have boundaries in all areas of their lives.

Trance intentions

1. Initiating the learning of communication skills.
2. Teaching extraction techniques.
3. Teaching boundaries.
4. Learning to be discerning about what is classified as an emergency or crisis.

You have a right to communicate when and how you wish (claiming communication rights)…at any time…you can even say "I'll get back to you on this" (de-escalating conflict)…take time and space to think about things (using the dissociation as a solution, paradoxical intent)…**going back to a communication when you're positively interacting** (direct post-hypnotic suggestion)…you can walk away from any situation at any time (permission to disengage from conflict)…everyone has a right to good boundaries in your family (indirect suggestion for personal boundaries)…friends…relationship (universal boundaries)… **you have a right to good boundaries in your family** (addressing her criteria of needs)…friends…relationship…**it's your world and you decide your boundaries** (ownership of terms of interactions)…there are few emergencies in life that demand your immediate attention…many may seem like an emergency but when you look from a distance they aren't (shrinking unimportant misperceived threats)…**learning the difference between the two** (initiating better communication skills)

In working with Janet, it seemed she had previously paid little attention to visual cues. We worked on body language in the session and her homework was to continue that learning by reading a body language book (Pease, 2017) and rehearsing the exercises from it at home in front of a mirror.

Session three was teaching her to control her emotions. I taught her a process to examine her own emotions when they happened and make changes. This is state-changing work.

> Tracie: *"Emotions are valuable and natural...we all experience all of them...when you feel your emotions are overwhelming...go to one side for a few moments and...***ask yourself these questions***:*

Emotional control protocol

- What are these emotions I am having?
- Why do I have these emotions?
- Are they appropriate at this time?
- Is the level of emotion right for me or too much or too little?
- Are these emotions right for these circumstances?
- What do I need to do now to control my emotions?

Trance intentions

1. Teaching emotional intelligence.
2. Gaining control by dissociation from overwhelming emotions.
3. Teaching self-analysis.
4. Teaching fast state changing.

Know how well you are doing (motivation by acknowledging effort and success)...**such great progression you have made** (indirect time-shifting suggestion, distancing from the past trauma)…when you become overwhelmed by emotion (global identification of distress)…**follow the emotional control protocol** (direct suggestion for taking action for emotional control)…look at yourself from a distance (objective perspective, desensitisation)…decide how you need to change fast…do this in a fast minute…**make it happen fast** (re-enforcement, direct suggestion for fast state changing)…take control… say to yourself…**I'm a strong woman…I'm intelligent** (ego strengthening)…**I'm free** (cancelling the victim status)… practise this again and again and again…**you get better and better and better at changing your experience fast** (stacking future-paced success)…just like you learnt to use a keyboard or ride a bicycle…practise practise practise

I do not generally use regression with assault victims as it is simply too re-traumatising for them, unless there is a vague history of chronic abuse and we need to change those memories.

The first three sessions were about creating a sense of safety, boundaries, and emotional control to stabilise Janet's personality. Only then did we go on to moving past the sexual assault and tackling the rape and trauma issues.

The most important part of helping trauma victims is teaching them emotional control and state shifting (Goleman, 2021). Without that, all the analytical, cognitive or behaviour therapy in the world will likely not be sufficient for recovery (see Appendix A, item 42).

The last time I saw Janet she was starting to date the young man who was interested in her. The friend who paid for the sessions contacted me a few years later to tell me Janet had married, moved 500 miles away and was expecting a child.

CASE STUDY: LOUIS

Louis, a 32-year-old man, came from a wealthy family. His father was an American businessman and his mother was from European aristocracy. As a child he had spent most of his time in an exclusive mountain area in a low tax zone, apart from boarding school after 12 years of age.

His father travelled a lot, was bisexual and had affairs with men. The mother oversaw all domestic arrangements, and Louis's education. Reportedly there had been very little sex between the husband and wife. Their sex life was basically not active.

His mother first came into Louis's room late at night when he was 11, put her hand under his bedding and started to masturbate him. She told him it was their secret, and he should not tell anyone because they would get into trouble.

> Louis: "I was conflicted because I liked what she was doing but I was confused as to whether she should be doing it with me. I didn't know how to stop her or if I wanted her to stop."

His mother climbed on top of him when he was 14 to have intercourse with him. That continued until he was 18 and left for university.

Little is taught to therapists about women who sexually abuse children. Research, however, shows us that it is far more common than generally thought, but it is considered far too controversial to discuss in public (Saradjian, 1996).

Here, I shall discuss the legal quagmire of health professionals' reporting duties. First, this happened in the past in another country. Second, as far as I knew, no one was being abused now. Third, since my client is an adult, I would be breaching confidentiality by contacting the authorities in his country of origin without his permission.

Therefore, in this case, at this time, I had no legal obligation to report the historical abuse. It was also his request for me not to do that. If as a health professional you are unsure about your legal obligations, you should always take supervision. You must also have guidance from your professional association's code of conduct and ethics.

Louis: *"I had several affairs and married my wife when I was 25. It was a society wedding and the night before, I told her what had happened between my mother and myself. Naturally, she was shocked and only consented to continuing the wedding if I promised to break all ties with my mother, have no contact and emigrate to another continent."*

Tracie: *"You now say you have two boys aged eight and 10. Are you happy you emigrated and cut those ties with your family of origin?"*

Louis: *"Yes, I've fully realised now I'm a father, that I was abused. Recently my father has been trying to establish contact with us. He says he doesn't understand why we want nothing to do with them. He thinks it's because he was bisexual, slept most of the time with men, and now lives with his male partner. I'm haunted about what to do. You're a sex therapist Dr Tracie – what should I do?"*

Therapists must be very careful about giving advice in these situations. Urging Louis to disclose could lead to his mother being charged and going to prison. He would have to relive that history again, plus what happened would become public knowledge. What may seem morally and legally right is not always mentally and emotionally good for the client. The number one priority was that I had to put the client's wellbeing first.

Louis associated his mother with sexual abuse and his father with being absent from his childhood. His sexual clusters seemed to be satisfied in his marriage which he considered normative. His sexual clusters around sex with his mother were still conflicted.

Trance intentions

1. Enabling him to make a decision that works for him.
2. Bring him into the present time to make that decision.

Well Louis...on this decision I can't advise you...but we can help you make a decision you and your family can live with...**just sit back and relax in my safe office closing your eyes**...look up inside your mind...seeing yourself as the man you are today (time shifting away from the abuse)...happily married...two beautiful children...running your own business (truisms)...**you are creating a good happy life every day** (affirming survival instinct, indirect suggestion for him to make decisions that support his present stable life)...protecting yourself...wife....children...**your today family is paramount** (activating Maslow's second level of criteria of needs, protection and safety from the world)...I know and you know you know how to do that (confusion, trance deepening)...you know how to continually do that...**protecting yourself and your now family today** (re-enforcement suggestion, raising that principle as his supreme value and priority in his superego)...

make that be your number one value in making your decision (direct suggestion, bombardment)...**you can play a film on a screen inside your mind**...what it might be like if you disclose the sexual abuse that happened (establishing that it was abuse, future possibility, projection, as if scenario)...you can also play in your mind on a parallel screen what it might be like if you don't disclose what happened (alternative future possibility projection)...take your time and compare the two (five minutes for him to compare the two)...**only you know all the factors in making this decision**...it's an important decision you make for you and your family and is the best decision for today (weighing up possibilities and probabilities)...**you know you can make the best decision you can** (creating confidence in his decision-making)...perhaps you make the decision today...tomorrow or next week (allowing resistance, illusion of choice, post-hypnotic suggestion for making the decision within a week)... your unconscious mind can weight up all the pros and cons (re-enforcing the call to action)...and at some stage you will wake up and know you have made the right decision for you and your family (post-hypnotic suggestion for eliciting unconscious resolution)...**you can be at peace with that decision**

It is important not to force people into a decision there and then, as that is oppressive and puts people under pressure just to decide, without considering all the consequences. The unconscious mind, like the conscious mind, can require time to calculate what is best for that person.

Many decisions are made when we are asleep and dreaming in the REM dream cycle. We have tens, if not hundreds, of dreams in a night, weighing up all the possibilities of our lives. This helps us calculate what is right for us today, tomorrow and in the distant future.

The second time I saw Louis, he told me he was happy with the decision he had made and which his wife agreed with.

Tracie: *"Are you happy in your life now?"*

Louis: *"Well, yes."*

Tracie: *"Do you believe you have dealt with what happened and it does not disturb your daily life or that of your family today?"*

Louis: *"To be honest, I sometimes think I did something wrong and got away with it. The problem is we both enjoyed the sex at the time. In fact, the sex could be really good. I'm so split about it and at times that drives me crazy. I've never told anyone that before."*

Tracie: *'Would you like to change that?"*

Louis: *"Yes, okay."*

Trance intentions

1. Retriggering safety anchor.
2. Metaphor for survival.
3. Shifting culpability to the mother.
4. Psychodynamic conflict resolution.

Thank you so much for your honesty...and trust...and of course everything we discuss is completely confidential...close your eyes and go inside safe in my office...**you are again safe now in my office** (time, space distancing from the abuse)...I know in your country of origin there are wild wolves... you told me you missed the wolves (initiating his survival instinct)...that's nature isn't it...and sometimes those wolves steal sheep even if it's dangerous for themselves (equating people to doing dangerous and wild things)...**wolves are wild** (initiating his survival instinct)...it's part of their survival... they may get shot at...chased...and have to hide at times... **they are wolves and survival is everything** (paralleling his journey with wolves surviving)...those wolves no matter what happens they begin again (indirect suggestion for psychic reinvention, metaphoric comparative to human behaviour)... they will do what they need to survive...**perhaps you can think of yourself as a wolf** (indirect suggestion for survival and reinvention)... you need to survive and you need to have the best life you can...sex is a biological driving force...it's a biological driver...**your wolf and human sides have that biological drive for sex**...but sometimes mother wolves make mistakes (shifting culpability to his mother)...they can even make life-threatening mistakes...it's the randomness of nature (rendering his guilt invalid)...you are now however an adult wolf...**you know what's right** (superego processing)...**for you and your family today**...you know new things now and have new skills (time shifting away from the past)...the mistakes your mother made are not your mistakes (cancelling his guilt, shame and culpability)...**you look to the present and the future as a strong wolf** (orienting him to his present life)... you have your own pack...your own territory...your own life... you live by different codes around the nature of things today (dissociating from the mother's actions)...**you have evolved**... **you survived and live peacefully**

Louis was raised in the mountains. He was fascinated by wolves and missed them. Mountain people often fear and love wolves. Most of all, they respect their ability to survive and give them a special totemism and mythological meaning associated with strength (Heacox, 2015). They co-exist with them.

Wolves do not like or dislike, they do what is best for survival. In the coldest of winters when there is no food, they cannibalise dead wolves' bodies. This implies his mother was surviving in the dysfunctional ways she knew without better knowledge. It is an indirect suggestion for unconscious logic and processing.

In betrayal trauma theory, incest survivors can suffer amnesia for events whilst trying to maintain attachment to the related abuser (Lawson, 2018). There can also be an unconscious conflict between libido and the superego in victims enjoying sexual sensations, and at the same time experiencing guilt (Cowan, 2020).

Louis was not in trauma over the incest, just trying to come to terms with it, so it was important not to overlay pathologies on to what happened. Three things probably saved him: distancing himself from his mother at boarding school, university, and marriage, which was a form of physical dissociation. This taught him compartmentalisation and objectivity, reducing the risk of PTSD.

Again, our job as hypnotists is not to re-traumatise people with their histories but to support the strategies they can use today for a good life.

In aligning Louis with the strength of his beloved wolves, he found peace in his incestuous sex history and the loving, respectful man he became.

The peace he found allowed him to decide to have contact with his father, but never his mother. He chose not to disclose the details of the conflict with his mother to his father (see Appendix A, item 43).

CASE STUDY: JENNY

Jenny was a 35-year-old woman with her own fashion retail business. She described herself as a party girl who was always out clubbing and going to fashion shows. She saw that lifestyle as part of her job.

She wore a fashionable low-cut t-shirt with no bra, even though she had large breasts. When she sat down her short skirt fully exposed her underwear.

Previously married in an abusive, violent relationship, she was now separated and had a current restraining order against her ex-husband, who had spent time in jail for violent crimes. She had two children under seven who were in long-term foster care. Jenny had voluntarily surrendered them because she would lose her temper with them. She said she loved them but did not know how to be a mother and could not trust herself.

She presented with the complaint that her life and moods were very unstable. With that, she said that she was highly promiscuous and sometimes would sleep with four or five different men a week and often take cocaine with them.

Jenny: *"I don't feel respected. Guys just see me as someone they can have sex with. Many can turn up at the shop knowing I'll sleep with them at a moment's notice. I'm a bike – they can get on and ride me. I don't particularly enjoy sex, I don't feel anything when it happens, but I just do it if guys ask."*

Tracie: *"How old were you when you first lost your virginity?"*

Jenny: *"I was nine when my dad first had sex with me."*

Tracie: *"And how long did that go on for?"*

Jenny: *"Well, it never stopped. He still comes to me for sex now. The last time was two weeks ago."*

Timms (2008) proposes that sexual abuse happens in one in three females and one in five males before the age of 18. The abuse can produce promiscuous sexual behaviour and emotional disturbances in adulthood in some people. The anxiety that occurs in childhood can give rise to a series of adult addictive behaviours.

It was clear how confused Jenny was around boundaries, sex, and relationships. Basically, she had no clear boundaries. Her mother had been a heroin addict and simply ignored her father abusing her. In reality, Jenny did not really understand that her father was an abuser or had any idea how to stop him.

Her mother had been a complicit co-abuser by not challenging her husband's abuse of Jenny. To keep the peace, and her successful husband continuing to supply money for the heroin, she sacrificed Jenny to her husband for sex. Added to that, as a teenager Jenny's grandfather and uncle also used her for sex.

She was taught that she was a sex object, there to facilitate the sexual needs of the men around her. This was her early imprint around her own self-image and worth. Female objectification as a sex object is not only common but standard throughout the world today, and translates into adult women undervaluing themselves (Kellie, 2019).

When a father and mother both use a child as a sex object, the child grows up with no template of how to have a wholesome, rewarding, healthy relationship. Being a sex object becomes their norm and, in many cases, the abused person carries that negative self-image and submissive character into adulthood.

Wenninger (1998) reports female survivors of child sexual abuse experience higher levels of negative self-image in relation to their body, reduced satisfaction of sexual performance, and lower self-esteem in adulthood. These are clearly signs of a delay in maturity and development of sexual confidence.

The absence of self-care, safety and genuine affection can become replaced by the equation that inappropriate sex equals self-validation or subjugation to other people's will. For Jenny, the more sex she had, the more she perceived herself to be validated, whilst at the same time feeling she was being used.

It cannot be said she had Stockholm Syndrome (Jülich, 2005) around her abusers because it was more a matter that she was simply trained to be available for sex with male family members and men in general.

Jenny: *"I try to have relationships, but they always end in disaster because I see the men as using me and I get frightened or angry. I'm also attracted to bad men who, in the end, beat me up. I'll scream, shout, and throw things until they get violent. The worse the man treats me, the more I'm attracted to him."*

Tracie: *"If I teach you how to behave in a more adult way, and create deeper rewarding relationships, will you do everything I say?"*

Jenny: *"Depends what you ask me to do."*

Tracie: *"Well, I'm not going to negotiate about that with you (negotiating with such behaviours would mean being subjugated as a therapist by the self-abusing part of her psyche)…you've come to me with a story out of a horror movie (acknowledging her distress)…and I know the way for a better life* *for you (reparenting)...**you can completely trust me** (permissive direct suggestion)...my role as a therapist is to help you have a better life (establish therapeutic momentum)...**you will be making massive changes** (direct suggestion)."*

Jenny: *"Okay, I'm in." (when a client displays impulsivity towards therapeutic gain as a therapist, I utilise it.)*

She associated sex with abuse and violence. Her sexual clusters were around facilitating men, but not herself as she had never been taught boundaries.

Trance intentions

1. Safety anchor and creating locational safety.
2. Bring her out of the flight/fight/freeze response.
3. Acknowledging her ability to be caring.
4. Resource mining.
5. Identifying preservation instincts.
6. Initiating boundaries and feminism.
7. Initiating self-caring.
8. Comparative suggestion that she deserves the respect that all other women rightly deserve.
9. Separation from abusers.
10. Behavioural Pavlovian response to reject unwanted sexual advances.
11. Future pacing a good life.
12. Momentum to change her life.

Close your eyes and safely rest in that comfortable chair...take deep breaths and very slowly (reducing hyperventilation)... slowly in through your nose...and slowly out though your mouth letting it go...**very very slowly** (bringing her down out of the panic response)...with your mouth slightly open (eliciting parasympathetic breathing)...**continue to breathe slowly as slowly....slowly...your body deeply relaxes** (contingent suggestion, slow breathing leads to body relaxing, leading to coming out of the fight, flight or freeze response)... how slowly you can breathe now (interrogative suggestion to induce Alpha brain wave activity)...**knowing you are always safe and protected in my office and when you hear my voice** (locational and auditory safety anchors)...and always will be (future pacing safety)...**safe...here...now...always... my voice** (post-hypnotic suggestion, direct suggestion, pure Milton Erickson)...you are a mother and in order to keep your children safe you surrendered them for fostering (implying she does know how to care for someone)...it was a selfless (silent indirect suggestion that she already knows what caring involves)... caring act of a loving mother (truisms)...**you know how to be a kind, respectful, loving mother** (direct suggestion, eliciting the superego in controlling the personality)...it's the instinct of a lioness...hiding her cubs when danger is around... it's nature...caring...love and kindness...**by nature you know how to be that caring...loving mother** (eliciting primal instincts)...as a lioness you would do anything to protect your cubs (modal operator of probability, activating protective mechanisms, 15-second break for unconscious processing).... **now** (preparatory conjunctive, bringing her into the present)... **that lioness inside you will protect Jenny** (intra- and post-hypnotic suggestion)...keep her safe with good boundaries (silent suggestion)...keep her protected...**show Jenny protection...love...caring** (associating boundaries with self-care)...just as you deserve as a woman...just as any woman deserves...just as all women deserve (stacking suggestions to initiate feminism)…a lioness makes her own way (indirection suggestion to separate from abusers)…a lioness takes care of herself…protects herself…**you are strong and protecting yourself no matter who you come in contact with** (post-hypnotic direct suggestion, eliciting self-protection)…the lioness always protects…and she begins with protecting herself…you will say…**no…no…to unwanted men's sexual advances** (governor, Pavlovian response, because the abuse is ongoing we need to use a modal operator of necessity)… **bring out your lioness** (eliciting self-protecting, resource scanning)…the lioness will withdraw to heal (distancing from abusers)…**as you will now one day at a time** (chunking down for manageable goals, direct suggestion) …sorting out your life and making your own way…a good way…a good life…**a life that is always of your own making** (indirect suggestion for continual self-protection, self-efficacy)…you're in charge… **no one** (suggestion for excluding abusers from her life, governor)…**no one…bosses you around**…or makes you do anything you don't want to…the lioness protects you…**you are an independent woman**…who protects…cares…and loves herself first (stacking resources)…**for the moment you say no to sex** (governor, rehearsal technique, giving her space to work on herself)…take a breath in your life…give yourself space to…**learn…grow…take care of yourself**

We agreed Jenny would have no contact with her family for now, nor have sex with anyone during the initial therapy.

> Tracie: *"You're going to be confused to begin with (direct suggestion for confusion in order to create new learnings)…this is what happens as everything changes…**stay with the plan.**"*

People who come into therapy, who are presently being abused, are not operating good boundaries for so many reasons. They may not know they have options, what boundaries are, how they apply to them, and do not have cultural power or a sense of self-agency.

Disengagement from the abuser requires locational separation, severing of communication, enlisting help, and sometimes going into a shelter of some kind, and possible legal protection orders (see Appendix A, item 44).

Jenny already had an established life and business which she could not leave. We had to build on the resources she already had. But she learned to say 'no' to sex with her abusers and men with whom she was not involved.

She even decided to report the childhood abuse to the police. Her relatives petitioned her to withdraw the complaint, but she became resolute she would see it through. Eventually she took out a court order to keep those relatives away from her.

After a year's therapy every three weeks, Jenny formed a relationship with a garment import supplier. She told him her history and I had to teach her how to have a respectful relationship. She secured her divorce from her first husband, a year later she married the new man, and only had sex with him after they were married.

Sagon (2023) reported how those who were in stable, romantic relationships showed higher psychological wellbeing and lower levels of psychopathology test scores. Whilst there is heteronormative and cultural bias, it does suggest that good attachment styles can offer profound spousal support.

After Jenny got married, she got her children back to live with her and continued to have no contact with her family of origin. She learnt to be a woman who demanded safety and respect and that it was not negotiable. In therapy she remapped her attachment styles and gave birth to her own feminism.

CASE STUDY: BARTIE

Bartie was a 45-year-old gay man living on his own, working as a tarot card reader. He was effeminate in mannerisms but preferred to describe himself as just camp.

Although he identified as gay, he had had no relationships in his adult life and had a great deal of reticence in trusting, either lovers or relationships.

Bartie: *"I came from a small town, well, a village really in the north of England, where I was obviously gay. In the early 1960s, it was illegal. As a young teenager I was bullied at school. When I was 15, I went to London and worked in a hairdressing salon as an apprentice. I had a small bedsit in Shepherds Bush."*

Tracie: *"How did that go?"*

Bartie: *"It went great. It was an exclusive salon in the West End where being camp was a plus rather than a drawback. The clients were wealthy, educated, often aristocrats, who were naturally avant garde. My sexuality was never an issue. I loved it and got quite confident."*

Tracie: *"So, how can we help you today?"*

Bartie: *"I got so confident that when I was 18, I decided to visit my parents in my old country town for the weekend. Big mistake. I was dressed very*

*fashionably and camper than ever. In the pub on
the Saturday night there were boys I'd gone to
school with."*

He started to shake, could not look at me and started to cry.
When he was ready, he carried on.

Bartie: *"They even bought me drinks and chatted to me.
When the pub closed, eight of them were waiting
for me at the bus stop. One of them punched me,
called me, "Little fairy poofter from London",
pushed me, ripped off my clothes and raped me
behind the bus shelter."*

He broke down again.

Tracie: *"You can take your time. You're safe here. In your
own time." (allowing him to tell his history)*

Bartie: *"Two of them kicked me and held my face down on
the ground and a third started to rape me. I don't
know how long it was but each one of the eight had
sex with me, one after the other. Then they just left
me there."*

Tracie: *"I can't imagine how that was for you. I'm so sorry
that happened to you (sometimes people want
someone to say sorry for what happened to them,
empathy not sympathy). You didn't deserve that
happening to you. No one deserves that happening
to them, ever."*

Bartie: *"Anyway – a local policeman in a patrol car drove
past and noticed my clothes by the bus stop. He*

drove me to the hospital. I had so much anal damage that I was bleeding everywhere. I had to have stiches. The policeman collected the rest of my things from my parents, and I never went back there. I never went back to that town ever again."

Tracie: "That must have been upsetting for your family as well.

Bartie: "They were never told what happened. No charges were pressed because it would be too hard to prove. I only ever saw my mother once again in London years later."

Tracie: "What do you need at this time?"

Bartie: "There's a friend. I've known him for 15 years. He's gay. He's very kind and fun to be with. He always spends time with me at Christmas and on my birthday. Paul's his name. Anyway, he's indicated he might like it if our friendship become something more."

Tracie: "Is that good news for you?"

Bartie: "I've consulted the tarot cards, and the star card came up, which means hope. The Empress card also came up, which means ready for love. But the warning card didn't come up. I like him very much and love him as a friend, but I can't get over my fear that something horrible will happen."

Walker et al. (2005) found that when males do report sexual assault, they are often not believed. They also encounter shaming and blame, so very few make a report to authorities.

For men the after-effects of sexual assault include emotional and mood disturbances, sleep difficulty, sexual difficulty, anxiety, fear, addiction, PTSD and an increased sense of vulnerability.

Bartie associated sex with the danger of being attacked again. His sexual clusters were mostly connected to his sense of poor self-esteem, lack of worthiness and that he felt he was always unsafe in such situations, because he could not protect himself against other men.

Trance intentions

1. Placing him as the expert on his own future.
2. Ego strengthening.
3. Reframing sex as a form of love.
4. Mining for trust resources.
5. Drawing his attention to the respect and kindness from Paul.
6. Teaching how to chunk tasks into smaller pieces for desensitisation to sex and systemic manageable progress.

Alright you can know you are safe right now and when you hear my voice…and I can never give you advice on whether to have a relationship with Paul or anyone else (implied directive that he has to make the decision)…**make yourself comfortable in that chair with your eyes closed peacefully** (direct suggestion for peace, depotentiating panic)…as your body relaxes I want to tell you I don't know anything about the tarot cards (indirect suggestion that he already knows his answer)…it seems that you know a great deal about them (ego strengthening and buying into his belief system)…**love of course is food and we all need to eat** (including him in the need for love with rest of the human race, allowing him to have a relationship)…**especially**

when a dish is very pleasant (associating a relationship with pleasure)...there are such lovely things in life...things like... **respect...kindness...love**...isn't it good to experience those things (interrogative suggestion, transderivational search, trance deepener, he has already experienced those with Paul)... but of course the most important one is respect...r-e-s-p-e-c-t...**respect for yourself and others** (indirect suggestion for recognising his value system)...and when you see that...it feels very nice and safe (association between Paul and safety)... you can remember how kind and caring you were to your hairdressing clients (recalling past ability to trust)...**you made them feel safe**...you can know how kind and caring you are to your tarot clients (establishing he is already doing trust again)...you make them feel safe...**so you know about how to help someone feel safe** (validating present resources)... just like you do with your clients today...just imagine the effort Paul has put into being there on your birthday and Christmas (suggestion for doing due diligence around Paul's behaviour)...helping you have a good time...**making you feel safe...respected...special** (associating Paul with safeness and being special)...you can recognise the trust, caring and respect he is showing you...**because you are someone special** (ego strengthening)...to begin with however making yourself feel safe (silent suggestion, self-responsibility for feeling safe, chunking down)...because that's respectful...a kind thing to do for you...**you can remember to look for respect**...kindness... fun...which expresses love...love is what you can observe someone is doing...**you can eat from the fruits of life** (indirect generalised suggestion to expand his experiences)...enjoy the sweetness of a loving time (indirect suggestion for engaging with Paul)...perhaps...and this is only a suggestion (allowing resistance, preparing for an upcoming direct suggestion)...**you**

320

can take it one step at time with Paul or anyone else (making his journey manageable, avoiding overwhelm)...and when you see respect and kindness builds trust (contingent suggestion, chunking up)...trust and kindness can deepen love (stacking the elements for feeling safe)...**and you can show kindness, caring, patience with Paul and of course yourself** (direct suggestion to engage in a two-way process of building mutual trust)...sex can be beautiful and loving when you allow that to happen (modal operator of possibility, post-hypnotic indirect suggestion to engage in sex, causal link)...**and you can perhaps enjoy sex as another expression of love** (repetitious suggestion re-enforcing the associations between respect, kindness, caring, love, and sex)...so you can slowly build respect...kindness... fun...trust...and love...one step at a time under your own control...**because you know how to make yourself and others feel safe** (indirect call for action, fun cancels the panic response)

Bartie's PTSD meant he needed to chunk everything into manageable, digestible tasks for his progress towards engaging in sex. It is a form of systematic desensitisation. When combined with behavioural hypnotherapy, and solution-focused therapy, recovery is faster, and the client becomes more resilient and willing to engage in sex.

Recalling he already knew how to express respect, love and caring helped him build trust in Paul in the present time. It also calls on Bartie to display the same qualities, helping him move away from self-traumatisation and victimisation towards altruism.

I suggested that they had very short sex exposure sessions together once week to get used to each other under the new circumstances, and to avoid overwhelm. Each of them could call time at any period during the session by using a code word.

And Bartie had a trigger warning word that he could use if something became too intense and overwhelming. Over the months Bartie learned to use these words less and less during their sessions.

Paul knew about Bartie's history and rape experience and was empathic with the routine for progressive exposure. Bartie reported that Paul had told him it was a fantastic idea, and he was fully on board.

Slowly over several months Bartie learned to let Paul in emotionally and it deepened their relationship. The key for igniting his sex life was to base it on the foundations of respect, kindness, and fun. He had to build his sex life on something more than libido, with large doses of desire and connection.

After a year they had a trial period of moving in together. Bartie had to measure and record his progress in a daily diary that we discussed in monthly sessions.

When they were more comfortable with each other as a couple, only then did we tackle PTSD in therapy. I worked this way around for Bartie to experience progressive, wholesome connections first, to give him the confidence that he could resolve the PTSD. Sometimes we must change therapy around to suit the individual client's needs. Bartie already had someone in his life who wanted to be close to him, so I believed it was wise to nurture that relationship first.

Whilst hypnotherapy is highly effective, it is important for the therapist to also work psychotherapeutically in such sexual trauma cases – in fact in all trauma cases (see Appendix A, item 45).

14 Sex and Disability

There is a fine line between disability and differently abled. Those who are differently abled have a right not to be pathologised, if that is how they see themselves. Those who struggle with physical or mental disadvantage can, however, gain many social and legal benefits from being classified as disabled.

Disabled people can struggle with many issues including self-image, physical or mental difficulties, prejudice, bullying, violence, social disadvantage, reduced access to resources, socioeconomic disadvantage, harassment, and social, legal, and institutional controls placed on their lives by others.

Callen (2020), in reviewing the disability civil rights movement of the 1960s and 1970s, and the ensuing scope for research projects, calls for a reclassification of the normative and non-normative paradigm. Although I think we have to be careful here in that those classified as disabled do frequently require special care and consideration that the average citizen does not. Removing certain disability classifications would harm many less abled people's access to resources.

Bahner et al. (2024) warns about the disadvantages of the desexsualisation of disabled people by supposed 'normative' structural ableist narratives. This can also cause conscious and unconscious disability prejudice within disabled people, damaging sexual desire and function. Bahner advises that a positive, constructive dialogue, narrative and attitude around disability and sexuality be adopted on the person's own terms. This requires us as health professionals not to over-pathologise those who do not wish to bear that label.

Shakespeare (2018) talks about the disadvantage of ageing and deterioration of health in disabled people. This gives rise to a double barrier in that non-normative ageism can come into play. Sexual desire might not change but declining physical and mental capacity and non-normative classification of the person as being aged and disabled creates reduced access to sex.

The spectrum of disability here to consider is vast, as any physical or mental disadvantage can cause disability, including genetic variance, disease, trauma, PTSD, mental illness and encountering unusual life events.

Each case must be assessed on the individual's own disadvantages and their effects upon sexuality and sexual function. Blanket hypnosis or hypnotherapy cannot facilitate the client as each treatment needs to be formulated uniquely for that person and their situation.

CASE STUDY: ALASTER

Alaster, a 37-year-old man, experienced bipolar disorder and was taking a plethora of anti-psychotic, anti-depressant, and sleep medications prescribed by his psychiatrist. That was the same psychiatrist who diagnosed him 10 years earlier.

Alaster also drank a bottle of wine a day and regularly took the drug ecstasy at weekends, connecting with women for sex on a dating app. Just lately he had been more depressed than usual, so his psychiatrist had increased his medication. He still, however, held a paying job in an accountancy firm where he had worked for several years.

Alaster: *"I just can't get it up anymore at 30 and I'm really depressed about it."*

Tracie: *"Firstly, let's talk about the elephant in the room. What discussions do you have with your psychiatrist about your alcohol and drug use?"*

Alaster: *"None, we never talk about it. He knows what I do but his attitude is as long as it keeps me happy."*

Tracie: *"When did you last have a psychotic episode?"*

Alaster: *"Ten years ago before I started the medication when I was coming down off a three-day bender on E's. I'd always been moody or manic."*

Tracie: *"I know your psychiatrist reviews your medication, but have you ever had any other kind of therapy?"*

Alaster: *"No. He says I don't need it but to just keep taking the medications. I really had to press him to get the referral to see you."*

Tracie: *"I would really like to help you, Alaster, but, and it's a big but, we have got to do the health math. You can't cheat the accounting process and expect all the figures to add up at the end of your calculations."*

Alaster: *"I don't understand."*

He associated drugs and alcohol with having sexual satisfaction. His sexual clusters were around getting as much sex as he could, no matter the cost to himself. As his body failed him, and the ED became obvious, his anger propelled him further into substance and medication dependency.

Trance intentions

1. Math metaphors to engage him in his own model of the world.
2. Confronting his alcohol and drug use.
3. Establishing scientific authority.
4. Using scientific logic to initiate intra-psychic conflict resolution.
5. Creating self-esteem and efficacy.
6. Promoting a healthy diet and exercise.

Look at and listen to me…(law of focused attention)…let me frame it as an equation you can understand (suggested presupposition he would understand)…take away alcohol and ecstasy…**you get better erectile function** (post-hypnotic suggestion, conditional suggestion trading with his unconscious)…add anti-depressants, anti-psychotics and some sleep medications and you get a higher probability of erectile dysfunction…add therapy and you will be able to… **manage your sex life better** (direct suggestion)…reducing those medications under supervision…when done carefully (conditional bargaining)…**can help restore erectile function** (it is important here to use a modal operator of possibility for there may be substantial physical dysfunction)…of course this equation is…**based on facts and solid science** (validation, as an accountant he works with facts)…but you have to do the math (challenging his delusions)…**accepting changing your life is now your best odds** (direct suggestions)…of course you won't know until you try it (behavioural challenge).

> Alaster: "You don't sugar coat it, do you Doc?"
>
> Tracie: "I'm not a sugar therapist…I'm a science-informed health professional…I can give you the facts

*(establishing authority)…**you can calculate the odds** (suggestion for parts negotiation)…your unconscious knows I'm right (transderivational search, trance deepener, he must resolve the conflict to check the statement)…and it can tell your conscious mind too…**when you have done the calculations.**" (bind as he cannot know the answer until he has resolved the conflict)*

I worked with Alaster to stop alcohol and ecstasy for over six weeks using the methods from my book *Stop Drug and Alcohol Addiction: A Guide for Clinical Hypnotherapists* (O'Keefe, 2018). He stopped recreational substance abuse before we began treatment for the ED, or so he consciously thought. With persuasion, the psychiatrist agreed to lower the dose of his medications. His brother, who lived in Alaster's house, monitored him each day for his mood and stability.

As therapists we face a patient's complex history when we see that previous or concurrent practitioners have been negligent or abusive. Smith (2012) discussed how many patients are given psychiatric medications without being properly assessed. This goes further in that many medications are maintained for no good reason after a short-term crisis ceases.

We can see here the psychiatrist did not properly assess Alaster and the original psychosis appeared to be induced by recreational drug use. Also, the psychiatrist told him he did not need therapy and ignored his alcohol and drug use. Instead he simply kept prescribing and taking a consultation fee. All of this will have undoubtedly contributed to the patient's ED.

Two months later:

Alaster: "I'm really angry at you."

Tracie: "Which part of you is really angry at me...it can't be all of you because you're sitting in my office (acknowledging the part of him that agrees with me and our approach)...**you came here on your own today**...and you seem to be happier and certainly look much healthier (validation of progressive success)...**keep on doing the work**" (direct suggestion)

Alaster: "The part that used to get me off my face to pick up women."

Tracie: "Oh, that part...hasn't it learnt yet that as you change it will be easier to communicate with women and (interrogative challenge)...**you will have better erections** (post-hypnotic direct suggestion)...how's your moods?" (creating amnesia for the resistance by sudden conversational change)

Alaster: "I don't really know. I've not been without drugs for about 15 years. So, I've got nothing to measure it by."

Tracie: "Have you crashed or burned?"

Alaster: "I've come close to crashing sometimes but managed to pull myself out of it."

Tracie: "Do you know how frigging (jolt mechanism) awesome that is (ego strengthening) ...you've come off drugs and alcohol and are reducing your meds...**and you've had no psychotic episode**" (indirect suggestion for self-validation)

People have psychotic episodes for many reasons and in Alaster's case, it was obviously post-drug-induced psychosis. Unless he was taking recreational drugs again, he would be unlikely to have another episode.

Alaster: *"Going to the gym, and on your crazy, crackpot, plant-based diet, taking all the supplements and managing work okay."*

Tracie: *"So let's recap...you're not shit-faced...not screaming...or threatening to cut your wrists (when a client focuses on the negative, reframe the negatives as absolute to create a positive state, negative reframing)...**exercising...eating like an athlete...going to work...making money** (bombardment suggestions, stacking good habits)... having a holiday from sex (sexual abstinence was essential during substance withdrawal as an early setback could have undermined treatment)...you can...**hear (Ai+)...see (Vi+)...and feel (Ki+)... the foundations for a stable happy life**...that will facilitate better sexual function (equating sobriety with a better sex life)...maybe some women might think...**you're a nice guy** (ego repair)...and not that you just want to put your cock in their vagina...as nice as that may be."*

Alaster spoke street slang. To lead him, I matched and mirrored him, including language, which is called code switching. Whilst many therapists may think this is risky and damaging their professional image, I do not. I constantly monitor a client's reactions every second in therapy to anything I suggest, and all our communications.

I have spoken at length before about the damage to sexual function from psychiatric medications, party drugs and alcohol and have seen countless cases where this has happened. Turabian (2021) adds to that by postulating that such drugs initiate long-term biological damage that can turn a mental health emergency into a lifelong, chronic, physical and mental dysfunction.

In cases like Alaster, we must move slowly and constantly observe the patient because he also became addicted to those prescription medications. His own self-regulating physiological and mental functions began to decline because the body did not have the demands on it to create auto-homeostasis. I needed to use third-party reporting, in this case his brother, to gain clinical objectivity as Alaster himself may be delusional (see Appendix A, item 46).

Trance intentions

1. Ego strengthening.
2. Time shifting by putting his past trouble behind him.
3. Self-regulation.
4. Progression of his personality towards maturity.
5. Reaffirming sobriety.
6. Reassociation to his body and its natural functions.
7. Reassociating sex with fun.

Alright I want you to simply close your eyes…relax in that chair…and be safe at the sound of my voice once again (triggering existing safety anchor)…**I want you to congratulate yourself** (creating and strengthening self-efficacy)…the brillant changes you have made already in your life…your responsibility (creating auto-regulation)…no one else's…**your triumphs** (ego strengthening)…your life…your responsibility…

no one else's...**time to move on and go forward** (direct suggestion)...you began as a child...grew into a teenager with all the experimentation...**now you're a man**...your life...your responsibility...no one else's...**party drug and alcohol free is the best way forward for you** (post-hypnotic direct suggestion)... your life...your responsibility...no one else's...**everything begins in your body** (associating him into his body)...your life...your responsibility (re-enforcement suggestion)...no one else's...**as you see yourself looking after your body now** (Vi+, contingent expectation of a reward)...the best ways you can (indirect suggestion for treatment compliance)...it looks after you the best ways it can...growing up and being a man (indirect suggestion for responsible behaviour)...**a proud man...beautiful man...a sexual man...enjoying life...your sex life...your responsibility** (bombardment suggestions)... no one else's...**enjoying sex** (direct suggestion)...as you're clean and sober (conditional suggestion that sobriety equals better sex)...feeling nature's power coming back into your body...**and sex becomes fun again** (direct suggestion, memory recall to a time when sex was fun, resource mining)...you can enjoy sex...enjoy erections (hidden suggestion)...you may even enjoy relationships...**feel nature's power coming back into your body now**...it's your right...it's a force for living with nature's power (moving away from substance dependence)... **feel nature's strength coming back into your penis now... good erections when you want them** (direction suggestion, time dependent)...enjoying sex...enjoying life...**enjoying being in a good place** (global suggestion for physical and mental function)

In Alaster's case, coming off the anti-depressants and anti-psychotics was not an option. He had travelled the road to being a psychiatric patient and he guarded that diagnosis as a possession and part of his identity, at least for the time being. He had become addicted to his diagnosis and medications.

To push him to come off those medications would have been a mistake at that time as it could have created overwhelm for him and led to treatment failure. Whether he would have ever experienced a psychotic event again was simply academic. Sometimes we must guide a client to a place where they can be and manage, not where we think they could, should or ought to be.

The damage from those psychiatric drugs and recreational substances, however, had taken its toll on his brain, hormonal activation system, and his sense of self-efficacy and agency.

The ultimate treatment solution for Alaster was to remain clean and sober, reduce psychiatric medications, take the herb Yin yang huo (horny goat weed) (Shindel, 2010), 2 x 500mgs B3 per day (Liu, 2020), 10mgs lithium orate per day, use Cialis, and remain on a wholefood, plant-based way of eating to raise testosterone (Allen, 2000), with daily self-hypnosis. This helped him to be far more stable and restore erectile function.

CASE STUDY: NIALL

Niall was a 28-year-old gay man and had been mute and profoundly deaf (below 95dB) his whole life. It has been known historically as 'deaf-mute'. He could lip read, use sign language, and write on a pad. The term 'mute' can be considered derogatory by some who just use the term 'deaf'.

Today, some non-speaking people write on their phones to communicate with hearing people, and the phone turns text into voice. Although at times it can be quicker to write on a notepad.

A neighbour who had previously come to see me made the initial appointment. Niall came to see me because I have had deaf friends during my life and when I was younger I lived with a deaf foster brother. I am also known in the gay community.

Whilst I had almost forgotten my sign language, having not used it for a long time, Niall's lip-reading skills were excellent. Sign language can also be very fast, and hearing people can have problems keeping up with what is being said.

It is important to remember the deaf culture is a society within itself, and when we hearing people go into it, we are the ones who are disabled by our lack of understanding. We must educate ourselves on how to behave with deaf people (Paul, 2010).

All too often, hearing health practitioners behave in ableist ways when seeing deaf clients (such as becoming impatient with the client or looking at them as if they are not intelligent) without even realising we are behaving that way (Bogart, 2019).

Tracie: "How can we help you?"

Niall (writing): "I'm gay but I find it difficult hooking up with hearing men in the gay community."

Tracie: "Why do you find it difficult?" (It is important not to use colloquial abbreviation when speaking to deaf people and to make sure you are facing them directly)

Niall (writing): "I see they get shocked at me not being able to speak to them. Make all sorts of faces. It puts me off during sex. I think they are being disrespectful."

Tracie: "Does it happen when you sleep with gay, deaf men?"

Niall (signing): "Gay deaf community too small. Run out of men." (He signed and we both laughed).

Tracie: "When you slept with gay, deaf men did it happen?"

Niall (signing): "No, we both speak ASL (Australian Sign Language)".

Tracie: "I am going to tell you, as a hearing and speaking person, that deaf people can sometimes make hearing people feel inadequate and nervous. All the expressions are bigger and at times hard to understand."

Niall (signing): "Yes, hearing people can be really slow." (We both laughed)

Tracie: "My second language is French, but I have not been in France for many years, so I would be very slow, and often do not understand, even though English and French share 30% of their words. We may share expressions with deaf languages, but it's called ASL for a reason – because it's a different language."

Niall (signing): "But the faces they make."

Mime is part of deaf language. It is pretty universal between different deaf languages and based on face and body language. During hypnosis a hypnotist must use the mime language because you need to stay working visually and kinaesthetically.

Deaf people can read your lips, face and body language, all at the same time. When going into an artificial somnambulistic trance, their eye movements can remain active. Confusion occurs when communicating with hearing people because we have less control of our facial expressions, which are often incidental rather than purposeful and it may at times be a form of parapraxis. Do not use indirect suggestions, or modal operators of possibility or probability, as they get lost in translation. Always use modal operators of necessity.

Niall associated hearing men with being disrespectful during sex. His sexual clusters were linked to him being not understood visually during sex so he could maximise his enjoyment.

Trance intentions

1. Moving him to second position.
2. Miming trance instructions as well as mouthing them.
3. Creating empathy for sex partners.
4. Moving him back to first position, being in control of the sex situation.
5. Restoring sex as fun.

Look at me…imagine you are a hearing person (moving him to second position)…you cannot understand what a deaf person is saying (shaking my head looking confused and waving my hands about)…you are afraid…you are unsure…confused… **you are frustrated** (tonal marking becomes visual marking)… you make faces…sometimes silly faces…you are embarrassed and confused (second position Ki- experience)...you lose control…and now imagine you are naked at the same time (fractionation of second person's perceived distress)...**you Niall can be kind to that person** (reassociation to first position, direct suggestion)… patience…take your time…help them…**be the leader and show them what to do** (direct suggestion)…be the guide to gay deaf sex (self-empowerment)…imagine how well that will go…you be the teacher…you lead…you take control… **you feel good in control** (Ki+)…you look good in control (Vi+)…you enjoy sex (direct suggestion, global suggestion)… you put the man at ease…it is a book…it is a film (miming the game of charades)…**Niall's guide to gay deaf sex for hearing men** (taking him out of the victim status and putting him into the guide identity)…and sex is fun…**sex is lots of fun for you both**

Since I could not send Niall home with an auditory hypnotic recording to listen to daily, we made a video and I put him on a learning self-hypnosis program, using my book *Self-Hypnosis for Life* (O'Keefe, 2000).

There is a phrase in deaf and disability culture, 'Does he take sugar?' It carries the assumption that the person cannot think for themselves or speak for themselves (see Appendix A, item 47). It is insulting and diminutive. A better attitude to take is engaging with the person and showing them how to do tasks for themselves.

Added to that was the list of self-affirmations Niall made to use in self-hypnosis and put up in large writing on his bedroom wall.

- I am a confident, gay, deaf man
- I am a good lover
- I am a kind lover
- I enjoy sex and have fun
- I teach my partners how to have sex with a gay, deaf man
- I like having sex with hearing men, helping them have a good time
- I feel good when I have sex with hearing men

Notice how all these are in the present tense so they are intra-hypnotic auto-suggestions, not post-hypnotic suggestions. We are all in a life trance and Niall needed to be self-creating having a good sex life. People come into the office living one trance and need to leave living another life trance (Wolinsky & Ryan, 2007).

I saw Niall for a second session a month later.

Niall (signing): *"I am having so much sex now and it is your fault." (We laughed and he was happy with the outcome. What he had really done is reframe his role in that sexual equation)*

CASE STUDY: CONNIE

Connie was 51, married for 30 years, lived in suburbia, and had two adult offspring who had left home. She did not work anymore, and her husband was a reasonably successful computer engineer.

Connie: *"Five years ago I had a double mastectomy, and they also took out several lymph nodes. Just for insurance against further cancer, I had a full hysterectomy and my ovaries removed. Now my arms swell a lot and I look like the marshmallow man."*

Tracie: *"And did you have breast implants?"*

Connie: *"No, because they took so many nodes, my surgeon advised me not to, in case they blocked the flow of the lymph. And I'm still on tamoxifen."*

In 2020, 2.3 million people were diagnosed with breast cancer and there were 685,000 deaths (World Health Organization,

2024). There were 7.8 million people alive who had been diagnosed within the preceding five years, and 0.5-1% of men get breast cancer.

Heyne (2021) reported an Epidemiological Multicenter Study in Germany, finding that 31% of female cancer patients reported sexual problems, and in the male group 40.5%. Both the cancer and all forms of treatment, plus the trauma of diagnosis, can cause sexual problems.

This causes physiological dysfunction, and damages self-image and sexual confidence. Not only is health suddenly taken away, but a person's sense of their own sexual attractiveness and value can be diminished.

Tracie: *"And what's your status now?"*

Connie: *"I have a scan every six months and at the moment I'm in remission. I always say, 'At the moment'."*

Tracie: *"What can we do for you do today?"*

Connie: *"I feel ugly. I've got no breasts. I've got scars, fat arms, my vagina's dry, my skin's dry, I can have hot sweats at any time, particularly during sex, I'm losing my hair, and I've put on a lot of weight. Barry, my husband, says I'm just as beautiful as I always was. Having sex is much more difficult for me now. I feel very awkward, clumsy, and unattractive."*

Tracie: *"You've sure got a lot going on inside your head. And what do you need from therapy?"*

Connie: *"Barry, he's the best. I couldn't have wished for a better husband, but all this is making him sad. He's not saying anything, but I know. What do I do?"*

Tracie: *"What do you want to do?"*

Connie: *"I want to make it all go away and be like it was."*

Connie now associated her cancer diagnosis with her being less than she was, and completely sexually undesirable. Her sexual clusters were that, whilst she said her husband was the best, living, even in remission, had caused her to dissociate from her relationship with herself, her body, and her husband.

Trance intentions

1. Fast hand drop induction.
2. Awareness of the good things in her life.
3. Focusing on being present.
4. Listening to her husband's compliments.
5. Affect bridge to previous good feelings around her self-worth and modelling that today.
6. Reassociation to her body.
7. Adaption and planning around sexual needs.
8. Weight loss to aid mobility.
9. Being a sex goddess.

Sit back in the chair and I'm going to take your hand and your unconscious can hold it in mid air (catalepsy, instant artificial somnambulism)...when I push it down you can go down deep deep into a hypnotic trance with your eyes closed (contingent suggestion)...**go deep deep into a trance now** (I pushed the hand down to her lap, fast induction, direct suggestion)... **sleep and go deep down now all the way inside your mind** (simultaneous suggestions to the conscious and unconscious mind)...time changes and no one can stop time...life changes and no one can stop life...**be aware how very precious life**

is each day (validating her still being alive)...**each hour**...
each minute...**each second**...be aware how beautiful life can
be when you focus on the beauty (reframing)...**inside your
mind enlarge the beautiful things in your life each day**
(direct suggestion, submodality manipulation, fractionation,
positive hallucination)...**focus on your beautiful life**...inside
your mind shrink the negatives (direct suggestion, reverse
fractionation, negative hallucination)...don't give them oxygen
keep it for yourself...**change your focus quick to what you have
now** (intra-hypnotic direct suggestion, the speed overcomes
procrastination)...you're still alive...you're cancer free...you
have two adult children...and one grandchild (stacking life
benefits)...**so much good to focus on**...**focus on your beauty
when you have sex** (direct suggestion)...opening your eyes and
looking to me (artificial somnambulism)

> Tracie: "*You know when I lost most of my breasts after
> an accident in my 50s, I really thought I would
> miss them. I was a 42DD, and they were always
> going somewhere before me. Now I can put my
> bras on backwards and not notice. But it gave me
> a certain physical freedom to work out more and
> focus more on self-care (encouraging modelling)...
> so what benefits have you got from the change
> (analytical challenge)...can you understand that?*"
> (interrogative suggestion)

> Connie: "*Okay, yes.*"

> Tracie: "*I'm not the person I was when I had those larger
> breasts...I thought it was too dangerous for me to
> have implants...I'm someone else now...change
> is inevitable (suggestion for adaption) ...and you*

can't stop change...***it's okay to be someone else
when life changes*** (*permission to change*)...*do
you accept that tell me*" (*interrogative suggestion,
nodding my head*)

Connie: "*Okay.*"

Tracie: "*I'm still beautiful. I'm still sexy...**and you are too.**"
(*It is an associated binding statement as she cannot
disagree. Therefore, she must apply the same logic
to herself*)

Close your eyes...see inside your mind your husband Barry
saying you are beautiful (Vi+, Ai+)...hear inside your mind his
words (Ai+)...**own that beauty it's a gift**...part of the precious
gift of living (validation by association)...feel what it feels like
when he says that to you at 30 years of age (regression, affect
bridge, Ki+)...you know the feeling of being beautiful already...
**remember that feeling of being beautiful in your body all the
time** (Ki+ & Ke+, post-hypnotic suggestion, reassociation to
her body)...you can remember that feeling at any time (post-
hypnotic suggestion, global suggestion)...you can remember
that feeling in your body here today (bombardment suggestions,
intra-hypnotic suggestion, present-day orientation)...**you can
remember that feeling of being beautiful when you have sex
with Barry** (post-hypnotic suggestion, future pacing)...and
that's okay....**it's really okay and as beautiful as it was before**
(non-specific reference to a past sense of being beautiful,
modelling her former self)...open your eyes and looking at me
(remaining in artificial somnambulism)

Tracie: "*When I was young I could do all sorts of things...
dancing six nights a week with two shows on*

*Saturdays, skateboarding, acrobatics, ice skating and have time for sex…(information overwhelm, confusion, artificial somnambulistic trance deepening)…I'm not young anymore so I must be mindful of my activities…**and the time and energy we give to them** (indirect suggestion for mindfulness around sex)…close your eyes and go deeper inside…**as things change you can change**… you can be more mindful during sex…being mindfully beautiful in the moment…**sex mindfully beautiful** (word salad causing referential index search, deepening trance, forcing reassessment of sexual interactions)…as sex has changed for you… **you can be mindful around sex** (re-enforcement suggestion)…planning is good…having a plan A…B…C…D…etc…you can be adaptable… **change positions**…have lymphatic drainage before sex…lose weight (silent suggestion)…**always talking to Barry during sex**…listen to him telling you…**you're beautiful** (direct suggestion)…the man who loves you (silent suggestion)*

Lymph vessels have no muscles to pump fluid along, unlike veins and arteries. When nodes are removed, the system's fluid backs up and can cause lymphedema. This can cause tissue perfusion and limbs to swell (Gillespie, 2018).

Connie's homework included regular low-intensity daily exercise to assist lymphatic drainage because movement moves the lymph along the system (Baumann, 2018). Added to that was regular lymphatic drainage massage, using a mechanical lymphatic drainage suit at home, Indonesian cinnamon (Padang cassia) for glucose metabolism (Zelicha et al., 2024), water foods, and foods high in potassium for diuretic action, horsetail tea (diuretic), and 2 litres of water a day to avoid dehydration, which can include juices. Join a gym for stretching, aerobic and resistance exercise, building arm and solar plexus muscle strength.

Also adopting a wholefood, plant-based diet, no grains or processed food, lots of celery, melon, cucumber or green juices. Improving kidney function is one of the main treatments in lymphedema.

Talking to her husband about sex, the best pillows, and positions to use that are comfortable for both of them.

Using a vaginal lubricant.

Keeping a wet flannel on the end of the bed in case she had hot sweats during sex.

Going away for a romantic four-day weekend.

It was six weeks before I saw Connie again. She had lost 10 kilos and had a weekend away at the beach with her husband.

Connie: *"We connected. It was like it used to be when we were courting, and sex was good. I realise now that I've been so obsessed with the cancer, and what it did to me, that I wasn't paying attention to Barry and what we have together."*

Tracie: *"That sounds really exciting." (suggesting forward motivation)*

Connie: *"One of my friends died. We used to have chemo together. I went to her funeral, and I could hear her saying to me, 'Don't waste the time you've got Connie'."*

Tracie: *"Listen to that voice...It's the voice of wisdom...* **enjoy the time you have like we all need to** *(converting the voice to a positive affirmation)... love and sex are food...eat at the banquet for life...* **let love in...be a goddess** *(appealing to the higher self and bypassing the conscious self-critic)...* **be Aphrodite."** *(goddess of sex and love)*

I saw Connie four more times over six months. At the end of that time, she got a diagnosis of metastatic cancer, but she decided not to have chemo and radiation again, but to pursue a naturopathic route of treatment.

Connie: *"I'm going to fight this with everything I have. I've got too much to lose."*

Connie had readjusted her perceptions of herself and her value within her relationship and embraced her own personal power (see Appendix, item 48).

CASE STUDY: LUCY

Lucy was born with spina bifida myelomeningocele, which is a neural tube defect of the spine formation prebirth. The severe neural damage meant she had never walked, and used a wheelchair.

Lucy: *"I'm 18 and getting married. My friends think I'm nuts and am too young. I always wondered if someone would want to marry me, but he does."*

Tracie: *"Tell me about him."*

Lucy: *"His name is Danny. He's 40, has a print shop, and has been married before, divorced, has three sons who live with his ex-wife, and his eldest son is two years older than me. I met him when he did some printing for a charity when I was raising funds for spina bifida. He didn't charge us for the printing. I always tell people that. I've been dating him for a year."*

Lucy was a chatterbox and natural communicator, who smiled a lot, keeping good eye contact.

Tracie: *"So, how can we help you today?"*

Lucy: *"There is one thing that worries me. There are times when I can have urinary incontinence. I pee myself. It comes with the condition for some of us. Danny and I have never had sex so I'm afraid of what might happen when we do."*

Streur (2022) tells us that people affected by spina bifida can experience incontinence during sex which can be highly distressing, along with reduced sexual sensitivity. It can also produce reduced sex drive and pain during intercourse for women.

Tracie: *"Do you masturbate, and does it happen then? Do you have much pain? You don't mind me asking these questions, do you?"* (interrogative overload, trance induction)

Lucy: *"I do masturbate sometimes and sometimes it does leak. I'm sort of used to the pain. It's very unpredictable."*

Lucy associated sex with pleasure but also possible embarrassment due to incontinence. Her sexual clusters were like most teenagers, wondering if she would be good enough once her real self was exposed.

Trance intentions

1. Linking safety to her wheelchair that goes with her everywhere.
2. Focusing on her likeability.
3. Focusing on what Danny is doing.
4. Rising balloon induction.
5. Recognising her body's competence.
6. Creating oxytocin when thinking of Danny.
7. Self-efficacy for working out the logistics of sex.
8. Chunking down to manage one situation at a time.
9. Linking sex with fun, not anxiety.
10. Being in a wheelchair, her difficulty is resisting gravity, so I used metaphors for defying gravity to elevate the sexual experience inside her mind.

As you sit in your chair in my office you can make yourself comfortable (contingent suggestion)...what I notice about you is that you like people and put people at their ease (resource mining)...**think about all the reasons Danny likes and loves you** (intra-hypnotic suggestion, referential search, trance deepening)...with every breath you breathe in a little air moves underneath your right hand...**each time you breathe in your right hand just lifts very slightly into the air** (a physical induction was appropriate as it gave her confidence in her body and trance)...like a balloon full of helium just watching it slowly lifting your hand into the air (validation of trance by observation)…**that's right**…you're right…you can know the right thing to do and the right thing to think…be aware how that balloon is helping your hand defy gravity…**just like the song I think I think I'll try defying gravity**…lifting higher and higher up to the eye level (lapse of 2 minutes)…see how clever your body is and close your eyes…when I banana that hand can drop down to your lap and you can go deeper into a deep deep trance…**banana** (word salad interference in conscious analytical thinking as I push the hand down)…**you feel good when you talk about Danny** (direct suggestion)…you seem to think of him as a kind and caring man…and you say he is…**isn't that a very good thing** (interrogative generalised suggestion to re-enforce her view of him)…he's only ever known you in a wheelchair…he's obviously aware of any complications of your condition…**and you tell me he wants to marry you and love you**…you seem very pleased about that (silent suggestion)… you seem very happy…people work things out in marriage one thing at a time…**sex is an adventure that you can both enjoy** (eliciting couples co-operation)…working out the mechanics and logistics of sex between you…positions…timing… comfort…adaptability…communication…preferences...who likes what…fun…**focus on the fun** (producing serotonin, oxytocin, endorphin)…defying gravity…telling him what's good for you (silent communication)…**sex equals fun adventure and connection** (contingent suggestion)

Her complaint was, "There is one thing that worries me." So, the worry about incontinence was the problem. As therapists we must not be ableist. She had been in the wheelchair with her condition her whole life, knowing far more about how to handle her condition than I possibly could. My job was simply to help her get over the worry.

Barrett's (2023) study found people with spinal cord injury (SCI) can experience internalised societal views and stigmatisation, diminished sexual confidence, navigating communication problems, the need to manage relationship dynamics, and the lack of support.

The worst of these is internalising societal views of disability. Lucy was a problem solver and needed support to boost her confidence to work out how sex was going to work between her and Danny (see Appendix A, item 49).

They agreed not to have children and seemed to get on very well with Danny's sons. After the marriage I encouraged them to hire a few bondage rooms so they could try sex swings, slings, stools and chairs to decide what they might like to try at home.

In the last session, three months after the marriage, I saw them both. Lucy said, "We've been defying gravity and trying that tantric stuff you recommended. Who knew I'd be into that?" (She laughed)

Danny was quite a quiet man and smiled every time he looked at her.

15 Good Sex

Sex is different for everyone as we all have different physiology, physical experiences and sensitivities, physical capabilities and restrictions, mental capabilities and experiential, sociological or religious governors, values, beliefs, perceptions, understandings, psychological gestalts, memories, fears and opportunities.

The lenses through which we all experience sex are multifocal and dependent on time, place, and circumstances. So, when working with people, it is essential to always consider the whole individual, and work towards what is good and rewarding for them.

Just as we can fall in and out of love, we can also fall in and out of love with sex, or sex with specific individuals. As we age, our life circumstances change, so sex must always change and can never remain the same.

No one size ever fits all, just as no one hypnotic, psychotherapeutic, or sex therapy technique can be used with all clients. As sex therapists we must devise a treatment specifically for every individual to maximise therapeutic outcomes.

CASE STUDY: PATTY

Patty: *"I want good sex, so can you hypnotise me to have good sex?"*

Tracie: *"What is or would be good sex for you, Patty?"*

Patty: "My husband's an alright bloke but sex is boring. He's good-looking and has a great body. Works out at the gym. He's always busy with his business, so sex is rushed."

Tracie: "Has it always been like that?"

Patty: "I married him because he got me pregnant. Sex was sort of okay at the beginning, but not earth-shattering. Since we had three kids it's just got boring."

Tracie: "Have you discussed this with him?"

Patty: "I really don't want to hurt his feelings cause he's a good bloke, and apart from the sex, the marriage is good."

Tracie: "Have you ever had earth-shattering great...really great sex...can you tell me about it...what did you do...how it felt...what was it like?" (interrogative overload, artificial somnambulistic recall, resource scanning in the kinaesthetic modality, affect bridge)

Patty: "Oh yeah, the sex with my previous boyfriend for two years was great. We did it just about everywhere, anytime. It felt great. I'd come again and again and again, but I dumped him because he kept cheating on me."

Tracie: "Are you saying the unexpected is thrilling for you and sexually exciting? Does that turn you on?"

Toledano et al. (2006), in putting forward a sexual arousal and desire inventory for testing women, saw that they had significantly higher scores with pre-arousal sexual fantasies. This was suggesting pre-arousal and arousal fantasies were highly important to women's sexual satisfaction.

Patty: *"Sometimes yes. After all, variety is nice, no same old, same old. And some spice would be nice."*

Tracie: *"Let's take stock. You've been married to Ricky for 10 years, and as far as you know he doesn't cheat. You have three children, a house with a mortgage, he brings in the money, plays with the kids on Sundays, and you think your sex life is unexciting?"*

Patty: *"That's about it. I read* Fifty Shades of Grey *(James, 2015) and it seems like everyone else is having hot sex, but me."*

Tracie: *"When couples come together there is what is called the honeymoon period for about two to three years, when everything is new and shiny. Providing financially for children and families is a lot of hard work and one of the partners usually experiences the most stress from doing that. I'm wondering if you could take on the role of the sex guide and organiser in the relationship."*

Patty: *"That sounds like work."*

Tracie: *"Well, in some ways it is...and in some ways it isn't (matching to lead)...when you get what you want that can be worth it (incentivising)...**imagine yourself trying many of those things in that book in private** (using her existing references)...see yourself organising the time for sex for you both."* (Vi+) empowering her)

Patty was a sexually bored housewife in a marriage to a nice man. She associated great sex with random, chaotic coupling. Her sexual clusters were around just making do and not disturbing the husband who she saw as a stable provider.

Trance intentions

1. Acknowledging her existing sexual references.
2. Eliciting oxytocin when thinking about Ricky.
3. Initiating sexual communication between the couple.
4. Time management.
5. Creating self-efficacy in that she can create the sex life she wants.
6. Initiating couple's communication.
7. Tasking her with enlivening and protecting their sex life.
8. Initiating fantasy sex, pre-arousal, and play acting.
9. Suggestion to act out a variety of fantasies.

Close your eyes and go inside comfortably…spend time deep inside your mind…**you already know about the sex you enjoy don't you** (interrogative trance deepener, regression, acknowledgement of past resources)…you're already happy with so many aspects of Ricky's behaviour as a husband (reducing the problem)…you say he ticks many boxes (fractionation of satisfaction)…**you can add spice to the dish of sex and marriage** (building on existing sex)…start talking about sex between you…having good discussions (framing the sex discussions and negotiation as positive)…**protecting private fun time for sex between you** (direct suggestion, reframing sex as fun)…I wonder what games you both will play (presupposition of variety and mutual participation, pre-arousal imagery)…**whetting his**

appetite and yours (double meaning for sexual appetite and vaginal lubrication, initiating the SRC)...turning fantasy into reality...different role playing...positions...games...bringing you both together (suggesting oxytocin production)...you will organise a more full sex life (direct, post-hypnotic suggestion)... **deepening your relationship and bonding around sex** (time scanning and future seeding auto-suggestion)...how many things from the book will you try (interrogative suggestion)... asking him what he would like to try...**creating good exciting sex** (direct suggestion for proactive sexual enjoyment)...a handsome man and beautiful woman making love (ego strengthening)...playing out your fantasies...playing out his fantasies...**creating adventurous hot sex in your marriage regularly** (post-hypnotic suggestion)

Patty had no complaints about the rest of her marriage, except Ricky working so much, and not paying enough attention to lovemaking. Her husband did not know she was unhappy about the lack of spontaneity and passionate sex. She had never addressed these issues with Ricky, but instead created the fear of missing out (FOMO), inside her mind, about the great sex other people were having.

San Martin et al., in a 2012 European survey, found that males' sexual performance was closely linked to their sense of sexual confidence. It was important to encourage Patty to elevate her husband's sexual ego by her organising sex, as opposed to finding fault with his performance. The carrot is always more powerful to get the donkey up the hill, than the stick.

Her actions began to awaken his appetite for variety and adventure in their sex life. By allotting and protecting the time for sex, she was no longer competing with his business for his attention.

The second time I saw her was two months later.

Tracie: "What's changed?"

Patty: "You've got to be effing kidding me. Pardon the language. Who knew inside my nice husband was a beast."

Tracie: "Got some spice and sugar then?"

Patty: "Oh yeah. He told me he didn't know I'd like the kink stuff. On top of the washing machine on the spin cycle, when the kids are at nursery, and in the back seat of the car before we got to the restaurant. We even went to a BDSM sex party. If I wasn't on the pill, I'd be pregnant again."

Tracie: "So what changed?"

Patty: "I listened to the recording every day that you gave me. It occurred to me I had to act and reinvent our sex life. We've never talked so much in bed and everywhere else."

Tracie: "That's a good thing...most people don't talk about sex...so they have no idea what the other person is thinking....good fun sex times go to waste for a lack of communication...**now you are communicating speaking the sex language** (counteracting the FOMO by putting her in the driver's seat)...what you are doing is really smart (ego strengthening)... you're both creating the hot sex between you that you wanted (validation of change)...**you do that between you**" (suggestion for bonding, oxytocin, association with the husband helps initiate the SRC)

Like any couple after they have had children, the pressures of child rearing can obliterate or subdue their sex life. Sex can become mundane, and couples come to it tired, just trying to fit it into their schedule. The quantity and quality of sex in a relationship or lack of it can have a direct correlation with life satisfaction scores (Flynn, 2016).

Patty's story told us she felt disempowered and undesired. The sex drive was still present for both partners. Putting her in charge of the sex schedule allowed her to protect their lovemaking time, and be more flirtatious and inventive.

I did not need to teach her more about sex as she already came with her own concept of her ideal sex life. Patty and Ricky were already having sex and she simply wanted it to be more exciting and rewarding.

Dewitte et al. (2020) point out that mismatched libidos are a major problem, which is generally under-researched. Some couples may have the intellect, time and resources to talk out the problem toward a solution, but many do not.

People, particularly with young families, are highly stressed due to the demands of modern-day life, so they need direction and actions to bridge the gap, rather than existential insights (see Appendix A, item 50).

Mersy & Vincell (2023) discuss many factors around the causes of mismatched libidos. From a hypnotic perspective, however, we as hypnotists need to provide shortcuts, motivating clients through suggestion, to expedite change in a relationship's sexual dynamics.

CASE STUDY: CLIVE

This was a single 24-year-old man in motor car sales from a Pentecostal church background. Clive had previously had two short-term girlfriends, but never gone as far as sex with them. His success in his work, he acknowledged, was partly due to his church contacts.

Clive: *"It's like a brotherhood. You scratch my back and I'll scratch yours. There are successful women, but most in the church are wives and mothers. If I get married, I don't know how to have good sex."*

Tracie: *"And what do you want from a relationship?"* (His major dialogue had been centered around relationships)

Clive: *"I've been so busy getting myself established with a career and house that I purposefully stayed away from sex and serious relationships. My dad told me to 'get your life sorted first'. There're some rumours in the church that I might be gay, but I'm not. I like women and have fantasies about having sex with them, but I have no experience."*

Tracie: *"What do we need to help you with today?"*

Clive: *"I know so much about cars. Where to buy them. How to sell them. What way to make the best profit. I got my own car lot this year so I'm making big money, but I've never had sex."*

Religious beliefs about sexual practices, including those of the Pentecostal church, are widely diverse, independent, and ethnographic. They are, however, based on the central Christian doctrine that espouses sex before marriage is a sin. Wareham (2022) clearly states the religious exemption to sex education in schools maintains misogyny, homophobia, and can lead to a sexually uneducated youth.

Tracie: "You seem to be doing a lot of things right for you... you've bought a house...own your own business... and are part of the community (establishing a sense of competence)...you seem like a young man who knows what he is doing (finding his hero's journey, not a problem)...there's a right time to start having sex...**the time that is right for you will be the time that is right for you** (future pacing success)...are there guidelines in your church that direct you?"

Clive: "Yes we aren't supposed to have sex before marriage."

Tracie: "Do you follow all the church's guidelines?"

Clive: "Pretty much. It's all I've ever known. All my family are in the church, and we refer to the church as family."

Tracie: "Will you marry within the church?"

Clive: "I think I will."

Tracie: "Do you masturbate?"

Clive: "About three times a week."

Tracie: "Well, everything seems to be in working order (normalising his sex journey)...then today is probably about you...**moving on to form some kind of relationship** (direct suggestion)...within the church that might lead to marriage (feeding his own plan back to him)...**do you think that's**

the next step for you (interrogative suggestion)…
and only then would you put sex with a woman
on the menu?" (using his value system, conditional
suggestion)

I did not see Clive for a year when he came back into clinic,
engaged to a young woman in the church and was due to be
married within four months.

Tracie: "Have you come for the sex talk now?"

Clive: "Yes, I need to know what I'm doing on the night,
and I don't want to discuss it with anyone in the
church."

Tracie: "Well, there is no embarrassment here…I talk
about sex with people like you several times a
week…it's just nature…that's how we got here
(humour, smiling, breaking the ice)…**firstly you
can be comfortable talking about sex** (direct
suggestion – suggestion softened with a modal
operator of possibility to avoid resistance)…it's
like selling (bridging competency in one skill to a
new skill)…the more you do it the more familiar
you are with the process…**it will even become
fun very quickly** (post-hypnotic, direct suggestion,
future pacing, converting anxiety to fun)…
you sell each car differently because every car is
different…you study the car to begin with to
make your pitch…**you will now be studying
sex**…is that okay?" (seeking therapeutic
alliance)

Clive: "I'm in the hot seat doctor."

He associated sex with being dichotomous – no sex before marriage and sex and relationships being bound up with marriage. His sexual clusters were that his values, beliefs and actions were in line with his religion.

Trance intentions

1. Associating sex with healthy excitement.
2. Associating sex with the deepening of their relationship.
3. Eliciting the belief that sex needs to be good for both of them.
4. Widening the possibilities of sex beyond his church values.
5. Initiating learning about sexual skills.
6. Associating sex with spiritual fulfilment.

Close your eyes and imagine…God gave you an imagination (using his beliefs to initiate trance induction)…you're moving towards your wedding day…**you're really excited about sex** (fractionating existing excitement)…such a wonderful time in your life…you've found a good beautiful woman (using his value system, presupposition he finds her sexually attractive)… **you're getting married then making sweet love** (post-hypnotic suggestion, contingent suggestion that one leads to the other)…it's good to discover sex together (inducing oxytocin at the thought of his future wife)…it's good to enjoy sex together…**you are both creating a good sex life together** (sexual co-operation)…learning…practising…playing…the joy of sex (reducing anxiety, increasing serotonin)…**can you wonder what wonderful adventures you will both discover together** (interrogative suggestion for it to be an adventure)… how many ways can you please your wife with sexual practices (interrogative suggestion to increase his sexual repertoire, particularly foreplay)...**can you wonder what will you really enjoy** (bombarding three interrogative suggestions causes transderivational search and trance deepening, presupposition he will enjoy sex)...**you will be very excited on your wedding night** (post-hypnotic suggestion to initiate stage 1 of the SRC)... you will also be very knowledgeable about sex as you have studied what to do...**confidently you can take your time to make love slowly** (post-hypnotic suggestion to initiate stage 2 of the SRC)...the joys of marriage...the joys of sex...**the joys of making babies** (initiating stage 3 of the SRC)...it's all part of building a life together and for your own family...it's nature... it's fun...it's divine...**blessed are the joys of sex as you lie together afterwards** (initiating stage 4 of the SRC)...

I sent Clive on a quest of learning about sex. This included reading books such as *The Original Kama Sutra Completely Illustrated* (Vatsyayana et al., 2012), *What Women Really Want in Bed: The Surprising Secrets Women Wish Men Knew About Sex* (Gentry, 2010), and listening to the audio book *The Joy of Sex* (Comfort, 2017).

In such cases it is important not to overload people with study but to sufficiently equip them with skills, of course depending on their abilities. I also shared with him my experiences of what women like in bed as a woman and someone who is married to a woman. Even though Clive was Pentecostal, he was also of a generation that were used to gay marriage. Ultimately, he took away from all this what was right for him.

He used his recording once a day over the next months. I saw him once more three months after he was married. Not only had the wedding night been a success, but he and his new wife were also enjoying sex as a couple.

I had advised no alcohol around sex, but it turned out he did not drink at all, so that would not be a problem for him. Also, to take very good care of their social life so that as a couple they had regular times when they had fun together.

As instructed, Clive had shared the educational material with his wife and had discussions about their sex life regularly. Demystification of sex and sharing your sexual experience with intimate partners allows people to adjust their sex life to what suits them (see Appendix A, item 51).

Whilst the internet is full of information about sex, much of it is poor quality and frequently incorrect. Some people from religious cults and sects also often do not have access to the internet to find any information.

I saw Clive two years later to help him with making a decision about buying another car lot. The couple had a baby, and she was pregnant with their second child. He reported the marriage and sex were both going well.

CASE STUDY: DAVID

David was a 33-year-old healthy man who worked in a furniture store warehouse. He was married, with two children aged five and three. His wife worked part time in the same furniture store.

They had been teenage sweethearts, started dating at 15, and had gone to school together. Their families of origin were friends, and it had been expected they would end up together, so they got married in a big church wedding at 21. Before they had children, they saved for the deposit for a house in the suburbs near both their parents.

They were, from a sociological perspective, 'Mr and Mrs Average'.

David: "I love June but when we have sex I think about other women. She doesn't know that, and if she did, I'm sure it would really hurt her. It's the only way I can come."

Tracie: "Has it always been like that?"

David: "Basically yes, except for the first few times when I was really nervous, and I couldn't think about anything."

Tracie: "And when was the first time?"

David: "When we were 18."

Tracie: "Have you had sex with other people?"

David: "Oh no, and I don't think June has either."

Tracie: "The first thing I notice is you seem to be suffering from the 'We' disease. You respond in the plural as if you are both joined at the hip. You've been together since you were very young so have no other dating experience."

David: "Well, that's because we're just comfortable with each other. Share the same backgrounds. We came from similar families."

Tracie: "Yes, it's all a bit expected...**you're too comfortable together** (dislodging his status quo)...it can happen in couples who have been together for a long time or who started dating very early in life."

David: "I don't understand." (confusion, transderivational search, going into artificial somnambulistic trance, he is open to suggestion)

Tracie: "Well, the first stage of sex is about excitement and
           we call it arousal...the waking up of libido and
           lust...**you get excited about having sex with each
           other** (post-hypnotic suggestion)...since it's different
           every time you don't know what you're getting....
           so like any mystery present...**you get all excited
           about what you are going to or might get**" (post-
           hypnotic suggestion)

David: "Oh I get excited alright. It's the next bit of staying
           excited about having sex with my wife that I have
           problems with. I have to start thinking about
           someone else to come."

Tracie: "We call this the plateau stage when...you are
           actually having intercourse with your wife (indirect
           suggestion)...so you are telling me you lose focus at
           this stage (identifying the problem)...**we can help
           you have more fun and focus with that**" (moving
           to solution-focused thinking, using fun to dissolve
           his anxiety)

David's problem was in coming towards climax and ejaculation,
he dissociated from his body and relied on fantasies to move
him towards resolution. He ceased to be erotically present
during ejaculation.

His association surrounding climax had not fully transferred
to focusing on June. The sexual clusters were split between June
and the fantasies he had used as a teenager. He was a vacant
lover.

This happens in two types of situations. Firstly, when there
is a history of trauma, particularly PTSD (Bird, 2021), which
did not seem to be the case for David.

Secondly, when sex is too mundane, and a person seeks what they think is a more exciting opportunity elsewhere inside their fantasies. Surveys show that 50-60% of people acknowledge fantasising about other people during sex (Grace, 2023; Hariton & Singer, 1974). However, it is also a sign of erotic disengagement during sex if it is always necessary to orgasm.

Trance intentions

1. Bringing him into the present when having sex.
2. To provide him with options other than dissociation during sex and fantasising about other women.
3. Introducing excitement via variation of their sexual experiences.
4. Reframing his erotic focus to stay on his wife during the SRC.
5. Linking their arousal and plateau stages to feed off each other.
6. Metaphor for paying more attention to his wife's sexuality.
7. Position his wife as the stimulus to climax.

Sex is different for everyone...every time you have sex it's different (truisms, causing him to search for referential index, trance deepening)...the magic of sex can be when...**you are fully present during sex** (post-hypnotic, direct suggestion, time seeding)...because sex is always different excitement can be a key element...it's exciting when you don't exactly know what you will be getting (simile suggestion, converting anxiety into pleasurable anticipation)...**having some mystery and variety lights the fire of desire** (initiating fantasies)...think about it...if you don't know what you're getting for Christmas it's more exciting because there's anticipation and surprise...**it's individuals coming together for a good time when having sex** (generalisation, cancelling co-dependency) perhaps you can imagine how...perhaps you can focus on...**you can sense sex as very exciting with your wife** (direct suggestion for erotic attachment and engaging the senses)...the many ways you could do that...**looking at her beauty during sex** (Ve+)...seeing her during sex...**listening for her breathing getting more rapid as she gets more excited** (Ae+)...responding to her physical excitement...**responding to the sex in her in the moment** (Ke+, post-hypnotic suggestion for him kinaesthetically staying present in his body)...matching her sex with your sex (suggestion for erotic feedback loop)...matching her passion with your passion (fractionating of erotic stimulus)...**matching her desire with your desire** (bombardment suggestions)... close your eyes now...I want you to imagine you are a miner... you've worked one particular mine for a very long time...**you're searching for the most precious gems in the world**...you know what precious looks like (he already has fantasies that bring him to ejaculation) you've found some pockets of gems but you walk past a particular seam every day and have never really mined it...**you can give it all your attention now** (indirect suggestion for paying attention to his wife)...as you focus on what you're doing you find the most exciting discovery of all (contingent suggestion, elevating her erotic status above other women in his mind)...the more you stay present with June the more exciting it becomes...all your attention on June...**she's so beautiful and exciting to you** (fractionation, time seeding, direct suggestion)..and as you are having a really good time... staying present with June...eventually there comes a good time to come (using his language)...**you find her so exciting that you orgasm thinking of June**

In David's case he had no other sexual experiences apart from with June. The relationship was too domestic and co-dependent to provide him with a high level of stimulation to ejaculate during sex, so he dissociated to a 'grass is always greener on the other side of the fence' option to ejaculate.

A person can fall in love with and find a chair leg sexually exciting if there are sufficient pleasurable associations made with the object. We know this from fetishism.

The barrier people often face when dissociating from their sexual partners is not being present, and a lack of commitment and focus. When fantasies create these problems, they are no longer sexual pleasures, but pattern interrupters that give birth to a lack of engagement with their partner.

As hypnotists we help people create their desired neural network associations in the brain that activate hormonal and neurological catalysts for the SRC. Whether that is by direct suggestion, indirect suggestion, inference, or metaphor depends on how the hypnotist can get their message past the client's critical defence mechanisms. These misperceived, often conscious and unconscious defence mechanisms create the problem and maintain it until a new stimulus reconfigures the psychodynamics.

In David's case, since he had no experience of sex with anyone else, he was being stimulated by his own teenage sexual fantasies about women during masturbation. As he came to his marriage bed a virgin, he continued to rely on the familiarity of those previous fantasies to bring him to orgasm and failed to transfer to a full erotic attachment to his wife.

Since sex renders us at our most vulnerable, reducing our awareness to dangers in the environment, we can develop high filters to sexual experiences. This is why I used suggestion bombardment to stimulate change in David's unconscious that controls psychobiological programming and activity.

All those suggestions point towards the same desired change, but some may meet resistance. However, the multiplicity of suggestions heightens the probability of change taking place. If a child does not want to eat their greens, you hide them in a sausage and do not tell them.

In hypnosis, treatment failure generally is the result of not making the right suggestions for that client, at the right time, in the right way, and not due to the absence of hypnotisablity or suggestibility. This is because the hypnotic state is a naturally occurring state of mind for all people, and clients expect to accept suggestions when they come to see a hypnotist.

David started connecting and attaching erotically with his wife and stayed present during intercourse, using her in his mind as a stimulus to take him towards ejaculation. Every day he listened to a hypnosis recording I made for him, and he enjoyed the deepening of their sexual relationship (see Appendix A, item 52).

When I saw him six weeks later, he said, "I'm seeing June differently now. It's like I am seeing her sexually for the first time. It's completely changed our sex life."

CASE STUDY: FOXY AND HECTOR

This was a couple in their 30s who were both professionals. She was an antique clothes dealer, and he was a hairdresser. They dressed very fashionably, had a large social life and neither of them wanted children.

Foxy: *"I see it this way. You only live once, so try to have a really good time. Don't waste it."*

Hector nodded his head, looking at her with a wide smile, "Yeah, that's right, Foxy."

They were a sort of double act, feeding off each other but still independent.

Tracie: "And how can we help you both today?"

Hector: "Well, sex is good. Life is good. (He looked to Foxy for confirmation, and she smiled at him and nodded.) Only we're not as adventurous in bed as we'd like to be."

Tracie: "Can I get you both individually to do an exercise, please. I'm giving you each a clipboard with blank paper and a pen. Write down the five things you want from therapy today. No conferring."

It is important in these situations to cross-check personal goals to find out if the couple are communicating well, and to check that one partner is not being coerced by the other into sex they do not want.

They read out their lists:

Hector:

1. I want her to be my sex goddess.
2. I want to satisfy her more than anyone else has.
3. More time away from work.
4. Making more time for lovemaking.
5. I want sex to last longer.

Foxy:

1. I want exciting sex.
2. For him to sometimes demand sex from me.
3. I want to do sex in different places.

4. At times I want risky sex in places where we could be discovered.
5. I want to switch roles at times.

Tracie: "Interesting. Hector, I am wondering if your
          list is also about deeper connection. And Foxy,
          yours seems to be more about spontaneity and
          excitement. Both lists seem to be about connection.
          What do you both think?"

It is imperative for couples to have clear, co-operative, mutual goals, and to constantly check with each other that they feel comfortable with those goals in therapy, so it goes well.

Foxy: "Yes, they are different, but I want both of us to
         feel satisfied." (Hector looked at her, smiled, and
         nodded towards me)

This was a couple that appeared to have good attachments, and associated each other with sexual pleasure. Their sexual clusters were about adventure, and they were seeking to further those experiences.

Trance intentions

1. Promoting communication around sex.
2. Implementing boundaries so both of them feel safe.
3. Building on their existing creativeness.
4. Variation in sexual scenarios.
5. Reflecting their fantasies back to them.
6. Suggesting multiple sexual scenarios.

Mmmm you seem to be very good communicators with each other and of course that's going to be...**a great communication asset in your sexual adventures** (building on mutual skill sets)...could you hold hands as your chairs are next to each other (creating oxytocin, associating the sexual adventure with each other)...sit back in the armchairs...**close your eyes and be respectfully safe together** (putting in boundaries dependent on mutual agreement)...think about how many different hairstyles you Hector have created...think about how many outfits you Foxy have put together...**you're both experts in creating fantasies** (indirect suggestion to use their imagination in their sex life)...moods...style...atmosphere and role playing...a different hairstyle and outfit causes you to take new adventures...you're both creators of dreams and adventures together (utilising existing resources)...**I wonder if you wander around the many roles you play during sex and erotic games** (interrogative suggestion for sex fantasy variations)...just like actors you change roles according to the story you are experiencing...**so many stories and adventures you can create** (expanding sexual repertoire)...sometime a goddess to be worshipped...and sometimes a sex-hungry man who wants to have sex with his wife on the kitchen table (feeding back their goals)...**changing roles and playing with the adventures**...sometimes not knowing where the adventures will lead when you begin them (suggestion for continuous sexual adventures and development)...always different...always changing...like the thousand stories of Scheherazade...**sometimes the dominant one and sometimes not** (role interchange)...planning your storylines...and seeing where they take you...one to one thousand stories of...**sex...lust...desire...love...and...pleasure...adoration...passion...possession...excitement...special times...role playing...**

370

adventure...spontaneity...and...connection...satisfaction... **creating memories** (bombardment suggestions)...and during those adventures...you see things so well (Vi+ & Ve+)...hear things with delight (Ai+ & Ae+)...**and your skin and body become hypersensitive** (Ki+ & Ke+, direct suggestion)...and the tales you will tell each other...**fantasy becoming reality**... in many different places at many different times...**so many fantasies you can enjoy** (attaching pleasure to variety)... in everyday life you might be ordinary people (cancelling hypersensitivity outside sex)...**in your private sex lives you're sex adventurers** (suggestions for clear division between the two lives)

Homework

1. Listen to the 10-minute hypnotic recording each day, holding hands side by side.
2. Protect the time for sex play.
3. Start two beautifully crafted handwritten books in which they both write. The first is a sex fantasy book in which they can write their sexual fantasies and what they would like to try together.
4. The second book was about recording each time they had pursued those sexual fantasies, writing 5 things that were good and two things they might like to add the next time.
5. To read *My Secret Garden* (Friday, 2008), about women's sexual fantasies, *Men in Love: Men's Sexual Fantasies* (Friday, 1998), *The Triumph of Love Over Rage* (Friday, 1998), Urban Tantra (Carrellas, 2017), and *The Explorer's Guide to Planet Orgasm* (Sprinkle & Stephens, 2017).
6. Move to plant-based eating.

Here I am feeding back to them the amalgamated lists they wanted in suggestion form. It was important not to be too specific about the sex they should have, because that would shut down many of their potential sexual adventures.

Most people are not sexually adventurous as they encase themselves in social constructs that equate sexual variety with moral degradation, and engage in self-hypercriticism, as opposed to healthy exploration of their sexual self. This is why I always teach people to follow the tantra (see Appendix A, item 53).

Many people are so stressed by the demands of their lives, which they believe they cannot escape, that sex becomes unimportant.

Sex, as well as other parts of our lives, is never based on reality; it is based on our own constructed perceptions of reality. Influencing the perceived reality of sex via hypnotic and psychosexual therapy is immensely powerful and expediates therapy.

Life, social constructs, personal perceptions, and sexual permissibility are always changing, so our therapy must also always be changing as we hone our own psychosexual therapeutic skills.

As sex therapists doing this work, we need to have been or are a sexual adventurer. Our conscious and unconscious communications and experiences profoundly influence the outcomes of the hypnotic process and suggestion.

I never hide that I have had a vast and varied sex life – it is in the public domain. People are coming to consult me for help with their sex lives. I believe it is important that I've done the practical as well as the theory, so I can help them. Encourage your clients to be sexually adventurous, explore their fantasies, and have fun during sex (see Appendix A, item 54).

A therapist being coy simply encourages repression, and being overly authoritative steals the power from the client, so we must play the continual game of balance in our approach. But most of all, as sex therapists, we need to display our love and respect for sex, because it is just nature.

As hypnotherapists we must operate with a high level of skill, conviction, and belief that the client can change, when we create therapy that is just right for them. We are the magic makers, not script readers, who help people make their own sexual adventures.

Afterword

I never know what clinicians will take away from my work when they study what I share. If you only learn one or two techniques from this text it can change someone's sex life as they learn to enjoy one of nature's greatest gifts to us as human beings: sex.

Whatever you learn I urge you to practise it again and again until you refine that therapeutic skill so you can get the result that clients need. Not all my cases over the past several decades were successful but the more I practised, the more I refined my skills. And of course, we learn just as much from our failures as we do from our successes.

I hope throughout this work you have got a sense that I have loved sex both personally and clinically, and used that appreciation to purvey the help I have administered. When you love sex, your unconscious language infuses the client's unconscious experience with enthusiasm.

My first greatest piece of advice to you is to study the text several times. The more you study it, the more will be revealed. Also get out into the world of sex: attend lectures, bondage parlours, brothels and wherever sex takes place. Experiential often surpasses academic learning.

My second piece of advice is to read every hypnotherapy book you can get your hands on and learn from those who use hypnosis everyday of our working lives. Then practise... practise...practise.

Finally, become a hypnosis and sex geek because that is what people pay you to be and even the simplest change you help the client make can enrich their sex life.

Appendix A: Technique Reviews

These notes can help you understand some of the hypnotic and psychotherapeutic approaches I used with each case. I did not show you all the steps in the cases, just the ones I wanted to highlight for you to learn. These techniques are not replications of the cases I reported but suggested general guidelines that you might try in similar cases.

Chapter 6: Absences of sexual desire

1. **Religious beliefs-driven behavioural adjustment**
   Sometimes a person's religious beliefs lead to them becoming disconnected from their sexuality and prevent them from engaging in sex.

   A. Clearly define what the person's religious beliefs are around sex.
   B. Review that religion's text to see if the client's perceptions are distorted.
   C. Challenge the distortions for generalisations and misinterpretation.
   D. In trance, feed the client an alternative interpretation from their religion that supports a wholesome view of sex and its enjoyment to adjust their psychodynamic structure and cause a behavioural shift.

2. **Cancelling auto-suggested PTSD-induced anaesthesia and nerve blocking that causes dissociation from sexual sensations**

   People who experience trauma often dissociate from their bodies, blocking their libido and sexual feelings (creating anaesthesia) which creates a lack of desire.

   A. The trauma must be resolved and placed into the client's past.
   B. The client needs to learn to control the PTSD.
   C. In hypnosis, lead them to be aware of their present-day, incontestable bodily functions, actions, sensory experiences, and a sense of being in their body.
   D. Expand that sensory awareness into sexual feelings and urges, then fractionate those experiences.
   E. Task the client to use hypnosis every day for bodily integration.
   F. Task the client to journal those experiences daily as they witness the increase in sexual feelings and kinaesthetic sensory awareness.

3. **The need for health and fitness to promote sexual desire**

   Many people have a dysfunctional body due to an inappropriate lifestyle or disease that blocks sexual desire. Being healthy promotes a better sex life.

   A. Lead the person to remove all addictive substances including alcohol, recreational drugs, caffeine, fast food and tobacco.
   B. Review for any unnecessary or inappropriate medications.
   C. If you are not trained in these areas, co-ordinate with the appropriate professionals.

D.   If the client carries excess weight, put them on a weight reduction program.

E.   Get them to embark on an exercise program regularly, three times a week.

F.   Remove all electrical devices from the bedroom to avoid electromagnetic interference.

4.   **Nasal breathing to raise sexual energy (teach the client):**
Many people with sexual problems try to engage in sex whilst in the freeze state so they do not raise their sexual energy. Energy breathing raises sexual excitement. It can also be used during sex to reinvigorate sexual energy.

A.   Close your mouth, breathe only through your nose and look up.

B.   Breathe in and out deeply, very fast, with a quick inhalation and a quick exhalation. This is filling your lungs with oxygen.

C.   Continue doing this for one minute, fast and deep.

D.   One second breathing in and one second breathing out.

E.   Keep your shoulders down and smile wide with your mouth closed as you think about sex.

F.   Focus on the out breath.

G.   Breathe from the stomach as this also activates the pelvic floor muscles.

H.   Practise by placing your hand on your stomach, feeling it contracting towards your back and then expanding your stomach forward.

5.   **Cataleptic hands and creating positive hallucinations for redefining the importance of sex in a partnership (reframing exercise)**

People often become afraid of sex because they feel their performance and very existence is being judged. Changing the main focus in relationships to Agape (friendship) allows the person to feel more comfortable in exploring sex within a partnership.

A. Talk about how you are going to teach them the three kinds of love. Place their left hand upturned in front of their chest to the left.

B. Get the client to place Agape (friendship, respect, kindness, and consideration) in the open hand. At the same time look at the hand and direct their attention to the contents of the hand. They are initiating a positive hallucination.

C. Get the client to repeat back to you what is in the hand.

D. Move the hand directly in front of their chest, tracking it with your eyes and directing them to track it also.

E. Talk about the sex kind of love Eros (sex, lust, romance) which is pure instinct and has no cognitive filtering or processing. They are changing the hallucination. Get the client to repeat back what is in the hand, metaphorically seeing it as a non-thinking kind of love.

F. Put the right hand in mid-air in front of the chest to their right, upturned, tracking it with your eyes and directing them to track it also.

G. Talk about the third kind of love as Philia (blood relative, partner, spouse, best friend you have known all your life). They are changing their hallucination. Get the client to repeat back what is in the hand.

H. Ask the client to choose what is the most important kind of love to base a relationship on. At the same time look to their left at their chest level.

I. Continue to direct them back towards Agape as the basis for a sexual partnered relationship.

6. **Cross-fertilisation of sensory sexual experiences**
    Sometimes we need to teach people to build their sexual sensory experiences. We can use existing experiences of pleasure to teach them how to map pleasure in their sexual sensory experiences.

    A. Identify sensory memories of pleasures in one or more of the sensory modalities.
    B. With suggestion and voice tones, fractionate those pleasures in the client's eyes-closed trance.
    C. Use comparative suggestions that such levels of pleasure can occur in other circumstances (sex) in the same or other sensory systems and to try that out in trance.
    D. Observe and monitor if the suggestions are accepted or if there is resistance.
    E. Future pace the person in a sex rehearsal scenario to assess how well those suggestions worked for them.

Chapter 7: Erectile dysfunction

7. **Regression for recall of successful sexual experiences.**
    All men with secondary ED have unconscious memories of previous erectile function. Eliciting those memories and fractionating them can allow the client to reactivate a sense of erectile function.

    A. Put in an auditory safety anchor connected to your voice.
    B. Regress the client to three previous times when he had good erectile function.

C. With the second and third memory, fractionate them by 10 and then 100 times.

D. Join all three memories together.

E. Future pace that erectile competency of those memories into a future scenario sexual encounter via a rehearsal technique.

F. Then get the client to take a copy of those competencies of erectile success and install a copy of that success into their body and mind in the present time and throughout their timeline.

8. **Incompetent therapist technique**

Sometimes people are not being resistant to suggestions, they simply do not have the mental ability to follow them. So, we allow them to be better hypnotists for themselves than we are for them.

A. Tell them you are going to teach them to do self-hypnosis for themselves.

B. Ask them to copy what you do and do it in their own way.

C. Give them suggestions they can use for themselves for erectile competence and confidence or any other sexual experience.

D. Teach only direct auto-suggestions in the present tense to use in their daily self-hypnosis.

E. Direct the person to use and practise the technique with a recording you made at least twice a day.

9. **Daily circulating sexual energy breathing technique (teach the client)**

Sexual energy is more than what we do during sex and is what we do in our everyday lives. Daily breathing and meditation can raise our general sexual energy and how we pay attention to sex.

A. Sit quietly with your legs crossed on the floor, alone, and in a peaceful place.

B. Keep your back straight but relaxed.

C. Focus on your breathing and circulating your sexual energy up through the chakras.

D. Breathe deeply and slowly, in through your nose with your mouth closed, seeing the breath coming in through the base chakra and going all the way up through your chakras to the crown chakra above the top of the head. It takes several seconds to breathe in to a count of 10.

E. Above the crown chakra count 8, 9,10 levels as you see those higher levels inside your mind.

F. You are gathering up your sexual energy as you inhale and bringing it up your body.

G. Release the breath through the mouth in the air above the 10th level, allowing it to slowly fall all around you, like snowflakes, back to the base chakra, taking 10 seconds.

H. Repeat continually for five minutes once a day as you dissipate negative energy, clear your chakras, recycle your sexual energy and build it day by day.

I. The reason there are levels 8, 9 and 10 above the seventh chakra is because most people do not inhale fully when they breathe in. So when you breathe in, be aware of your rib cage expanding sideways and when you breathe out, your rib cage collapses. Keep your shoulders down and smile to produce serotonin.

10. **Time-delayed conflict resolution with psychodynamic conflict in internalised homophobia**

Some people are unable to accept their sexuality which puts them into a constant state of psychodynamic conflict.

A. Maintain a strictly non-judgmental and non-directive attitude to the client's conflict.

B. In trance, suggest the conflict might not be serving them and others by alerting them to a situation when it is self-defeating.

C. Suggest they could consider other options to their present-day position and invite them to consider what those might be over the next week or month.

D. Ask them to create conflict resolution by finding an option where all their sexual parts are in alignment.

E. Find leverage to motivate that resolution.

F. Indirectly suggest that when the parts are aligned sexual function can happen naturally.

11. **Advanced, age-related erectile performance adaption**

Advanced-ageing men can lose their physical ability to gain good erections. Helping them to adapt to those circumstances and maximise erectile opportunities can at times be the best option.

A. Encourage the client to expand their lovemaking skills beyond intercourse.

B. Consider the assistance of medication when necessary.

C. Use suggestions for sexual ego strengthening.

D. Use mind mechanics through stacking visual, auditory and kinaesthetic hallucinations to reconstruct his erectile confidence.

E. Suggestions for extended erectile function.

Chapter 8: Premature ejaculation

12. **Regression to traumatic first sexual encounter**

Sometimes PE is the result of early traumatic sexual encounters. It is useful to regress the person to identify that memory and reframe it within the context of their present-day experiences.

A. Put in safety anchor.

B. Acknowledge all the skills, competencies and success that the client already has today.

C. Regress the person to their earliest traumatic sexual experience.

D. Ask the client to identify the location, time and circumstances.

E. Ask the client to tell you what is happening.

F. Create a time shift orientation for them to place that incident in their past and be aware it is not happening in the present. Thereby inferring that the present gives opportunities for good sexual experiences.

13. **Circle pelvic muscles exercise for PE (teach the client)**

Learning to relax the pelvic floor muscles on cue considerably improves PE by retarding ejaculation.

A. Clench the anus muscles, pulling them inside you.

B. Clench the kegel muscles when you suck up everything inside you in the area behind your scrotum and penis. You naturally do this when you suddenly want to stop urinating.

C. Push down the PC muscles (bearing down) between your scrotum and anus.

D. Now relax your anus

E. Relax your kegels

F. Relax the PC muscle.

G. Create a circular exercise of tensing these muscles one after the other and then relaxing them one after the other.

H. Practise this 3 x daily.

I. After a week focus on relaxing these muscles in a circular exercise.

J. After another week focus on relaxing the muscles all at once.

K. When you want to delay or stop ejaculation, relax all three sets of muscles at once.

14. **Nasal breathing for extending intercourse and delayed ejaculation (for the client)**

Slowing the breathing down and focusing it in the nose delays ejaculation. It increases nitric oxide in the blood and lengthens the plateau stage 2 of the SRC.

A. Close your mouth and breathe only through your nose.

B. Breathe very slowly in with a long inhalation, and a long slow exhalation.

C. Breathe into the lungs, not moving the hips or lower body.

D. Particularly focus on exhalation.

E. Make no sound and keep your shoulders down.

F. Don't breathe from your stomach as this activates the pelvic muscles.

15. **Intercourse positions for PE (teach to the client):**

The biomechanics of intercourse are generally universal, and you can educate men around what positions help extend intercourse.

A. Do not thrust your hips during the plateau period (the time when you are having intercourse) until you are ready to ejaculate.

B. Use the one knee up position, continually bringing the partner towards you as you keep your back straight.

C. Use the supine position as you lay on your back and your partner is on top of you with you controlling how they bear down on you, creating slow coitus.

D. Use the position where you are on your knees, sitting on your feet and the partner is bearing down onto you.

E. Use the side-to-side position and push with your straight back, not thrusting with your hips.

F. Use the doggy position but draw the partner onto you, keeping your back straight without pushing with your hips.

16. **Focused attention during sex (teach the client):**
It is important during sex not to be distracted by other elements of your life. Being present aids physical control.

A. Organise your schedule so other parts of your life do not bleed into the time for sex.

B. Make specific times to have sex and protect those times to stop intrusive thoughts and interruptions and maintain boundaries around the time for intimacy.

C. Be fully present during sex, paying attention to yourself and your partner or partners.

D. Purposefully, consciously and mindfully slow sex down and take your time.

17. **Partners practising focused attention (teach the client):**
Rushed sex can lead to partners not being present in their

mind so they are relying solely on libido and not creating higher-level sensory experiences.

A. Ensure there are no distractions.
B. Clean the space of all electrical equipment including telephones.
C. Protect the time for sex.
D. Sanctify the space as a temple of lovemaking.
E. Play some nice music or use favourite smelling oils.
F. Spend time together smiling at each other and being relaxed before starting sex.

18. Treating ED via sensory reduction in the penis

Many men experiencing PE suffer high anxiety and hypersensitivity of the penis. Reducing that sensitivity with hypno-anaesthesia can help the second stage of the SRC.

A. Induce glove anaesthesia on a 1-10 Likert sensory awareness scale.
B. Give the man control of increasing or decreasing the sensitivity.
C. Use suggestions for transferring the anaesthesia to several different parts of the body to train them in sensory alteration, control and locational shifting.
D. Use suggestions for moving the reduction in sensory awareness and sensation into his penis when he needs to during intercourse.
E. Train him to increase sensory awareness at orgasm or ejaculation.

19. Overcoming separation-induced trauma ED

After separation from partners many men experience an existential crisis of being that creates PE.

A. Teach the person to allow himself to trust himself again.
B. Teach him that trust is the very foundation of a relationship with self and others.
C. Use trust-building exercises to allow him to begin to trust others again.
D. Future pace him in trance to trust partners and feel safe during sex.
E. Use ego strengthening for trusting himself to be able to extend the second stage of the SRC.

20. **Orgasmic diffusion**

Orgasms can happen in other parts of the body other than the genitals. Teaching the client to do this not only increases pleasure but can serve many purposes in helping them.

A. Fully explain that an orgasm is a mini seizure in the brain.
B. Get them to recall other heightened sensory experiences that are orgasmic in different sensory modalities.
C. Suggest the person experiences small sex seizure-like sensations in different parts of the body.
D. Rehearse them in changing the locations of these sensory seizures.
E. Task them to practise these skills at home.
F. Fractionate these pleasures of diffused orgasms as being equally as pleasurable as a genital orgasm.
G. Get them to rehearse these skills in trance in the clinic.
H. Teach them that at any time during sex they can experience diffused orgasm without a genital orgasm.
I. Get them to practise this during masturbation.
J. Teach them to use these mini orgasms during sex before striving for an ejaculatory orgasm.

21. **Realignment of personal criteria of needs to facilitate overcoming PE**

There is a difference between ego-driven statements and what a person is prepared to do to have sex as important in their lives. Helping the person to re-organise their criteria of needs to have sex as more important helps them be focused during sex.

A. Ask the client how they live their life and what their schedule is.

B. Assess their level of sex education and whether they are knowledgeable about sex to assess whether you need to engage in sex education.

C. In trance, invite the client to re-prioritise the importance of sex in their lives and relationships, suggesting setting time aside for sex.

D. Use suggestions for greater connection with partners and shared time for a sexual adventure.

E. Repositioning intercourse as dessert and the main part of lovemaking being foreplay.

F. Use suggestions for paying attention to sex and slowing intercourse down, sometimes stopping and resting then recommencing again after a resting period.

22. **Imposter syndrome induced PE**

Some men have low sexual self-image and self-esteem. They believe they are not good enough as lovers and someone will discover they are faking being a valid male and a worthy sexual partner.

A. Despite testosterone-driven, external bravado, males often have very fragile sexual egos which can be easily damaged via the threat of being thought of as 'less than'. Assess the extent of the man's sexual ego damage.

B. Use metaphor to help him reframe his value as a male to being fully worthy.

C. Refocus his attention away from the obsession with the almighty singular orgasm towards smaller orgasmic pleasures, enjoyment and deeper connections with partners.

D. Get him to practise this during stage 2 of the SRC.

E. Suggest he experiments with multiple orgasms without ejaculation.

F. Use ego strengthening to steer his self-identity towards being a competent lover, taking his time.

Chapter 9: Vaginismus

23. Resolution of disease induced pain during intercourse

A. Establish a very clear medical diagnosis of the infection or the organ disorder.

B. Initiate physiological treatment.

C. Life issues need to be resolved to reduce stress and increase healing.

D. Assess what makes the disorder worse or better.

E. If the pain is overwhelming, get the client to chunk each task down, one by one, to make the whole treatment more manageable for them.

F. If necessary, use hypnosis for pain reduction.

G. Use regression for resource mining to find previously used skills and competencies that they can use today, including feeling good about themselves.

H. Use bombardment suggestions for utilising those resources and adding new resources for healing and making life manageable today.

I. Continually use suggestions for self-care and re-integration into the body.

J. Use fractionation and stacking for every success the client achieves.

K. Feed back to them further suggestions about solutions that have previously worked for them.

L. Train them in vaginal dilation with themselves and their partner taking part if there is one. Eventually transfer that comfortability with dilation to intercourse.

24. Assistance in vaginal deformity vaginismus

A full gynaecological examination is required with a report. At times a second and third opinion may be sought for clarity.

A. If surgery is not required, then begin vaginal dilation with the client using their fingers and soft silicone sex toys, progressively stretching the vagina using lubrication, at the same time as masturbating.

B. Direct them to purposefully transfer the activity to penile insertion (but the man staying still) whilst she masturbates. The partner must be given instructions on how to facilitate the woman's needs.

C. The activity can progress to intercourse.

D. Assistance from a pelvic floor physiotherapist can be useful.

E. Suggestions for pelvic floor relaxation during dilation are essential.

F. Direct suggestion that the process is progressive and adherence to the treatments programs is essential.

G. Each success the client has needs to be fed back to them using fractionation suggestions for self-efficacy.

H. If treatment progress fails, a plastic or gynaecological surgery referral may be needed and the patient supported therapeutically through that process.

25. **Circle pelvic floor exercise for vaginismus (teach the client)**

Many women who experience vaginismus have never explored the ability to manipulate their own pelvic floor muscles, which are used during sex and intercourse.

A. Clench the anus muscles, pulling them inside you (the seat).

B. The kegels are when you suck up everything inside you in the area behind your vagina. You naturally do this when you suddenly want to stop peeing.

C. Push down the PC muscles (bearing down) between your vagina and anus.

D. Now relax your anus.

E. Relax your kegels.

F. Relax the PC muscle where you bear down.

G. Create a circular exercise of tensing these muscles one after the other and then relaxing them one after the other.

H. Practice this several times a day.

I. After a week, simply focus on relaxing the muscles around the anus, then the kegels and PC.

J. During dilation and intercourse relax those 3 sets of muscles continually.

26. **Assistance in stress-induced vaginal atrophy**

Stress causes bodily and vaginal muscles to tense and the woman can hold that tension in those muscles over long periods. This interferes with the hormonal system, which can arrest menstruation, ovulation and cause the vagina to shrink.

A. A full gynaecological examination is required with a report. At times a second and third opinion may be sought.

B. A full blood panel may indicate premature, early or natural menopause or amenorrhea. If the results are positive, either HRT or a naturopathic approach can correct hormonal irregularity.

C. It is important to understand the profound psychological changes and sometimes trauma that can occur at the cessation of menses and vaginal atrophy.

D. In premature cessation of menses, it is important to determine what may be the cause and to what extent that may be psychological.

E. Hypnotherapy can play a supportive role in natural menopause for personal adjustment and life transition.

F. In cases where psychological trauma, anorexia, disease, medications, addiction, radiation or chemotherapy may be involved, suggestions for restoring health need to be paramount.

G. Traumas need to be resolved and the client brought into living calmly and fully in the present time.

H. Stress management is a key strategy.

I. Initiate the regular daily use of dilators with lubricant. Using the pelvic floor relaxation exercise is helpful.

J. A pelvic floor physiotherapist can be of assistance.

27. Comfortable loss of virginity for women

When a virgin is unsure about what will happen during sex, she can experience pain at intercourse due to fear of an oncoming experience.

A. Determine if there have been any early attempts at sexual intercourse.

B. Sex education is paramount. What are the most comfortable positions that also open the vagina for her?

C. Emphasise confidence building in that she has the right to control the situation.

D. Use suggestions for slowing the process down so she can make good decisions for herself.

E. Associate intercourse with adventures and good experiences physically, mentally and even spiritually.

Chapter 10: Anorgasmia

28. Women discovering a first orgasm

A woman may have never experienced an orgasm. It is important to educate her on the diversity of orgasms.

A. Order a blood test to determine hormone levels. If they are low, consider HRT.

B. Demystify orgasms by exploring what an orgasm might be and that it is not what pornography positions it to be.

C. Use regression to recall many neurological sensory seizures and interpreting them as neurological orgasms, making sensory seizures accessible to the client.

D. Suggest appropriate and comfortable sex positions, and that control and demands of her body are solely her prerogative.

E. Rehearsing the tensing pelvic muscles circle exercise to gain control over her pelvic floor. Using them several times a day.

F. Starting with small pelvic floor orgasms as she tenses the pelvic floor muscles (anus, kegels, bearing down on the PC muscle) and thrusts her hips.

G. Get her to practise solo orgasms and increase the intensity of those orgasms. Emphasising practice for pleasure, not perfection.

H. Suggestions for good communications and directing her partner to do what is right for her to produce comfortable sex.

I. It is important to encourage the client to explore her sexual fantasies during trance while practising these exercises.

29. Circle exercise for anorgasmia in women (teach the client):

Many women are disengaged from their genitals. Just like exercising and controlling other muscles, a person needs to be aware of and control the pelvic floor muscles.

A. Clench the anus muscles, pulling them inside you (the seat).

B. The kegels are when you suck up everything inside you in the area behind your vagina. You naturally do this when you suddenly want to stop peeing.

C. Push down the PC muscles (bearing down) between your vagina and anus.

D. Now relax your anus.

E. Relax your kegels.

F. Relax the PC muscle.

G. Create a circular exercise of tensing these muscles one after the other and then relaxing them one after the other.

H. Practise this several times a day.

I. After a week, focus on tensing the muscles around the anus, then the kegels and push down on your PC.

J. When excited and approaching climax, bear down on the PC muscles and tense the kegels and anus, whilst thrusting your hips, all at once, creating a pleasurable seizure during masturbation or intensive sex play.

K. Remember, the more you practise, the more familiar you become with your sexual orgasmic pleasures. Learn exactly how these motions apply to you and practise intensifying those pleasures.

30. Anorgasmia with sensory-restricted males

Due to neurodiversity, genetic variance, trauma, disease or brain damage, some men do not experience heightened neurological sexual seizures.

A. Assess the reason for the lack of neurological experiential variances.

B. What help does the man need physiologically if that is necessary?

C. Teach him physiological sensory awareness by using mind mechanics and state shifting.

D. Teach him tantric breathing and chakra locational work, getting him to practise that daily at home. Use the language of raising sexual energy as he brings the energy up to and beyond the crown chakra (Sahasrara).

E. As he continues to construct and practice altered sensory awareness, frame peak sensory sexual experiences as orgasms.

31. Multiple orgasms for men

Some men exploring sex will want to try multiple orgasms that happen before ejaculation.

A. Explain that orgasm and ejaculation are two separate functions. Ejaculation in most men is seen as the end of sex. Post-ejaculation the vagal nerve initiates the parasympathetic nervous system for relaxation (stage 4 SRC).

B. Always emphasise orgasm is a simply a pleasurable sexual seizure.

C. Teach them the practice of extreme edging (approaching orgasm then stopping, resting and starting again). It can be repeated for many hours.

D. Breathe through the nose using long, very slow, nasal breathing, with no hip movement and relaxed pelvic muscles.

E. In trance, fractionate the near orgasm experience as an orgasm without ejaculation.

F. Install a safe word should the emotions become too intense and overwhelming so the man needs to ejaculate.

G. Orgasmic diffusion can also be used to stack different orgasms in different parts of the body before ejaculation.

32. Multiple female orgasms

Multiple orgasms are repeating sexual seizures – in any part of the body.

A. Regress for pleasurable orgasmic seizure experiences in any multiple sensory modalities.

B. Map these kinaesthetic pleasurable sensory experiences and use them as a format for sexual seizures.

C. Teach the pelvic circle exercise for anorgasmia for women.

D. Teach tantric breathing and the use of sexual chakra energy.

E. Upon climax, immediately repeat step J of the circle exercise for anorgasmia in women (item 29) again and again.

F. Get the client to use their sexual fantasies to help raise sexual energy.

G. Teach her not to let go fully into stage 4 of the SRC but to continue repeating the later parts of stage 3 to produce repeated orgasms.

33. Adjusting perceptions of cultural norms to allow diverse orgasmic experiences

A. People can only experience what their beliefs, values and cultural perceptions allow their bodies to perceive.

B. Investigate the client's personal values, beliefs and perception of sexual acceptability.

C. Identify the roadblocks to them being fully accepting of their body and sexual experiences. If those roadblocks are not obvious, use regression to uncover the source or psychological governor that is preventing orgasm.

D. Assess if the person's circumstances will allow them to fully embrace their sexuality. When and how could they change those circumstances?

E. What values, beliefs and perceptions do they need to change to fully accept their sexuality which would allow them to experience orgasm? Feed the answers back to them in the form of intra- and post-hypnotic suggestions.

F. Identify the time when this change can take place and they can enjoy orgasms, and ejaculation, then bring that change into the present time.

Chapter 11: Unwanted sexual behaviour

34. **Behavioural approach to operating psychological governors in unwanted sexual behaviours**
Behaviour that does not serve a person can be initiated by past experiences or cultural modelling. Reprogramming through direct suggestion can install new behaviours and displace old ones.

A. Identify the unwanted sexual behaviours.
B. Get the client to clearly state why they are unwanted and what dangers they pose.
C. Use suggestions for alternative behaviours.
D. Identify the trigger for the behaviour and provide a new suggested response (pattern interrupter ('When X happens you will do Y').
E. Use direct re-enforcement and bombardment suggestions to create a new Pavlovian response (pure behaviouralism).
F. Always identify a reward that follows the performance of the new behaviour.
G. The new response acts as a governor, blocking the old, unwanted response.
H. Test the new response is working in the session and in follow-up sessions.

35. **Cognitive approach to unwanted sexual thoughts**
When thoughts are not compatible between the person's sub-personalities, it causes psychodynamic conflict.

Becoming aware of the conflict and disturbing negative mind chatter can help people reassess their behaviours.

A. Assess whether those unwanted sexual thoughts are reasonable, the result of psychodynamic conflict or the result of behavioural programming. Are they harmful to the client or others?

B. It is important not to remove or block thoughts that are natural as it could cause physiological and psychological damage and sexual repression, which causes neurosis.

C. Provide the client with extra information to expand their perceptions of those thoughts. Expand the gestalts around thoughts and behaviours that could work for them. Reframe the situation so they have a choice of whether to pay attention to those thoughts or not.

D. Test if the client is happy with the change due to expanded cognitive awareness.

36. **Exposure therapy approach for unwanted sexual thoughts and behaviours)**

People are often afraid of what they do not understand or what they have not been exposed to. Constant exposure in trance can desensitise them to sexual material.

A. Clearly identify the disturbing sexual thoughts and behaviours. Feed them back to the client to clarify that you understand them.

B. Determine whether they are harmful to the client or others, or simply natural.

C. If those thoughts and behaviours are perfectly natural, do not attempt to eradicate them but acclimatise the client to them.

D. If they are harmful, take a behavioural or parts negotiation approach to change.

E. Psychodynamic conflict locks a person into restricted sexual thoughts, behaviours and choices. Identify the parameters of those restrictions.

F. Dilute the restrictions by exposing the client to new sexual thoughts and behaviours in trance, as trance reduces the activity of the amygdala, reducing the risk of a panic reaction.

G. Continually repeat the process intermittently to avoid resistance and overwhelm. This creates desensitisation for new material.

H. Deliver post-hypnotic suggestions for the client to expand their experience in the real world.

I. Test and measure the responses.

37. **Supportive approach to leave or change an unhealthy relationship where the client has self-destructive behaviours**

When clients are in physical and emotional danger, we must give them support and any information they need to stay safe.

A. Carry out a risk assessment (physical, mental and emotional) and a quality-of-life assessment.

B. If the clients or others are in danger, we have a duty to point that out and offer supportive alternatives.

C. Ask the client to consider all their options, no matter how unlikely. This can be done in eyes-closed trance or in artificial somnambulism, getting them to choose their best present option that is most rewarding.

D. Support them in carrying out that option by using suggestions for ego strengthening their ability to make those real-life choices and following through with actions.

E. Do not use obvious direct suggestion, as an abused person typically already feels overly dominated.

F. If they have already made the decision and are seeking support, get them to future pace their ability to follow through on their actions.

G. If necessary, give them information about services for abused people and when they are in danger consider your mandatory reporting options.

Chapter 12: Sex addiction

38. Resolving conflicting sexual trances

Sometimes people find themselves living more than one life trance (code switching), with one threatening the other. Parts negotiation for self-preservation can help equalise psychodynamic and life harmony.

A. Get the client to define the opposing trances and reflect them back on them so they begin to own and become uncomfortable with the incongruence.

B. By suggestion, offer them a better, congruent option that is emotionally appealing, other than the conflict. They may choose one themselves, but they often need guidance.

C. Suggest to them that all parts need to be to be congruent and present during sex in a wholesome way, seeking satisfaction and connection.

D. Suggest they take time to explore other options whilst the psychodynamic shift begins to take place.

E. In follow-up sessions, help them to clearly define and redefine what the new options will be.

F. Future pace and test and measure the outcome.

39. Learning to manage sexual self-independence in cases of sexual dependence

People can become sexually addicted to one or multiple people and they need to step back, reassess and re-negotiate the situation.

A. Clearly define the person's sexual addiction, stating with whom, when, where and how it takes place.

B. Use a My Friend John technique metaphor around another person who lost control and then found it again. This helps de-stigmatise guilt and loss of control.

C. Use suggestions for regression to review the journey of how they became addicted to the other person.

D. Invite a separation of themselves and others, enjoying sex with someone, but on their own terms.

E. Suggest a re-negotiation of the terms of the relationship on equal terms if the client is being dominated, or obsessed with the other person.

F. Use hypnotic dreaming for the client to work out the independent new terms and conditions of the relationship.

40. Screening for biological causes of sex addiction

Many people who experience sexual addiction are experiencing biological dysfunction and it is important to screen for that before presuming psychopathology.

A. Take a full medical history.

B. Order blood tests to look for hormonal anomalies.

C. Work with an allopathic medical practitioner or clinical naturopath.

D. What remedies can be applied if there are problems with LH, SBGH, testosterone, oestrogen, progesterone, TSH, T3, T4, DHEA, and cortisol.

E. Do not ascribe psychological causation when medical problems exist.

F. Teach risk assessment skills.

G. Assist with adjustment in trance, by installing behavioural boundaries to control the libido and direct it to healthier activities as well as constraining sexual behaviours.

H. Always remember as hypnotists that hypnotherapy can help adjust biological function, but also remember physiological dysfunction requires medical assistance.

41. **Resolving relationship conflict due to over-sexualisation of one partner**

Mismatched sexual needs in a relationship can cause resentment and affects the whole relationship. Using couples therapy can help partners find commonalities and re-negotiate the terms of their sexual engagement.

A. Consult both partners together, asking them to state their desired outcomes from therapy.

B. Check for the presence of coercive behaviours by observing the couple and comparing their lists of desired therapeutic outcomes.

C. Regress them both together to a time when sexual negotiation was working.

D. Feed that information back to them as strategies in the present day to reboot negotiations about what would work for both partners today.

E. Get them to future pace those strategies to restore harmony in the relationship, including compromise by all parties and the use of constant, respectful communication.

F. Use suggestions for reinstatement of sex as joyous and fun in the relationship.

Chapter 13: Recovery from rape and sexual assault

42. **Learning self-trust and installing boundaries again after sexual abuse**
All victims of sexual assault lose trust in themselves and others and need to learn to trust again.

A. It is important for people who experience sexual abuse to be screened for PTSD and dissociation.

B. All victims of sexual abuse feel their boundaries have been breached and they have been violated. Install a psycho-imaginary safe space to which only they have access.

C. Teach them the operation of personal boundaries, giving them the choice of with whom, when, where and why they interact with others.

D. Teach them to be a proactive communicator.

E. Teach emotional control and how to change their emotional state fast.

F. Use suggestions for ego strengthening, trusting themselves, initiating self-determination, whilst interacting with others.

43. Decisions on whether to disclose sexual abuse

Disclosing sexual abuse can have both benefits and, at times, be dangerous. The best judge of their circumstances is the person themselves, unless they are a minor or a ward of the court.

A. Attentively listen to them telling their story, allowing catharsis.

B. Use suggestions for present-tense stability.

C. Establishing that culpability is not with the victim.

D. Use a split screen technique to assess the possible outcomes of disclosing or not disclosing.

E. Use suggestion for unconscious resolution and comfort with whichever decision they make.

F. Use metaphor for survival and prosperity regardless of which decision they choose.

44. Leaving a present sexual abuse situation

As therapists. at times we must help people exit abusive circumstances. Most of all such people need support and guidance.

A. Use suggestions that large changes need to take place and seek therapeutic alliance to make that happen.

B. Bring them down out of high beta brain wave activity to alpha wave in their daily life to control the fight/flight/freeze response.

C. Use regression to mine for existing skills they will need to change their circumstances.

D. Acknowledge capabilities and existing skills.

E. Initiate self-care and boundaries as their number one criteria of needs.

F. Suggest a self-protective archetype for them to identify with during the separation.

G. Install a Pavlovian response to reject sexual abuse.

H. Promote independence and physical isolation away from the abusers.

I. Give safe place information for a refuge if appropriate.

45. Re-initiate the SRC in a gang assault victim

In gang sexual assault cases people always experience PTSD which must be treated to help them develop a sense of self-determination.

A. Use past tense language to distance the client from the event.

B. Reframe sex as being a wholesome expression of love in the present.

C. Teach the client to consider potential future partners by their actions and not just what they say.

D. Educate the client in communication skills.

E. Suggest self-determination in the present and future.

F. Teach reciprocity for respectful behaviour.

G. Use suggestions for the client to make others feel safe as well. Altruism always overcomes self-victimisation.

H. Teach desensitisation to sex by chunking down progressive exposure to present and future relationships into manageable acclimatisation.

I. Actively resolve PTSD.

J. Use ego strengthening by stacking the client's successes, feeding them back to them, and getting them to celebrate them and their progress.

Chapter 14: Sex and disability

46. Unwinding the complications of mental illness, disability and sex

People with mental illness have special needs and we must help them access that particular help to improve their sex lives.

A. Take note of all the complications of their diagnosis and medication and use Occam's razor to determine where the problems lie that you can help with.

B. Use metaphors to help them rewrite their daily story in an empowering way.

C. All addictive substances must be removed.

D. Encourage a healthy lifestyle.

E. Help them create very simple solutions and practical changes that they can manage, as their life may already be complicated.

F. Involve an interdisciplinary team or community help to monitor and support them.

G. Attach positive emotional components to the solutions, then fractionate them.

H. Check and measure the result, being flexible with what they can manage.

I. Ego strengthen by attributing all success to them.

47. Speaking the language of being differently abled

Differently abled people often feel misunderstood, ignored or looked down on by averagely abled people. Encourage the differently abled person to take charge of the communications.

A. Each area of being differently abled has its own language so learn how to communicate in that language.

B. Sex with averagely abled people can seem intimidating and frustrating when the differently abled person is misunderstood.

C. Use the second position perspective for the client to see how difficult it may also be for the averagely abled person to do the right thing.

D. Suggest the client takes charge and directs how sex would be good for them.

E. Use ego strengthening and self-affirmations to elicit confidence in that role.

F. Avoid using direct suggestions as it can come across as ableist privilege.

48. Body dysphoria due to disease and physical trauma-induced disfigurement

Physical trauma or disease affects people's ability to engage in sex because they can feel unattractive and unworthy. It is important to lead the person to focus on their worthiness and blessings.

A. Establish the extent of the disfigurement and how that impacts on the client's sexual self-image.

B. Acknowledge their distress and get them to acknowledge the blessing of their present life.

C. Reframe their perspective on how those who care for them and love them see them as a positive, beautiful force.

D. Use an affect bridge to regress them to when they felt whole.

E. Map those positive emotions and copy them into the present, fractionate them, and then future pace them.

F. Get the client to work out the practicality of how they will deal with their disabilities and sex in the future.

49. **Accommodating a person's lifelong disability as they embark on a sex life**

The first and early sexual experiences can seem daunting. This is magnified when a person is seen as physically or mentally different.

A. Get the client to consider a risk assessment for suitable partners to have sex with, in that the other person can facilitate the client's needs.

B. Fractionate the person's existing abilities and assets.

C. Suggest careful planning to stay safe with the scope to be adventurous.

D. Always encourage adaptability.

E. Use ego strengthening and confidence building in that the client creates sex as a good, fun, and rewarding experience.

F. Frame sex as a great and beautiful adventure for them and their partners.

Chapter 15: Good sex

50. **When one partner is bored with their sex life**

The pressures of life and bringing up a family can cause 'sex death bed' where sex is deprioritised and partners feel frustrated and unhappy.

A. Assess whether there have been any reasonable discussions between them about their sex life.

B. Put one partner in charge of organising time and space for sexual exploration and protecting that space.

C. Teach communication skills around sex, both in and out of the bedroom.

D. Encourage them to embark on a sexual adventure they have never tried before.

E. Give suggestions that all of this is done within the confines of mutually respectful and supportive behaviours.

51. Teaching young couples about sex

Most people are afraid of sex or certain sexual experiences due to lack of education, traumatic media stories or cultural constraints.

A. Sex therapy begins with us, as therapists, being comfortable with sex and discussing all its aspects. Our unconscious presents our own congruency or incongruency when communicating with clients.

B. In your communications, positively frame sex simply as being one of nature's beautiful and wholesome experiences.

C. Provide information for them about sex and how they may enjoy its many wonders, encouraging them to be proactively curious.

D. Teach them chunking so they can pursue one adventure at a time, so it does not become overwhelming.

E. Use trance work and suggestions to build their sexual confidence.

52. Transfer of the focus of sexual excitement

People can get attached to using a narrow focus of psychological sexual stimuli, people and objects to activate different stages of the SRC.

A. Teach the person that sexual focus on people or activities is as flexible as pointing a car in any direction.

B. Use mind mechanics for them to focus their libido and desire on new people or sexual activities.

C. Fractionate the levels of pleasure they can achieve in doing this.

D. Use positive re-enforcement suggestions to build their confidence in their new sexual associations and attachments.

53. Tantra sex principles (weaving) (teach the client):

It is important in teaching our clients about sex that we are practising what we are teaching. I teach many clients about tantric sex.

A. Put time aside for sex and protect that time to relax.

B. Sex can be with yourself or with others.

C. Be present and aware with no distractions, giving yourself and the other person your full attention.

D. Create a space and atmosphere that allows those involved to feel comfortable and excited.

E. See sex as natural, wholesome and wonderful.

F. Learn as much about sex as you can.

G. Take your time for lovemaking, running into hours of connection which does not always involve the genitals, orgasm or ejaculation.

H. Start by facing each other and staring straight into the other person's eyes, breathing together, calmly connecting and smiling, creating trust. Hold that for 5 to 20 minutes (increasing oxytocin).

I. Start using the sexual excitement breathing to raise the sexual energy.

J. Explore what your partner likes. For instance, stroking, massage, kissing, tickling, talking, cunnilingus, fellatio, nipple play, role playing, BDSM, or the use of sex toys. Become an expert in those skills as you raise the sexual energy up your chakras.

K. Be a great communicator during sex.

L. If you are engaging in fantasy sex, start acting it out (safely of course).

M. Remember, sex is pleasurable so enjoy it and even sometimes laugh.

N. As a male, bring your partner to ecstasy before intercourse.

O. Take control of your pelvic floor muscles, when to relax and when to tense them.

P. Know the different lovemaking techniques and intercourse positions.

Q. As a female, learn to extend your orgasms and produce multiple orgasms.

R. At times slow it down, stop and rest, then continue.

S. As a male, learn how to use edging to delay ejaculation while still having an orgasm.

T. Always be mindful of your breathing.

U. When it comes to intercourse, take your time as the aim is to enjoy connection, not to rush to climax.

V. Be mindful that orgasms can occur without ejaculation and in any part of the body (male and female).

W. When you want to ejaculate (male) raise your breathing, move your hips and raise the sexual energy up your body to release it from the crown chakra (Stage 3 SRC).

X. Spend time together after sex to connect and appreciate each other.

54. Couple embarking on sexual fantasies

Some couples are naturally sexually more adventurous and curious. When embarking on sexual fantasies they may need help and guidance.

A. Ask the couple to write separate lists about what they are seeking. This helps them clarify their goals. It also checks for congruence to see if there is any coercive behaviour.

B. Do not create a sterile clinical environment. People open up and feel safe in discussing sexual fantasies in a warm, friendly environment.

C. It is important for us as therapists not to suggest what that sexual exploration should be but to simply help people in trance create fertile ground for their curiosity. Suggesting what those explorations could be may cause resistance and shut down the client's curiosity.

D. Give them information about many different options through literature or a visual medium.

E. Get them to keep fantasy books where they can write down their fantasies and record their adventures. This structure helps them maintain safe boundaries through reflective cognition.

F. Use ego strengthening for them to have the confidence to move beyond a vanilla sex life.

G. Most of all, frame sex fantasies as adventurous and fun.

Glossary

Abreaction: A sudden negative reaction during the trance experience where the person may have a sudden release of disturbing thoughts, memories and feelings.

Affect bridge: Tracing a previous experience back in time by getting the person to reconnect with those kinaesthetic previous experiences. It is a form of regression.

Apposition of opposition: Directing the client to position two opposite behaviours and set of thoughts against each other to cause a psychodynamic and behavioural shift.

Arm levitation: Suggestion for an arm to raise under the control of the unconscious mind.

Artificial somnambulism: A hypnotic, waking, trance-like state that can be induced by hypnosis or can happen spontaneously.

As if scenario: Suggestion for future pacing imaginary possible future thoughts, behaviours, actions and experiences to see how they work out.

Associated binding statement: The hypnotist states a fact and suggests that another associated statement is therefore true.

Auto-anaesthesia: Self-suggested anaesthesia that people can be trained to produce in hypnosis. It may also be the result of dissociation during trauma.

Auto-hypnosis: When a person leads themselves into an altered state of trance.

Auto-suggestion: Self-suggestion.

Behavioural incentive: Suggestion for a reward after having done a certain action.

Binding statement: One statement is true, therefore the second statement must be true.

Blanket hypnosis: The practice of using a narrow range of hypnotherapeutic techniques for all people.

Bombardment fractionation: Repeated similar suggestions to re-enforce or multiply the intensity of a concept, idea or experience.

Boredom technique: This is when the hypnotist consistently produces information that might not be of interest to the person's conscious mind or is monotonous. It can be used as a trance induction or trance deepener.

Bridging resources: A suggestion that resources from one part of a person's life can be used in other circumstances.

Call to action: A suggestion, command or inference that the client now needs to take action.

Catalepsy: The body or parts of the body become immobile, stiff, or wax-like.

Cataleptic hand: Placing the hand stiff and immobile in mid-air which requires unconscious control to rest it there, so it is a trance induction, deepener and used to ratify trance.

Causal link: As one thing happens, something else will happen at the same time or directly afterwards. One causes the other to happen.

Challenging a statement: Providing additional information to place a statement in the context of no longer being viable. It is a reframe.

Challenging incongruence: Feeding back the information the person provided that contains opposing statements. This forces the unconscious to re-evaluate the value of their statements.

Chunking down: Breaking thoughts and tasks into smaller processes to make each stage easier to complete.

Chunking up: The joining together of smaller competencies to create a more sophisticated and synchronous action.

Code switching: The process of the hypnotist changing their language and demeanour to match that to the style of the person they are working with. Also the practice of the client changing aspects of their personality.

Conditional bargaining: Suggestion that a person thinks or behaves in a certain way to facilitate a goal.

Conditional suggestion: A suggestion that something will happen if something else happens.

Confrontation shock technique: Reflecting back to the person elements of their own historical behaviour that they presently are unable to see. Holding up the mirror that causes cognitive and psychodynamic shift.

Contingent suggestion: A suggestion that when one thing happens, another happens simultaneously.

Desensitisation: Consistent exposure to a word, thought, behaviour or stimulus to lower resistance to a stimulus. A behavioural therapy technique providing progressive familiarisation to the stimulus to lower a phobic response.

Direct suggestion: A command to complete a task.

Disassociation from trauma: A suggestion to physically step away from a traumatic situation, reducing the stress response. This can even be a psycho-imaginary distancing.

Emotive driver: Suggestions that guide, motivate and channel a person's emotion in a particular direction.

Esoteric generalised suggestion: A suggestion that has no basis in science cannot be processed or interfered with by the analytical mind. It therefore has to be processed emotionally.

First position: Seeing and experiencing the world from a subjective point of view.

Fractionation: Suggestions for multiplying an existing experience so it becomes more intense for the person.

Future pacing: Getting the person to imagine a different behaviour in the future, test it, and see how it works for them.

Gathering resistance: Suggestion that allows the person to have some resistance or self-control.

Global suggestion: A generalised suggestion that will apply to different actions and situations.

Glove anaesthesia: Reduction of sensory awareness in the hand by suggestion.

Hidden suggestion: A less emphatic suggestion which nevertheless carries a message into the unconscious by avoiding conscious resistance. It may even be a direct suggestion, but because the client is trained to listen to the emphasised suggestions, there is less resistance to a hidden suggestion.

Hetero-hypnosis: When another person leads someone into an altered state of trance.

Hobson's choice: Offering one or more choices that all lead to the same outcome.

Holding up the mirror: Feeding back to the person their reported story and experiences so they can observe it from a more objective perspective to gain more clarity.

Hypnotic anaesthesia transference: Suggestion to move hypnotic anaesthesia to different parts of the body.

Hypnotic authority: There are times when a hypnotist needs to establish their position as the guide, so the client can follow their instructions.

Hypnotic bind: Constructing language or communication that locks a person into certain actions e.g. "It's clear to listen to me you need to breathe."

Hypnotic catalepsy: Suggestion that a limb or the body becomes rigid and immobile in the trance-like state.

Hypnotic dreaming: A time when the person is in trance and can work out a solution or find new solutions by just being allowed to dream.

Hypnotic governor: A series of suggestions to limit a person's behaviours and experiences within certain margins.

Hypnotic indirect bind: A permissive indirect suggestion to create an experience e.g. "The funny thing about hearing someone is that it might mean you're still breathing."

Hypnotic reassociation to the body: Using suggestions for the person to physically enter back into their body after trauma-induced dissociation has happened.

Hypnotic regression: During trance suggestions induce the person to go back in time to a previous or multiple experiences inside their mind.

Hypnotic therapeutic alliance: There is no hetero-hypnosis unless the hypnotherapist establishes a co-operation between themselves and the person being hypnotised.

Hypnotically induced amnesia: The creation of amnesia by suggestion or sudden conversational change.

Ideomotor response: The body's response to a suggestion or question. It can be the nod of the head, twitch of a finger or movement in the toes. Be sure it is not simply a neurological spasm.

Implied directive: This is a verbal context that frames a message for the expectation that something will happen.

Indirect suggestion: An implied suggestion that something might happen is used to lower resistance to the outcome.

Inferred meaning: A statement that infers something else will be true, which is a form of indirect suggestion.

Installing boundaries: Suggestions for the creation of the edge of behaviours beyond which the person should not go. A hypnotic governor installs and protects the boundaries.

Instant artificial somnambulism: Suggestions that lead the client into artificial somnambulism without an official trance induction.

Interrogative loading: Providing so many questions that the person can no longer remain conscious to process the information. It is a confusion technique.

Interrogative overload: A series of questions, one directly after the other, without allowing the chance for the person to respond, causing confusion and transderivational search. Can be used to initiate artificial somnambulism of eyes-closed trance.

Interrogative truism: A loaded question to which there is only one possible answer.

Interspersal suggestion: The same or similar suggestions made at different periods during a therapeutic trance.

Intra-hypnotic suggestion: Suggestion that causes an action to happen whilst in the trance state.

Law of association: Suggestion that ideas are linked together so when one is true, the others are likely to be true.

Law of concentrated attention: Focusing the attention on a suggestion is likely to produce a cognitive and behavioural change or experience.

Law of delayed effect: The use of post-hypnotic suggestion to cause an event or action to happen later at an appointed time or due to encountering a stimulus.

Law of dominant effect: A suggestion that induces a stronger emotion makes a new behaviour more likely than the old behaviour that induces a weaker emotion.

Law of probable effect: Continuous exposure to suggestions and induced cognitive change will result in experiential and behavioural change, establishing a new normal.

Law of reverse effect: Suggestion telling someone not to do something motivates them to do that action. Or that something cannot happen, so the person tries to make it happen.

Linked behaviours: Linking two or more behaviours together.

Location dissociation: Suggestions, direct or indirect, that the client distances themselves from the original place of trauma.

Locational adjustment: Suggestions that the person experiences different sensations, thoughts and feelings in a different location.

Locational anchor: A suggestion that a particular experience is associated with a particular place.

Locational focal shift: Suggestion to change the focus of attention to different parts of the body.

Locational safety anchor: Suggestions for associating a place with a sense of safety.

Locking the gate: Using 'yes' sets and 'no' sets to cross-check a psychological change has taken place, due to the responses to 'yes' and 'no' questions.

Matching and leading: Copying and mirroring a person's communication or body language to be in sync with them and then changing your communication to lead them.

Meta challenge: Challenging the person to step outside their present perspective and look at their experience from a different position or viewpoint to reframe a statement or communication.

Mind mechanics: Suggestions for multiple sensory systems experiences, stacking them one on top of the other to cause experiential, thought and behavioural shift. e = external perceptions and i equals internal imaginary experiences. + = positive hallucinations and - = negative hallucinations e.g.: Vi- visual internal negative hallucination; Ai- auditory internal negative hallucination; Ki- kinaesthetic internal negative hallucination; Oi- olfactory internal negative hallucination; Gi- gustatory internal negative hallucination; Ve+ visual external positive hallucination; Ae+ auditory external positive hallucination; Ke+ kinaesthetic external positive hallucination; Oe+ olfactory external positive hallucination; Ge+ gustatory external positive hallucination.

Modal operator: A linguistic classification of language from the Milton model that includes verbs such as 'I must' (necessity) 'I could' (probability), 'I can' (possibility).

Modelling: The process of getting the client to copy your behaviours or the behaviours of a person who is performing in a way that the client would like to perform.

My Friend John technique: Suggestion by metaphor about someone who is in a similar situation.

Negative hallucination suggestion: A suggestion for not seeing, hearing, feeling, smelling, tasting something being present or happening, when it is happening.

Negative reframing: Reverse engineering the client's negative statements as incredulously ridiculous to incite them to develop different positive thoughts and behaviours.

No set: Establishing 'no' responses to a singular or multiple questions. "You don't want to do that do you?"

Nudging suggestion: A series of suggestions that progressively lead the person towards ever-increasing goal-identified experiences.

Official trance: Induction suggestions to the person that the hypnosis will now take place, even though instant artificial somnambulism may have already taken place outside their conscious awareness.

Paradoxical intent: Using the mechanism of symptoms to activate a solution behaviour.

Parts negotiation: Suggestions for positioning opposing sub-personality-driven thoughts and behaviours so they can or are forced to negotiate a solution for congruent behaviours.

Pavlovian response: Training someone to take certain actions on encountering a particular stimulus. It trains a person's stimulus/response reaction to become automatic.

Permissive directive: A statement that suggests new options that would take a person towards their goals, but does not tell them directly to take them. It is a strongly hidden suggestion, even though it may be emphasised tonally.

Permissive suggestion: A suggestion using modal operators of possibility such as 'might', 'possibly' or 'can'. Used to lower resistance to suggestion.

Positive hallucination suggestion: A suggestion for seeing, hearing, feeling, smelling, or tasting something being present or happening, when it is just in the imagination.

Post-hypnotic suggestion: A suggestion that the person completes a task, or has an experience later, at no appointed time, or at an appointed time.

Preparatory conjunctive: A linguistic conjunctive word, with pauses on each side, to create anticipation that the next suggestion is important.

Presupposition: A statement that assumes something will happen.

Pseudo-orientation in time: Taking the person forward in time to where the problem does not exist anymore. Getting them to gather the resources and skills that enabled that change and bring a copy of those back to the present time to make a change straight away.

Reassociation suggestion: A suggestion that a person physically returns back into their body after a dissociation has taken place. This is also necessary at the end of every hypnotic session to fully restore physical function.

Recontextualising: Framing a situation differently changes the way we look at problems and opportunities.

Regression by metaphor: Using a story or parable to imply regression.

Re-enforcement suggestion: A suggestion that comes after previous suggestions to re-enforce the message. It may be a different suggestion but it will contain the same message.

Reorientation to the present: Bringing someone back to focus on the present time after they have been in regression or projected to the future imaginary tense.

Resistance: Unco-operative hypnotic and communicative behaviour and failure to follow suggestions.

Resistance allowance: Setting a person up to resist a command but in a limited way so they complete the task to a satisfactory level. It is a hidden suggestion to cause an action to take place whilst allowing the person to have some resistance.

Resource mining: Getting the person to search their unconscious mind to find previous resources, thoughts, behaviours, skills or experiences they can use in the present day. This is initiated either through an interrogative suggestion or regression in trance.

Reverse fractionation: Suggestions for reducing the intensity of any particular experiences.

Reverse logic: A contradiction of an assumed logical statement to cause an examination and displacement of that assumed logic. It can be used to cause a cognitive and behavioural shift.

Safety anchor: Suggestion for the installation of a Pavlovian response to create a safe experience: "When you hear the sound of my voice you get an instant sense of safety." The stimulus can be in any of the sensory systems.

Seeding possibility: Statements that imply something could possibly happen. It may be the use of several statements that re-enforce an idea.

Second position: Seeing and experiencing the world from another person's point of view.

Self-affirmation: A suggestion a person makes to themselves that then becomes true. In other words, auto-suggestion.

Self-reflection: Considering your own thoughts, behaviour and position.

Sensory control suggestion: A suggestion to control experiences in any of the five sensory systems.

Sensory reduction suggestion: A suggestion to reduce the intensity of any sensory experiences.

Shock technique: Feeding back to the client their dysfunctional behaviour in such a way that it causes them to become highly uncomfortable with that behaviour, inciting change.

Silent suggestion: A suggestion that is not tonally emphasised, but the unconscious takes note of it due to sensory monitoring. It is a form of indirect suggestion, even though it may contain a direct command.

Simile suggestion: Using similar suggestions, one after the other, to re-enforce a command.

Split screen technique: Suggesting two imaginary screens in trance that either use moving pictures or single stills to compare the experience of one screen against another.

Spontaneous regression: The person experiences a sudden change of focus of attention onto past experiences. It can happen through suggestion or naturally.

Stacking: Suggestion for layering one experience on top of another so the weight of the multiple experiences causes a shift of thoughts, behaviours and experience.

State changing: Suggestion for suddenly changing a behaviour and thoughts by immediately changing the emotional state.

Sub-modalities: The discrete elements and characteristics of a sensory modality. For example: loudness, shrillness and timbre of sound.

Suggestion re-enforcement: A suggestion that re-enforces the meaning of a previous suggestion.

Superego: Freud's concept of the regulating part of the psyche that enforces moral principles and values.

Third position: Observing yourself, experiences and interactions from an objective perspective – known as the observer position.

Time distortion: The expansion or contraction of the perception of time during trance, initiated by suggestion.

Time scanning: Searching for memories and seeding resources throughout the person's timeline, and throughout different levels of their psyche.

Time shifting: Moving someone from one time frame to another where a present, past or future-paced statement suddenly changes the time reference of the communication.

Tonal direction and marking: The use of the hypnotist's voice tone, loudness, softness, force, fastness, or slowness, and where the voice is physically directed in space to imply meaning.

Tonal marking: The hypnotist using the force and tone of their voice to emphasise certain communications.

Trance deepener: Suggestion or action that conveys to the person that their sense of being in trance is deepening.

Trance logic: People understand, speak and act literally in trance, often not interpreting grammar or the subtleties of grammar.

Trance ratification: This is a challenge question or statement where the person is asked to examine their experience to register that it is different from the normal waking state. It may be an ideomotor response. It is validation of the hypnotic state.

Transderivational search: Confusing or challenging communications cause the client to go inside to search, clarify or validate information. Use in trance inductions and causing experiential change.

Transderivational search by proxy: Indirect suggestion techniques to cause the client to go inside to search for or validate information. It is a hidden directive.

Truism: A statement that is undisputably correct.

Validation by association: Suggesting an association between two people to validate a statement.

Visual leading: The hypnotist uses their body language or mime as a form of suggestion.

Visual marking: The hypnotist uses their visual communications to emphasise certain other communications.

Word salad: Milton Erickson's use of incorrect grammar or jibberish to cause confusion, including transderivational search, used in trance induction or deepening.

Yes set: A person's affirmative ideomotor response and communication indicating they agree with something or have completed a task. It is compliance communication e.g. "You want to do that, don't you?"

References List

Chapter 1 References

Allan, C., Winters, G. M., & Jeglic, E. L. (2023). Current trends in sex trafficking research. *Current Psychiatry Reports, 25*(5), 175–182. https://doi.org/10.1007/s11920-023-01419-7

Alvarez, A. (2005). When I was at school … *The Guardian.* https://www.theguardian.com/education/2005/oct/12/publicschools.schools

Becker, B. (2022). The colonial struggle over polygamy: Consequences for educational expansion in sub-Saharan Africa. *Economic History of Developing Regions, 37*(1), 27–49. https://doi.org/10.1080/20780389.2021.1940946

Béguin, G. (2017). *Khajuraho: Indian temples and sensuous sculptures.* 5 Continents edition.

Boehm, E. E. B., & Walker, K. K. (2021). Chimpanzee sexuality. In T. K. Shackelford & V. A. Weekes-Shackelford (Eds.), *Encyclopedia of evolutionary psychological science.* Springer. https://doi.org/10.1007/978-3-319-19650-3_3407

Bumiller, E. (1997, June 13). Same-sex academies grapple with parents' concerns. *The New York Times.* https://

www.nytimes.com/1997/06/13/nyregion/same-sex-academies-grapple-with-parents-concerns.html

Conway, L. (2012, June 18). Aboriginal erotic rock art proves that – even 28,000 years ago – men had ONE thing on their minds. *MailOnline.* https://www.dailymail.co.uk/news/article-2161118/Aboriginal-erotic-rock-art-proves--28-000-years-ago--men-ONE-thing-minds.html

Cortoni, F. (2017). *Women who sexually abuse: Assessment, treatment & management.* Safer Society.

Courtois, C. A. (2010). *Healing the incest wound: Adult survivors in therapy.* (2nd ed.). W. W. Norton & Company.

De Beauvoir, S. (2011). *The second sex.* Vintage. (Original work published 1949)

Douglas, R. M. (2018). *On being raped.* Beacon Press.

Drescher, J. (2015). Out of DSM: Depathologizing homosexuality. *Behavioral Sciences (Basel), 59*(4), 565–575. https://doi.org/10.3390/bs5040565

Elliott, M. (1994). *Female sexual abuse of children* (M. Elliott, Ed.). The Guilford Press.

Encyclopædia Britannica. (n.d.). Honor killing. In *Encyclopedia Britannica.* Retrieved May 30, 2025, from https://www.britannica.com/topic/honor-killing

Freud, S. (1964). *The standard edition of the complete psychological works of Sigmund Freud.* (J. Strachey, Ed.). Macmillan.

Gauld, A. (1992). *A history of hypnotism*. Cambridge University Press.

Gordon, J. (2022, November 24). *Masculinity and misogyny in contemporary right-wing populism*. King's College London. https://www.kcl.ac.uk/masculinity-and-misogyny-in-contemporary-right-wing-populism

Haberman, M. (2022). *Confidence man: The making of Donald Trump and the breaking of America*. Penguin Press.

Johnson, S. (2024, September 11). Religious groups 'spending billions to counter gender-equality education'. *The Guardian*. https://www.theguardian.com/global-development/article/2024/sep/11/religious-groups-christians-islamists-catholic-billions-counter-gender-equality-sex-education-lgbtq-equal-rights

Lawton, L. (2022, March 27). *Ask me anything about sex in prison* [Video]. YouTube. https://www.youtube.com/watch?v=2fn2_zpV6PY

Lichfield, J. (2001, July 5). *Erotic cave paintings could be 37,000 years old*. Independent. https://www.independent.co.uk/news/world/europe/erotic-cave-paintings-could-be-37-000-years-old-9188709.html

Malla, K. (2023). *Sacred sexuality: The ananga ranga or the ancient erotic art of Indian love & sex* (R. Burton, Trans.). Indoeuropeanpublishing.com. (Original work translated into English 1885).

Masters, W. H., & Johnson, V. E. (1966). *Human sexual response*. Little, Brown.

Mehta, N. (2011). Mind-body dualism: A critique from a health perspective. *Mens Sana Monographs*, *9*(10), 202–209. https://doi.org/10.4103/0973-1229.77436

Moore, A. (2023, April 20). The rape survivor who spoke out: Ellie Wilson on the brutal reality of taking an attacker to court. *The Guardian*. https://www.theguardian.com/society/2023/apr/20/the-survivor-who-spoke-out-ellie-wilson-on-the-brutal-reality-of-taking-an-attacker-to-court

Propper, D. (2022, June 26). *G7 leaders mock Vladimir Putin over shirtless horse-riding picture.* New York Post. https://nypost.com/2022/06/26/g7-leaders-mock-vladimir-putin-over-shirtless-horse-riding-pic/

Russo, F. (2017, January 6). Where transgender is no longer a diagnosis. *Scientific American*. https://www.scientificamerican.com/article/where-transgender-is-no-longer-a-diagnosis/

Sasson, J. (2010). *Daughters of Arabia*. Transworld Digital. https://www.amazon.co.uk/gp/product/B004ASOW16

Schaller, S. L., Kvalem, I. L., & Træen, B. (2023). Constructions of sexual identities in the ageing body: A qualitative exploration of older Norwegian adults' negotiation of body image and sexual satisfaction. *Sexuality & Culture*, *27*(4), 1369–1402. https://doi.org/10.1007/s12119-023-10067-1

Simpson, P. (2021). 'At your age???!!!': The constraints of ageist erotophobia on older people's sexual and intimate relationships. In P. Simpson, P. Reynolds, & T. Hafford-

Letchfield (Eds.), *Desexualisation in later life: The limits of sex and intimacy* (pp. 35–51). Policy Press. https://doi. org/10.1332/policypress/9781447355465.003.0003

Sinozich, S., & Langton, L. (2014). *Rape and sexual assault victimization among college-age females, 1995–2013* (Report No. NCJ 248471). U.S. Department of Justice, Office of Justice Programs, Bureau of Justice Statistics. https://bjs.ojp.gov/content/pub/pdf/rsavcaf9513.pdf

Sperling, V. (2014). *Sex, politics, and Putin: Political legitimacy in Russia.* Oxford University Press.

Suntsova, M. V., & Buzdin, A. A. (2020). Differences between human and chimpanzee genomes and their implications in gene expression, protein functions and biochemical properties of the two species. *BMC Genomics, 21*(7), Article 535. https://doi.org/10.1186/s12864-020-06962-8

Tasca, C., Rapetti, M., Carta, M., & Fadda, B. (2012). Women and hysteria in the history of mental health. *Clinical Practice & Epidemiology in Mental Health, 8,* 110–119. http://dx.doi.org/10.2174/1745017901208010110

United Nations Educational, Scientific and Cultural Organization. (2023, November 16). *Comprehensive sexuality education: For healthy, informed and empowered learners.* Retrieved September 12, 2024, from https://www.unesco.org/en/articles/why-comprehensive-sexuality-education-important

Wang, Z., Chen, X., & Radnofsky, C. (2021, March 5). *China proposes teaching masculinity to boys as state is alarmed by changing gender roles.* NBC News. https://www. nbcnews.com/news/world/china-proposes-teaching-masculinity-boys-state-alarmed-changing-gender-roles-n1258939

Watts, A., & Elisofon, E. (1971). *The temple of Konarak: Erotic spirituality*. Macmillan.

Williams, R. (2022). *Macho men: How toxic masculinity harms us all and what to do about it.*

World Health Organization. (2024, April 10). *Adolescent pregnancy*. https://www.who.int/news-room/fact-sheets/detail/adolescent-pregnancy

Wylie, K. (2010). Sex education and the influence on sexual wellbeing. *Procedia Social and Behavioral Sciences, 5*, 440–444. https://doi.org/10.1016/j.sbspro.2010.07.119

Chapter 2 References

Ajmal, N., Khan, S. Z, & Shaikh, R. (2019). Polycystic ovary syndrome (PCOS) and genetic predisposition: A review article. *European Journal of Obstetrics & Gynecology and Reproductive Biology: X, 3*, Article 100060. https://doi.org/10.1016/j.eurox.2019.100060

Allen, N. E., & Key, T. J. (2000). The effects of diet on circulating sex hormone levels in men. *Nutrition Research Reviews, 13*(2), 159–184. https://doi.org/10.1079/095442200108729052

Besong, E. E., Akhigbe, T. M., Ashonibare, P. J., Oladipo, A. A., Obimma, J. N., Hamed, M. A., Adeyemi, D. H., & Akhigbe, R. E. (2023). Zinc improves sexual performance and erectile function by preventing penile oxidative injury and upregulating circulating testosterone in lead-exposed rats. *Redox Report: Communications in Free Radical Research, 28*(1), Article 2225675. https://doi.org/10.1080/13510002.2023.2225675

Barba-Müller, E., Craddock, S., Carmona, S., & Hoekzema, E. (2018). Brain plasticity in pregnancy and the postpartum period: Links to maternal caregiving and mental health. *Archives of Women's Mental Health, 22*(2), 289–299. https://doi.org/10.1007/s00737-018-0889-z

Brike, H., Ekholm, O., Højsted, J., Sjøgren, P., & Kurita, G. P. (2019). Chronic pain, opioid therapy, sexual desire, and satisfaction in sexual life: A population-based survey. *Pain Medicine, 20*(6), 1132–1140. https://doi.org/10.1093/pm/pny122

Caplin, A., Chen, F. S., Beauchamp, M. R., & Puterman, E. (2021). The effects of exercise intensity on the cortisol response to a subsequent acute psychosocial stressor. *Psychoneuroendocrinology, 131*, Article 105336. https://doi.org/10.1016/j.psyneuen.2021.105336

Cappelletti, M., & Wallen, K. (2016). Increasing women's sexual desire: The comparative effectiveness of estrogens and androgens. *Hormones and Behavior, 78*, 178–193. https://doi.org/10.1016/j.yhbeh.2015.11.003

Choi, H.-I, Ko, H.-J, Kim, A.-S, & Moon, H. (2019). The association between mineral and trace element concentrations in hair and the 10-year risk of atherosclerotic cardiovascular disease in healthy community-dwelling elderly individuals. *Nutrients, 11*(3), Article 637. https://doi.org/10.3390/nu11030637

Chow, E., Friedman, D., Yasui, Y., Whitton, J., Stovall, M., Robison, L., & Sklar, C. (2007). Decreased adult height in survivors of childhood acute lymphoblastic leukemia: A report from the Childhood Cancer Survivor Study. *The Journal of Pediatrics, 150*(4), 370–375. https://doi. org/10.1016/j.jpeds.2006.11.036

Connell, K. M., Coates, R., & Wood, F. M. (2014). Sexuality following trauma injury: A literature review. *Burns & Trauma, 2*(2), 61–70. https://doi.org/10.4103/2321- 3868.130189

Cosgrove, D., Gordon, Z., Bernie, J., Hami, S., Montoya, M., Stein, M., & Monga, M. (2002). Sexual dysfunction in combat veterans with post-traumatic stress disorder. *Urology, 60*(5), 881–884. https://doi.org/10.1016/S0090- 4295(02)01899-X

Crafa, A., Cannarella, R., Barbagallo, F., Leanza, C., Palazzolo, R., Flores, H. A., La Vignera, S., Condorelli, R., & Calogero, A. (2023). Mechanisms suggesting a relationship between vitamin D and erectile dysfunction: An overview. *Biomolecules, 13*(6), Article 930. https:// doi.org/10.3390/biom13060930

Dhaliwal, A., & Gupta, M. (2023, April 10). PDE5 inhibitors. In *StatPearls*. StatPearls Publishing. https://www.ncbi. nlm.nih.gov/books/NBK549843/

El-Sakka, A. (2018). Dehydroepiandrosterone and erectile function: A review. *World Journal of Men's Health, 36*(3), 183–191. https://doi.org/10.5534/wjmh.180005

Fernández-Carrasco, F. J., Rodríguez-Díaz, L., González-Mey, U., Vázquez-Lara, J. M., Gómez-Salgado, J., & Parrón-

Carreño, T. (2020). Changes in sexual desire in women and their partners during pregnancy. *Journal of Clinical Medicine, 9*(2), Article 526. https://doi.org/10.3390/jcm9020526

Foruzan-Nia, S., Abdollahi, M., Hekmatimoghaddam, S., Namayandeh, S., & Mortazavi, M. (2011). Incidence of sexual dysfunction in men after cardiac surgery in Afshar Hospital, Yazd. *Iran Journal of Reproductive Medicine, 9*(2), 89–94. https://www.ncbi.nlm.nih.gov/pmc/articles/PMC4216441/

Fraiman, J., Erviti, J., Jones, M., Greenland, S., Whelan, P., Kaplan, R. M., & Doshi, P. (2022). Serious adverse events of special interest following mRNA COVID-19 vaccination in randomized trials in adults. *Vaccine, 40*(40), 5798–5805. https://pubmed.ncbi.nlm.nih.gov/36055877/

Fuchs, A., Czech, I., Sikora, J., Fuchs, P., Lorek, M., Skrzypulec-Plinta, V., & Drosdzol-Cop, A. (2019). Sexual functioning in pregnant women. *International Journal of Environmental Research and Public Health, 16*(21), Article 4216. https://doi.org/10.3390/ijerph16214216

Gabrielson, A. T., Sartor, R. A., & Hellstrom, W. J. (2019). The impact of thyroid disease on sexual dysfunction in men and women. *Sexual Medicine Reviews, 7*(1), 57–70. https://doi.org/10.1016/j.sxmr.2018.05.002

Ganapathy, A., Hari Priya, V. M., & Kumaran, A. (2021). Medicinal plants as a potential source of phosphodiesterase-5 inhibitors: A review. *Journal of Ethnopharmacology, 267*, Article 113536. https://doi.org/10.1016/j.jep.2020.113536

Geller, S., & Studee, L. (2006). Contemporary alternatives to plant estrogens for menopause. *Maturitas, 55*(Suppl. 1), S3–S13. https://doi.org/10.1016/j.maturitas.2006.06.012

Gewirtz-Meydan, A., & Lahav, Y. (2020). Sexual dysfunction and distress among childhood sexual abuse survivors: The role of post-traumatic stress disorder. *The Journal of Sexual Medicine, 17*(11), 2267–2278. https://doi.org/10.1016/j.jsxm.2020.07.016

Ghosh, S., & Klein, R. (2017). Sex drives dimorphic immune responses to viral infections. *The Journal of Immunology, 198*(5), 1782–1790. https://doi.org/10.4049/jimmunol.1601166

Guillermo, C., Manlove, H., Gray, P., Zava, D., & Marrs, C. (2010). Female social and sexual interest across the menstrual cycle: The roles of pain, sleep, and hormones. *BMC Women's Health, 10*, Article 19. https://doi.org/10.1186/1472-6874-10-19

Hall, W. (2009). Dietary saturated and unsaturated fats as determinants of blood pressure and vascular function. *Nutrition Research Reviews, 22*(1), 18–38. https://doi.org/10.1017/s095442240925846x

Haloul, M., Vinjamuri, S. J., Naquiallah, D., Mirza, M. I., Qureshi, M., Hassan, C., Masrur, M., Bianco, F., Frederick, P., Cristoforo, G., Gangemi, A., Ali, M., Phillips, S., & Mahmoud, A. (2020). Hyperhomocysteinemia and low folate and vitamin B12 are associated with vascular dysfunction and impaired nitric oxide sensitivity in morbidly obese patients. *Nutrients, 12*(7), Article 2014. https://doi.org/10.3390/nu12072014

Hamilton, L., Rellini, A., & Meston, C. (2008). Cortisol, sexual arousal, and affect in response to sexual stimuli. *The Journal of Sexual Medicine, 5*(9), 2111–2118. https://doi.org/10.1111/j.1743-6109.2008.00922.x

Harden, K. P. (2014). Genetic influences on adolescent sexual behavior: Why genes matter for environmentally-oriented researchers. *Psychological Bulletin, 140*(2), 434–465. https://doi/10.1037/a0033564

Helmeich, D., Parfitt, D., Lu, X.-Y, Akil, H., & Watson, S. (2005). Relation between the hypothalamic-pituitary-thyroid (HPT) axis and the hypothalamic-pituitary-adrenal (HPA) axis during repeated stress. *Neuroendocrinology, 81*(3), 183–192. https://doi.org/10.1159/000087001

Hernández-Blanquisett, A., Quintero-Carreño, V., Álvarez-Londoño, A., Martínez-Ávila, M., & Diaz-Cáceres, R. (2022). Sexual dysfunction as a challenge in treated breast cancer: In-depth analysis and risk assessment to improve individual outcomes. *Frontiers in Oncology, 12*, Article 955057. https://doi.org/10.3389/fonc.2022.955057

Higgins, A., Nash, M., & Lynch, A. (2010). Antidepressant-associated sexual dysfunction: Impact, effects, and treatment. *Drug Healthcare and Patient Safety, 2010*(2), 141–150. https://doi.org/10.2147/DHPS.S7634

Juster, R.-P., Hatzenbuehler, M., Mendrek, A., Pfaus, J., Smith, N., Johnson, P., Lefebvre-Louis, J.-P., Raymond, C., Marin, M.-F., Sindi, S., Lupien, S., & Pruessner, J. (2015). Sexual orientation modulates endocrine stress reactivity.

Biological Psychiatry, 77(7), 668–676. https://doi.
org/10.1016/j.biopsych.2014.08.013

Kaur, J., Leslie, S. W., & Singh, P. (2023). Pudendal Nerve
Entrapment Syndrome. In *StatPearls*. Retrieved May 30,
2025 from StatPearls Publishing. https://www.ncbi.nlm.
nih.gov/books/NBK544272/

Kobori, Y., Koh, E., Sugimoto, K., Izumi, K., Narimoto, K.,
Maeda, Y., Konaka, H., Mizokamo, A., Matsushita, T.,
Iwamoto, T., & Namiki, M. (2009). The relationship
of serum and salivary cortisol levels to male sexual
dysfunction as measured by the International Index of
Erectile Function. *International Journal of Impotence
Research, 21*(4), 207–212. https://doi.org/10.1038/
ijir.2009.14

Kostis, J., & Dobrzynski, J. (2019). Statins and erectile
dysfunction. *World Journal of Men's Health, 37*(1), 1–3.
https://doi.org/10.5534/wjmh.180015

Krzastek, S., Bopp, J., Smith, R., & Kovac, J. (2019). Recent
advances in the understanding and management of
erectile dysfunction. *F1000 Research, 8*, Article 102.
https://doi.org/10.12688/f1000research.16576.1

Lee, S. R, Cho, M. K., Cho, Y. J., Chun, S., Hong, S.-H, Hwang,
K. R., Jeon, G-H., Joo, J. K., Kim, S. K., Lee, D. O., Lee,
D.-Y, Lee, E. S., Song, J. Y., Yi, K. W., Yun, B. H., Shin, J.-
H, Chae, H. D., & Kim, T. (2020). *The 2020 menopausal
hormone therapy guidelines. Journal of Menopausal
Medicine, 26*(2), 69–98. https://doi.org/10.6118/
jmm.20000

Li, J., Sun, C., Cai, W., Li, J., Rosen, B., & Chen, J. (2021). Insights into S-adenosyl-l-methionine (SAM)-dependent methyltransferase-related diseases and genetic polymorphisms. *Mutation Research - Reviews in Mutation Research, 788,* Article 108396. https://doi.org/10.1016/j.mrrev.2021.108396

Lidawi, G., Asali, M., Majdoub, M., & Rub, R. (2022). Short-term intracavernous self-injection treatment of psychogenic erectile dysfunction secondary to sexual performance anxiety in unconsummated marriages. *International Journal of Impotence Research, 34*(5), 407–410. https://doi.org/10.1038/s41443-020-00399-z

Lin, H., & Wang, R. (2013). The science of vacuum erectile device in penile rehabilitation after radical prostatectomy. *Translational Andrology and Urology, 2*(1), 61–66. https://doi.org/10.3978/j.issn.2223-4683.2013.01.04

Lombardo, R., Tsamatropoulos, P., Piroli, E., Culasso, F., Janini, E., Dondero, F., Lenzi, A., & Gandini, L. (2010). Treatment of erectile dysfunction due to C677T mutation of the MTHFR gene with vitamin B6 and folic acid in patients non-responders to PDE5i. *The Journal of Sexual Medicine, 7*(1), 216–223. https://doi.org/10.1111/j.1743-6109.2009.01463.x

Mahoney, C., Reid, F., Smith, A., & Myers, J. (2023). The impact of pregnancy and childbirth on pelvic sensation: A prospective cohort study. *Scientific Reports, 13,* Article 1535. https://doi.org/10.1038/s41598-023-28323-7

Majeed, H., & Gupta, V. (2022). Adverse effects of radiation therapy. In *StatPearls*. StatPearls Publishing. https://www.ncbi.nlm.nih.gov/books/NBK563259/

McCarthy, M. (2014). Testosterone therapy is associated with raised risk of myocardial infarction, US study finds. *BMJ*, 348. https://doi.org/10.1136/bmj.g1297.

Millar, B., Starks, T., Rendina, H., & Parsons, J. (2018). Three reasons to consider the role of tiredness in sexual risk-taking among gay and bisexual men. *Archives of Sexual Behavior, 48*(1), 383–395. https://doi.org/10.1007/s10508-018-1258-8

Mondillo, C., Varela, M., Abiuso, A., & Vázquez, R. (2018). Potential negative effects of anti-histamines on male reproductive function. *Reproduction, 155*(5), R221–R227. https://doi.org/10.1530/rep-17-0685

Moon, K., Park, S., & Kim, Y. (2019). Obesity and erectile dysfunction: From bench to clinical implication. *World Journal of Men's Health, 37*(2), 138–147. https://doi.org/10.5534/wjmh.180026

Morelli, M., Gambardella, J., Castellanos, V., Trimarco, V., & Santulli, G. (2020). Vitamin C and cardiovascular disease: An update. *Antioxidants (Basel), 9*(12), Article 1227. https://doi.org/10.3390/antiox9121227

Mousavi, M., Mahmoudi, M., Golitaleb, M., Khajehgoodari, M., Hekmatpou, D., & Vakilian, P. (2018). Exploratory study of andropause syndrome in 40-65 years in Arak: A cross-sectional study. *Journal of Family and Reproductive Health, 12*(3), 142–147. https://www.ncbi.nlm.nih.gov/pmc/articles/PMC6571447/

Mozafari, M., Khajavikhan, J., Jaafarpour, M., Khani, A., Direkvand-Moghadam, A., & Najafi, F. (2015). Association of body weight and female sexual dysfunction: A case control study. *Iranian Red Crescent Medical Journal, 17*(1), Article e24685. https://doi.org/10.5812/ircmj.24685

Nia, L., Iravani, M., Abedi, P., & Cheraghian, B. (2021). Effect of zinc on testosterone levels and sexual function of postmenopausal women: A randomized controlled trial. *Journal of Sex & Marital Therapy, 47*(8), 804–813. https://doi.org/10.1080/0092623x.2021.1957732

Panjari, M., Bell, R., Jane, F., Wolfe, R., Adams, J., Morrow, C., & Davis, S. (2009). A randomized trial of oral DHEA treatment for sexual function, well-being, and menopausal symptoms in postmenopausal women with low libido. *The Journal of Sexual Medicine, 6*(9), 2579–2590. https://doi.org/10.1111/j.1743-6109.2009.01381.x

Park, Y., Kim, Y., & Lee, J. (2012). Antipsychotic-induced sexual dysfunction and its management. *World Journal of Men's Health, 30*(3), 153–159. https://doi.org/10.5534/wjmh.2012.30.3.153

Pincus, S. M., Mulligan, T., Iranmanesh, A., Gheorghiu, S., Godschalk, M., & Veldhuis, J. D. (1996). Older males secrete luteinizing hormone and testosterone more irregularly, and jointly more asynchronously, than younger males. *Proceedings of the National Academy of Sciences of the United States of America, 93*(24), 14100–14105. https://doi.org/10.1073/pnas.93.24.14100

Pinheiro, A., Raney, T. J., Thornton, L., Fichter, M., Berrettini, W., Goldman, D., Halmi, K., Kaplan, A., Strober, M., Treasure, J., Woodside, D. B., Kaye, W., & Bulik, C. (2011). Sexual functioning in women with eating disorders. *International Journal of Eating Disorders, 43*(2), 123–129. https://doi.org/10.1002/eat.20671

Radenkovic, D., Reason, & Verdin, E. (2020). Clinical evidence for targeting NAD therapeutically. *Pharmaceuticals (Basel), 13*(9), Article 247. http://dx.doi.org/10.3390/ph13090247

Raghubeer, S., & Matsha, T. (2021). Methylenetetrahydrofolate (MTHFR), the one-carbon cycle, and cardiovascular risks. *Nutrients, 13*(12), Article 4562. https://doi.org/10.3390/nu13124562

Rajfer, J. (2000). Relationship between testosterone and erectile dysfunction. *Reviews in Urology, 2*(2), 122–128. https://www.ncbi.nlm.nih.gov/pmc/articles/PMC1476110/

Ramirez-Fort, M., Rogers, M., Santiago, R., Mahase, S., Mendez, M., Zheng, Y., Kong, X., Kashanian, J., Niaz, M., McClelland, S., Wu, X., Bander, N., Schlegel, P., Mulhall, J., & Lange, C. (2020). Prostatic irradiation-induced sexual dysfunction: A review and multidisciplinary guide to management in the radical radiotherapy era (Part I defining the organ at risk for sexual toxicities). *Reports of Practical Oncology & Radiotherapy, 25*(3), 367–375. https://doi.org/10.1016/j.rpor.2020.03.007

Rodriguez, K., Kohn, T., Davis, A., & Hakky, T. (2017). Penile implants: A look into the future. *Translational Andrology and Urology, 6*(Suppl. 5), S860–S866. https://doi.org/10.21037/tau.2017.05.28

Rubin, D., Ross, J., & Grad, Y. (2020). The frontiers of addressing antibiotic resistance in Neisseria gonorrhoeae. *Translational Research, 220*, 122–137. https://doi.org/10.1016/j.trsl.2020.02.002

Shoily, S., Ahsan, T., Fatema, K., & Sajib, A. (2021). Common genetic variants and pathways in diabetes and associated complications and vulnerability of populations with different ethnic origins. *Scientific Reports, 11*, Article 7504. https://doi.org/10.1038/s41598-021-86801-2

Singh, M., Bathla, M., Martin, A., & Aneja, J. (2015). Hypoactive sexual desire disorder caused by antiepileptic drugs. *Journal of Human Reproductive Sciences, 8*(2), 111–113. https://doi.org/10.4103/0974-1208.158619

Skolnick, A., Schulman, R., Galindo, R., & Mechanick, J. (2017). The endocrinopathies of male anorexia nervosa: Case series. *AACE Clinical Case Reports, 2*(4), e351–e357. https://doi.org/10.4158/EP15945.CR

Temkitthawon, P., Hinds, T., Beavo, J., Viyoch, J., Suwanborirux, K., Pongamornkul, W., Sawasdee, P., & Ingkaninan, K. (2011). Kaempferia parviflora, a plant used in traditional medicine to enhance sexual performance, contains large amounts of low-affinity PDE5 inhibitors. *Journal of Ethnopharmacology, 137*(3), 1437–1441. https://doi.org/10.1016/j.jep.2011.08.025

Tran, C., Yeap, B. B., Ball, J., Clayton-Chubb, D., Hussain, S. M., Brodtmann, A., Tonkin, A. M., Neumann, J. T., Schneider, H. G., Fitzgerald, S., Woods, R. L., & McNeil, J. J. (2024). Testosterone and the risk of incident atrial fibrillation in older men: further analysis of the ASPREE study. *EClinicalMedicine*, *72*, Article 102611. https://doi.org/10.1016/j.eclinm.2024.102611

U.S. Food and Drug Administration. (2019, July 12). *Drug trials snapshots: VYLEESI*. https://www.fda.gov/drugs/drug-approvals-and-databases/drug-trials-snapshots-vyleesi

U.S. Food and Drug Administration. (2024, January 12). *Drug trials snapshots: ADDYI*. https://www.fda.gov/drugs/drug-approvals-and-databases/drug-trials-snapshots-addyi

U.S. Food and Drug Administration. (2019, June 21). *FDA approves new treatment for hypoactive sexual desire disorder in premenopausal women* [Press release]. https://www.fda.gov/news-events/press-announcements/fda-approves-new-treatment-hypoactive-sexual-desire-disorder-premenopausal-women

van Basten, J.-P. A., van Driel, M., Hoekstra, H., & Sleijfer, D. T. (2000). Erectile dysfunction with chemotherapy. *The Lancet*, *356*(9224), 169. https://doi.org/10.1016/S0140-6736(05)73187-1

Walter, K. N., Corwin, E. J., Ulbrecht, J., Demers, L. M., Bennett, J. M., Whetzel, C. A., & Klein, L. C. (2012). Elevated thyroid-stimulating hormone is associated with elevated cortisol in healthy young men and women. *Thyroid Research*, *5*, Article 13. https://doi.org/10.1186/1756-6614-5-13

Windsor, C., Hua, C., De Roux, Q., Harrois, A., Anguel, N., Montravers, P., Viellard-Baron, A., Mira, J.-P., Urbina, T., Gaudry, S., Turpin, M., Damoisel, C., Annane, D., Ricard, J.-D., Hersant, B., Dessap, A. M., Chosidow, O., Layese, R., de Prost, N., & AP-HP NSTI Study Group. (2022). Healthcare trajectory of critically ill patients with necrotizing soft tissue infections: A multicenter retrospective cohort study using the clinical data warehouse of Greater Paris University Hospitals. *Annals of Intensive Care, 12*, Article 115. https://doi.org/10.1186/s13613-022-01087-5

Witchel, S. (2018). Disorders of sex development. *Best Practice & Research Clinical Obstetrics & Gynaecology, 48*, 90–102. https://doi.org/10.1016/j.bpobgyn.2017.11.005

Chapter 3 References

Ahrold, T. K., Farmer, M., Trapnell, P. D., & Meston, C. M. (2011). The relationship among sexual attitudes, sexual fantasy, and religiosity. *Archives of Sexual Behavior, 40*(3), 619–630. https://doi.org/10.1007/s10508-010-9621-4

Bhatt, R., Martin, S., Evans, S., Lung, K., Coates, T., Zetzer, L., & Tsao, J. (2017). The effect of hypnosis on pain and peripheral blood flow in sickle-cell disease: A pilot study. *Journal of Pain Research, 10*, 1635–1644. https://doi.org/10.2147/JPR.S131859

Brownlee, K., Moore, W., & Hackney, A. (2005). Relationship between circulating cortisol and testosterone: Influence of physical exercise. *Journal of Sports Science and*

Medicine, 4(1), 76–83. https://www.ncbi.nlm.nih.gov/pmc/articles/PMC3880087/

Bruce, D., Harper, G. W., & Bauermeister, J. A. (2015). Minority stress, positive identity development, and depressive symptoms: Implications for resilience among sexual minority male youth. *Psychology of Sexual Orientation and Gender Diversity, 2*(3), 287–296. https://doi.org/10.1037/sgd0000128

Clawson, T., Jr., & Swadem, R. (2011). The hypnotic control of blood flow and pain: The cure of warts and the potential for the use of hypnosis in the treatment of cancer. *American Journal of Clinical Hypnosis, 17*(3), 160–169. https://doi.org/10.1080/00029157.1975.10403735

de Beauvoir, S. (2015). *The second sex.* Vintage Classics. (Original work published 1949)

De Bellis, M., & Zisk, A. (2014). The biological effects of childhood trauma. *Child and Adolescent Psychiatric Clinics of North America, 23*(2), 185–222. https://doi.org/10.1016/j.chc.2014.01.002

DeCou, C., Cole, T., Lynch, S., Wong, M., & Matthews, K. (2017). Assault-related shame mediates the association between negative social reactions to disclosure of sexual assault and psychological distress. *Psychological Trauma: Theory, Research, Practice, and Policy, 9*(2), 166–172. https://doi.org/10.1037/tra0000186

Dhawan, E., & Haggard, P. (2023). Neuroscience evidence counters a rape myth. *Nature Human Behaviour, 7,* 835–838. https://doi.org/10.1038/s41562-023-01598-6

Ember, C. R. (1978). Men's fear of sex with women: A cross-cultural study. *Sex Roles: A Journal of Research, 4*(5), 657–678. https://doi.org/10.1007/BF00287331

Erickson, M. H. (1980). *Hypnotic alteration of sensory, perceptual, and psychophysical processes* (E. L. Rossi, Ed.). Irvington Publishers.

Fejes, F. (2008). *Gay rights and moral panic: The origins of America's debate on homosexuality*. Palgrave Macmillan.

Fejes, N., & Balogh, A. P. (Eds.). (2013). *Queer visibility in post-socialist cultures*. Intellect.

Foa, E., Rothbaum, B., & Steketee, G. (1993). Treatment of rape victims. *Journal of Interpersonal Violence, 8*(2), 206–219. https://doi.org/10.1177/088626093008002006

Foucault, M. (1990). *The history of sexuality: Vol. 1. An introduction* (Reissue ed.). Random House. (Original work published 1978)

Glenn, A., Raine, A., Schug, R., Gao, Y., & Granger, D. (2011). Increased testosterone to cortisol ratio in psychopathy. *Journal of Abnormal Psychology, 120*(2), 389–399. https://doi.org/10.1037/a0021407

Gurgevich, S. (2007). *Relieve anxiety with medical hypnosis* (S. Gurgevich, Narr.). [Audiobook] Sounds True. https://www.audible.co.uk/pd/Relieve-Anxiety-with-Medical-Hypnosis-Audiobook/B004F2RKHA

Joel, D., Garcia-Falgueras, A., & Swaab, D. (2020). The complex relationships between sex and the brain. *The Neuroscientist, 26*(2), 156–169. https://doi.org/10.1177/1073858419867298

Kasos, E., Kasos, K., Pusztai, F., Polyák, A., Kovács, K., & Varga, K. (2017). Changes in oxytocin and cortisol in active-alert hypnosis: Hormonal changes benefiting low hypnotizable participants. *International Journal of Clinical and Experimental Hypnosis, 66*(4), 404–427. https://doi.org/10.1080/00207144.2018.1495009

Khoury, C., & Findlay, B. (2014). What makes for good sex? The associations among attachment style, inhibited communication, and sexual satisfaction. *Journal of Relationships Research, 5*, Article e7. https://doi.org/10.1017/jrr.2014.7

Krule, J. (2016, February 28). *STIs, shame, and the Sabbath: What it's like to learn about sex as an Orthodox Jew.* Vice. https://www.vice.com/en/article/sex-shame-and-shabbat-orthodox-jews-reflect-on-how-they-learned-about-sex/

Law, B., Siu, A., & Shek, D. (2012). Recognition for positive behavior as a critical youth development construct: Conceptual bases and implications on youth service development. *The Scientific World Journal, 2012*(1), Article 809578. https://doi.org/10.1100/2012/809578

Lefroy, E. (2022, June 16). *Over 20% of parents won't talk to their kids about sex: Poll.* New York Post. https://nypost.com/2022/06/16/over-20-of-parents-wont-talk-to-their-kids-about-sex-poll/

Mahon, M., & McGorrery, P. (Eds.). (2020). *Criminalising coercive control: Family violence and the criminal law.* Springer. https://doi.org/10.1007/978-981-15-0653-6

Masters, W. H., & Johnson, V. E. (1966). *Human sexual response.* Little, Brown.

National Sexual Violence Resource Center. (2015). *Statistics about sexual violence*. https://www.nsvrc.org/sites/default/files/publications_nsvrc_factsheet_media-packet_statistics-about-sexual-violence_0.pdf

Neville, S., Adams, J., Montayre, J., Larmer, P., Garrett, N., Stephens, C., & Alpass, F. (2018). Loneliness in men 60 years and over: The association with purpose in life. *American Journal of Men's Health, 12*(4), 730–739. https://doi.org/10.1177/1557988318758807

Peterson, Z., Voller, E., Polusny, M., & Murdoch, M. (2011). Prevalence and consequences of adult sexual assault of men: Review of empirical findings and state of the literature. *Clinical Psychology Review, 31*(1), 1–24. https://doi.org/10.1016/j.cpr.2010.08.006

Rahardjo, H., Becker, A., Märker, V., Kuczyk, M., & Ückert, S. (2023). Is cortisol an endogenous mediator of erectile dysfunction in the adult male? *Translational Andrology and Urology, 12*(5), 684–689. https://doi.org/10.21037/tau-22-566

Reeves, R. (2022). *Of boys and men: Why the modern male is struggling, why it matters, and what to do about it.* Brookings Institution Press.

Sævik, K. W., & Konijnenberg, C. (2023). The effects of sexual shame, emotion regulation and gender on sexual desire. *Scientific Reports, 13*, Article 4042. https://doi.org/10.1038/s41598-023-31181-y

Scardino, M., & Scardino, A. (2014). Hypnosis and cortisol: The odd couple. *MOJ Immunology, 1*(2), 46–48. https://doi.org/10.15406/moji.2014.01.00012

Sharples, A., & Turner, D. (2023). Skeletal muscle memory. *American Journal of Physiology-Cell Physiology, 324*(6), C1274–C1294. https://doi.org/10.1152/ajpcell.00099.2023

Slominski, K. (2020, August 21). *How religion made modern sex ed.* The Immanent Frame. https://tif.ssrc.org/2020/08/21/how-religion-made-modern-sex-ed/

Smerecnik, C., Schaalma, H., Gerjo, K., Meijer, S., & Poelman, J. (2010). An exploratory study of Muslim adolescents' views on sexuality: Implications for sex education and prevention. *BMC Public Health, 10*, Article 533. https://doi.org/10.1186/1471-2458-10-533

Trickett, P., Noll, J., Susman, E., Shenk, C., & Putnam, F. (2011). Attenuation of cortisol across development for victims of sexual abuse. *Development and Psychopathology, 22*(1), 165–175. https://doi.org/10.1017/S0954579409990332

Vaknin, S., & Erickson Institute. (2010). *The big book of NLP, expanded: 350+ techniques, patterns & strategies of neuro-linguistic programming* (11th ed.). Inner Patch Publishing.

Walker, A., & Luther, A. (2023, May 7). Caring, chemistry, and orgasms: Components of great sexual experiences. *Sexuality & Culture, 27*, 1735–1756. https://doi.org/10.1007/s12119-023-10087-x

Wesche, R., Walsh, J., Shepardson, R., Carey, K., & Carey, M. (2019). The association between sexual behavior and affect: Moderating factors in young women. *Journal of Sex Research, 56*(8), 1058–1069. https://doi.org/10.1080/00224499.2018.1542657

Wobst, A. H. (2007). *Hypnosis and surgery: Past, present, and future. Anesthesia & Analgesia, 104*(5), 1199-1208. https://doi.org/10.1213/01.ane.0000260616.49050.6d

Wong, J., & Gravel, J. (2016). Do sex offenders have higher levels of testosterone? Results from a meta-analysis. *Sexual Abuse, 30*(2), 147–168. https://doi.org/10.1177/1079063216637857

Woods, N., Mitchell, E., & Smith-DiJulio, K. (2009). Cortisol levels during the menopausal transition and early postmenopause: Observations from the Seattle Midlife Women's Health Study. *Menopause, 16*(4), 708–718. https://doi.org/10.1097/gme.0b013e318198d6b2

Xi, Z., Suarez-Jimenez, B., Lazarov, A., Such, S., Marohasy, C., Small, S., Wager, T., Lindquist, M., Lissek, S., & Neria, Y. (2022). Sequential fear generalization and network connectivity in trauma-exposed humans with and without psychopathology. *Communications Biology, 5*(1), Article 1275. https://doi.org/10.1038/s42003-022-04228-5

Yapko, M. (2013). *Hypnosis and the treatment of depressions: Strategies for change.* Routledge.

Chapter 4 References

Aigner, M., Eher, R., Fruewald, S., Frottier, P., Gutierrez-Lobos, K., & Dwyer, S. (2008). Brain abnormalities and violent behavior. *Journal of Psychology & Human Sexuality, 11*(3), 57–64. https://doi.org/10.1300/J056v11n03_06

Al-Sughayir, M. (2005). Vaginismus treatment: Hypnotherapy versus behavior therapy. *Neurosciences Journal, 10*(2), 163–167. https://nsj.org.sa/content/10/2/163.short

American Medical Association. (2021). *ICD-10-PCS 2022: The complete official codebook.*

Anagha, K., Shafeena, T., Shihabudheen, P., & Uvais, N. A. (2021). Side effect profiles of selective serotonin reuptake inhibitors: A cross-sectional study in a naturalistic setting. *Primary Care Companion for CNS Disorders, 23*(4), Article 20m02747. https://doi.org/10.4088/PCC.20m02747

Asadi, L., Noroozi, M., Mardani, F., Salimi, H., & Jambarsang, S. (2023). The needs of women survivors of rape: A narrative review. *Iranian Journal of Nursing and Midwifery Research, 28*(6), 633–641. https://doi.org/10.4103/ijnmr.ijnmr_395_22

Briken, P., Matthiesen, S., Pietras, L., Wiessner, C., Klein, V., Reed, G., & Dekker, A. (2020). Estimating the prevalence of sexual dysfunction using the new ICD-11 guidelines. *Deutsches Ärzteblatt International, 117*(39), 653–658. https://doi.org/10.3238/arztebl.2020.0653

Brown, J. M., & Chaves, J. F. (1980). Hypnosis in the treatment of sexual dysfunction. *Journal of Sex & Marital Therapy, 6*(1), 63–74. https://doi.org/10.1080/00926238008404247

Bryant, R. A. (2021). *Treating PTSD in first responders: A guide for serving those who serve.* American Psychological Association.

Burton, D. L. (2003). Male adolescents: Sexual victimization and subsequent sexual abuse. *Child and Adolescent Social Work Journal, 20*(4), 277–296. https://doi.org/10.1023/A:1024556909087

Catanese, S. A. (2010). Traumatized by association: The risk of working sex crimes. *Federal Probation, 74*(2), 36–38. https://www.uscourts.gov/sites/default/files/74_2_9_0.pdf

Chivers-Wilson, K. (2006). Sexual assault and posttraumatic stress disorder: A review of the biological, psychological, and sociological factors and treatments. *McGill Journal of Medicine, 9*(2), 111–118. https://www.ncbi.nlm.nih.gov/pmc/articles/PMC2323517/

Cooney, L. (1999). Hypnotherapy and sexual offenders: The first steps towards empathy and healing. *Journal of Heart Centered Therapies, 2*(1), 59.

Corey, G., Corey, M. S., & Corey, C. (2023). *Issues and ethics in the helping professions* (11th ed.). Cengage Learning. https://link.gale.com/apps/doc/A65014124/HRCA

Crasilneck, H. B. (1982). A follow-up study in the use of hypnotherapy in the treatment of psychogenic impotency. *American Journal of Clinical Hypnosis, 25*(1), 52–61. https://doi.org/10.1080/00029157.1982.10404064

Crasilneck, H. B., & Hall, J. A. (1985). *Clinical hypnosis: Principles and applications* (2nd ed.). Grune & Stratton.

Dittburner, T., & Persinger, M. A. (1993). Intensity of amnesia during hypnosis is positively correlated with estimated prevalence of sexual abuse and alien abductions: Implications for the false memory syndrome.

Perceptual and Motor Skills, 77(3), 895–898. https://doi.
org/10.2466/pms.1993.77.3.895

du Maurier, G. (1922). *Trilby: A novel.* Harper & Brothers
Publishers. (Original work published 1894). https://
archive.org/details/trilbynovel00dumaiala

Erickson, M. H. (1982). *Innovative hypnotherapy* (E. L. Rossi,
Ed.). Irvington Publishers.

Fuchs, K. (1980). Therapy of vaginismus by hypnotic
desensitization. *American Journal of Obstetrics and
Gynecology, 137*(1), 1–7. https://doi.org/10.1016/0002-
9378(80)90376-2

Gauld, A. (1992). *A history of hypnotism.* Cambridge
University Press.

Haley, J. (2010). *Uncommon therapy: Psychiatric techniques of
Milton H. Erickson.* W. W. Norton & Company.https://
archive.org/details/historyofhypnoti0000gaul/page/n7/
mode/2up

Halliday, J. (2020, January 9). Police issue warning over posts
'identifying Reynhard Sinaga victims'. *The Guardian.*
https://www.theguardian.com/uk-news/2020/jan/09/
manchester-police-issue-warning-posts-identifying-
reynhard-sinaga-victims

Hambleton, R. (2002). *Practising safe hypnosis: A risk
management guide.* Crown House Publishing.

Hanevik, E., Røvik, F., Bøe, T., Knapstad, M., & Smith, O.
(2023). Client predictors of therapy dropout in a
primary care setting: A prospective cohort study. *BMC*

Psychiatry, 23, Article 358. https://doi.org/10.1186/
s12888-023-04878-7

Hassan, W. M. A. (2014). Hypnosis and clinical hypnotherapy
in the treatment of psychological and psychosomatic
ailments. *Medical Journal of Babylon, 11*(2), I–XV.
https://www.iasj.net/iasj/download/a840bcfdbd8568c5

Hlywa, E. (2008). Spontaneous and induced abreaction.
*Australian Journal of Clinical & Experimental Hypnosis,
36*(2), 176–190. https://www.hypnosisaustralia.org.
au/wp-content/uploads/AJCEH_Vol-36_No2_Nov08.
pdf#page=84

Hodder-Fleming, L., & Gow, K. (2005). Adult survivors of
childhood sexual abuse: Triggers to remembering.
*Australian Journal of Clinical and Experimental
Hypnosis, 33*(3), 1–23. http://www.hypnosisaustralia.org.
au/wp-content/uploads/journal/AJCEH_Vol33_No1_
MAY05.pdf#page=7

Hucker, S. J., & Bain, J. (1997). Androgenic hormones and
sexual assault. In W. L. Marshall, D. R. Laws, & H. E.
Barbaree (Eds.), *Handbook of sexual assault* (pp. 93–
102). https://doi.org/10.1007/978-1-4899-0915-2_6

Kumalasari, R., Tamtomo, I., & Prasetya, H. (2020,
November 18–19). *Hypnosis and sexual arousal: A
meta-analysis* [Paper presentation]. Universitas Sebelas
Maret 7th International Conference on Public Health,
Solo, Indonesia. https://theicph.com/wp-content/
uploads/2020/12/409-Ratna-Dewi-Kumalasari-Didik-
Gunawan-Tamtomo-Hanung-Prasetya.pdf

Långström, N., Babchishin, K. M., Fazel, S., Lichtenstein, P., & Frisell, T. (2015). Sexual offending runs in families: A 37-year nationwide study. *International Journal of Epidemiology, 44*(2), 713–720. https://doi.org/10.1093/ije/dyv029

Leavitt, J. (1991). *Split-screen imagery in forensic hypnotherapy. Medical Hypnoanalysis Journal, 6*(2), 77–80.

McConkey, K., & Sheehan, P. (1987). *A survey of the police use of hypnosis in Australia.* Criminology Research Council. https://www.aic.gov.au/sites/default/files/2020-05/16-86.pdf

McLeod, S. (2024, January 24). Anna O (Bertha Pappenheim): Life & impact on psychology. *Simply Psychology.* https://www.simplypsychology.org/anna-o-bertha-pappenheim.html

O'Connell, G. (2024). *3 reasons for the nationwide police shortage.* Brother Mobile Solutions. https://brothermobilesolutions.com/insights/article/3-reasons-for-nationwide-police-shortage-in-2022/

Otgaar, H., Howe, M., Peters, M., Sauerland, M., & Raymaekers, L. (2013). Developmental trends in different types of spontaneous false memories: Implications for the legal field. *Behavioral Sciences & the Law, 31*(5), 666–682. https://doi.org/10.1002/bsl.2076

Poon, M. W.-L. (2007). The value of using hypnosis in helping an adult survivor of childhood sexual abuse. *Contemporary Hypnosis, 24*(1), 30–37. https://doi.org/10.1002/ch.324

Poon, M. W.-L. (2009). Hypnosis for complex trauma survivors: Four case studies. *American Journal of Clinical Hypnosis, 51*(3), 200–213. https://doi.org/10.1080/00029 157.2009.10401676

**Ramírez, C., Pinzón-Rondón, A. M., & Botero, J. C. (2011). Contextual predictive factors of child sexual abuse: The role of parent-child interaction. *Child Abuse & Neglect, 35*(12), 1022–1031. https://doi.org/10.1016/j. chiabu.2011.10.004

Richardson, D. (2003). *Heart of tantric sex.* O-Books.

Rocha, G., & Téllez, A. (2016). Use of clinical hypnosis and EMDR in kidnapping and rape: A case report. *Australian Journal of Clinical and Experimental Hypnosis, 41*(1), 115–133. https://www.hypnosisaustralia.org.au/ wp-content/uploads/10330_AJCEH_2016_FINAL. pdf#page=119

Rosso, P., Di Bartolomeo, G., Piedimonte, A., Cavarra, M., Bellina, M., Ambu, A., & Gava, N. (2016). Ericksonian hypnosis in sexual rehabilitation of patients who underwent radical, nerve-sparing prostatectomy. *Contemporary Hypnosis & Integrative Therapy, 31*(1), 13–27. https://www.researchgate.net/ publication/315895990_Ericksonian_hypnosis_in_ sexual_rehabilitation_of_patients_who_underwent_ radical_nerve-sparing_prostatectomy

Saitz, T. R., & Serefoglu, E. C. (2016). The epidemiology of premature ejaculation. *Translational Andrology and Urology, 5*(4), 409–415. https://doi.org/10.21037/ tau.2016.05.11

Spanos, N. P. (1996). *Multiple identities & false memories: A sociocognitive perspective*. American Psychological Association.

Spiegel, H., & Spiegel, D. (1989). *Clinical hypnosis: Brief treatment with restructuring and selfmanagement*. Guilford Press.

The Holy Bible: King James version. (1991). Random House.

The Illustrated Holy Bible: King James version. (2023). Smart Books.

Thomas, C. G. (1973). Matriarchy in early Greece: The Bronze and Dark ages. *Arethusa, 6*(2), 173–195. https://www.jstor.org/stable/26307431

United Nations Educational, Scientific and Cultural Organization. (2023, November 16). *Comprehensive sexuality education: For healthy, informed and empowered learners*. Retrieved September 12, 2024, from https://www.unesco.org/en/articles/why-comprehensive-sexuality-education-important

WA Police Union. (2023). *Police officer suicides in Australia*. https://www.wapu.org.au/wp-content/uploads/2024/03/gale-attachment-report_sucicide.pdf

Ward, T., Hudson, S., Marshall, W., & Siegert, R. (1995). Attachment style and intimacy deficits in sexual offenders: A theoretical framework. *Sexual Abuse: A Journal of Research and Treatment, 7*(4), 317–335. https://doi.org/10.1007/BF02256835

Weiss, S. (2018, March 6). I went to a masturbation class in search of my biggest orgasm yet. *Harper's Bazaar*.

https://www.harpersbazaar.com/culture/features/a15893157/betty-dodson-masturbation-workshop-orgasms/

Wolffram, H. (2017). Crime and hypnosis in fin-de-siècle Germany: The Czynski case. *Notes and Records, 71*(2), 213–226. https://doi.org/10.1098/rsnr.2017.0005

Wood, H. (2019). Gender inequality: The problem of harmful, patriarchal, traditional and cultural gender practices in the church. *HTS Teologiese Studies / Theological Studies, 75*(1), Article 5177. https://doi.org/10.4102/hts.v75i1.5177

World Health Organization. (n.d.). *International classification of diseases 11th Revision (ICD-11).* https://icd.who.int/en

Yang, Q., Cai, H., Wan, Z., Chen, M., Yang, B., Xie, Y., Zhang, Y., Sun, X., Tang, J., Kuang, M., Liu, H., & Deng, C. (2023). Impact of cognitive behavioral therapy on premature ejaculation patients: A prospective, randomized controlled trial protocol. *PLOS ONE, 18*(12), Article 0295663. https://doi.org/10.1371/journal.pone.0295663

**Zeig, J., & Tanev, K. (2020). Marital hypnotherapy: A session with Milton Erickson with commentary. *International Journal of Clinical and Experimental Hypnosis, 68*(3), 263–288. https://doi.org/10.1080/00207144.2020.1762493

Chapter 5 References

Assalian, P. (2013). Psychological and interpersonal dimensions of sexual function and dysfunction.

Arab Journal of Urology, 11(3), 217–221. https://doi.
org/10.1016/j.aju.2013.07.007

Byrne, A.-L., Baldwin, A., Harvey, C., Brown, J., Willis, E.,
Hegney, D., Ferguson, B., Judd, J., Kynaston, D., Forrest,
R., Heritage, B., Heard, D., McLellan, S., Thompson, S., &
Palmer, J. (2021). Understanding the impact and causes
of 'failure to attend' on continuity of care for patients with
chronic conditions. *PLOS ONE, 16*(3), Article e0247914.
https://doi.org/10.1371/journal.pone.0247914

Defar, S., Abraham, Y., Reta, Y., Deribe, B., Jisso, M., Yeheyis,
T., Kebede, K. M., Beyene, B., & Ayalew, M. (2023).
Health related quality of life among people with
mental illness: The role of socio-clinical characteristics
and level of functional disability. *Frontiers in Public
Health, 11*, Article 1134032. https://doi.org/10.3389/
fpubh.2023.1134032

Erickson, M. H. (1980). *Hypnotic alteration of sensory,
perceptual, and psychophysical processes.* Irvington
Publishers.

Erickson, M. H. (2010). *Collected works of Milton H. Erickson:
Vol. 5. Classical hypnotic phenomena Part 1* (E. L. Rossi,
R. Erickson Klein, & K. Rossi, Eds.). Milton H. Erickson
Foundation Press.

Freud, S. (2010). *Beyond the pleasure principle* (C. J. M.
Hubback, Trans.). Kessinger Publishing. (Original work
published 1922)

Garcia, M. R., Leslie, S. W., & Wray, A. A. (2023). Sexually
transmitted infections. In *StatPearls*. StatPearls Publishing.
https://www.ncbi.nlm.nih.gov/books/NBK560808/

Grace, B., Wainwright, T., Solomons, W., Camden, J., & Ellis-Caird, H. (2020). How do clinical psychologists make ethical decisions? A systematic review of empirical research. *Clinical Ethics, 15*(4). https://doi.org/10.1177/1477750920927165

Hanevik, E., Røvik, F. M. G., Bøe, T., Knapstad, M., & Smith, O. R. F. (2023). Client predictors of therapy dropout in a primary care setting: A prospective cohort study. *BMC Psychiatry, 23*, Article 358. https://doi.org/10.1186/s12888-023-04878-7

Health Care Complaints Commission. (2023). *Expert guidelines.* Parliament of New South Wales, Australia. https://www.hccc.nsw.gov.au/ArticleDocuments/315/Expert%20Guidelines%20Registered%20HP%20-%20Nov%202019.pdf

Hu, F., Wu, Q., Li, Y., Xu, W., Zhao, L., & Sun, Q. (2020). Love at first glance but not after deep consideration: The impact of sexually appealing advertising on product preferences. *Frontiers in Neuroscience, 14*, Article 465. https://doi.org/10.3389/fnins.2020.00465

Hull, C. L. (2002). *Hypnosis and suggestibility: An experimental approach* (2nd ed.). Anglo American Book Company.

Kedia, G., Mussweiler, T., & Linden, D. E. J. (2014). Brain mechanisms of social comparison and their influence on the reward system. *Neuroreport, 25*(16), 1255–1265. https://doi.org/10.1097/WNR.0000000000000255

Lazar, B. S., & Dempster, C. R. (2011). Failures in hypnosis and hypnotherapy: A review. *American Journal of Clinical*

Hypnosis, 24(1), 48–54. https://doi.org/10.1080/0002915
7.1981.10403283

O'Keefe, T. (2008, March 2). *Why use contracts in
hypnotherapy?* Dr Tracie O'Keefe. https://tracieokeefe.
com/why-use-contracts-in-hypnotherapy/

Sadikaj, G., Moskowitz, D. S., & Zuroff, D. C. (2016).
Negative affective reaction to partner's dominant
behavior influences satisfaction with romantic
relationship. *Journal of Social and Personal
Relationships, 34*(8), 1324–1346. https://doi.
org/10.1177/0265407516677060

Sakaluk, J. K., Kim, J., Campbell, E., Baxter, A., & Impett, E.
A. (2020). Self-esteem and sexual health: A multilevel
meta-analytic review. *Health Psychology Review, 14*(2),
269–293. https://doi.org/10.1080/17437199.2019.1625281

Seh, A. H., Zarour, M., Alenezi, M., Sarkar, A. K., Agrawal,
A., Kumar, R., & Khan, R. A. (2020). Healthcare
data breaches: Insights and implications. *Healthcare
(Basel), 8*(2), Article 133. https://doi.org/10.3390/
healthcare8020133

Verrastro, V., Saladino, V., Petruccelli, F., & Eleuteri, S.
(2020). Medical and health care professionals' sexuality
education: State of the art and recommendations.
*International Journal of Environmental Research
and Public Health, 17*(7), Article 2186. https://doi.
org/10.3390/ijerph17072186

Walker, M. J. (2011). *Dirty medicine: The handbook*. Slingshot
Publications.

Willis, K. L. (2020). *Therapist effects on dropout in couple therapy* [Master's thesis, Brigham Young University]. BYU ScholarsArchive Theses and Dissertations. https://scholarsarchive.byu.edu/cgi/viewcontent.cgi?article=10211&context=etd

Wingrove, P. (2023, June 21). *Pharmaceutical trade group sues US over Medicare drug price negotiation plans.* Reuters. https://www.reuters.com/world/us/us-sued-block-program-that-gives-medicare-power-negotiate-drug-prices-2023-06-21/

Chapter 6 References

Abdelsamea, G., Amr, M., Tolba, A., Elboraie, H., Soliman, A., Hassan, B. A.-A, Ali, F., & Osman, D. (2023). Impact of weight loss on sexual and psychological functions and quality of life in females with sexual dysfunction: A forgotten avenue. *Frontiers in Psychology, 14*, Article 1090256. https://doi.org/10.3389/fpsyg.2023.1090256

Bird, E., Piccirillo, M., Garcia, N., Blais, R., & Campbell, S. (2021). Relationship between posttraumatic stress disorder and sexual difficulties: A systematic review of veterans and military personnel. *Journal of Sexual Medicine, 18*(8), 1398–1426. https://doi.org/10.1016/j.jsxm.2021.05.011

Calabrò, R., Cacciola, A., Bruschetta, D., Milardi, D., Quattrini, F., Sciarone, F., la Rosa, G., Bramanti, P., & Anastasi, G. (2019). Neuroanatomy and function of human sexual behavior: A neglected or unknown issue?

Brain and Behavior, 9(12), Article e01389. https://doi.
org/10.1002/brb3.1389

Cappelletti, M., & Wallen, K. (2016). Increasing women's
sexual desire: The comparative effectiveness of estrogens
and androgens. *Hormones and Behavior, 78*, 178–193.
https://doi.org/10.1016/j.yhbeh.2015.11.003

Craparo, G., Ortu, F., & van der Hart, O. (Eds.). (2019).
*Rediscovering Pierre Janet: Trauma, dissociation, and a
new context for psychoanalysis.* Routledge.

Doretto, L., Mari, F. C., & Chaves, A. C. (2020). Polycystic
ovary syndrome and psychotic disorder. *Frontiers in
Psychiatry, 11*, Article 543. https://doi.org/10.3389/
fpsyt.2020.00543

Fereydooni, K., Bazzazian, S., Pourasghar, M., & Jafar, P.
(2022). The effectiveness of cognitive hypnosis therapy
on women's sexual desire and marital satisfaction.
Journal of Preventive Counseling, 3(1), 71–88. https://doi.
org/10.22098/jpc.2022.1662

Frankenbach, J., Weber, M., Loschelder, D. D., Kilger,
H., & Friese, M. (2022). Sex drive: Theoretical
conceptualization and meta-analytic review of gender
differences. *Psychological Bulletin, 148*(9-10), 621–661.
https://doi.org/10.1037/bul0000366

Montejo, A., de Alarcón, R., Prieto, N., Acosta, Buch, B.,
& Montejo, L. (2021). Management strategies for
antipsychotic-related sexual dysfunction: A clinical
approach. *Journal of Clinical Medicine, 10*(2), Article
308. https://doi.org/10.3390/jcm10020308

Noordewier, M., Scheepers, D., & Hilbert, L. (2020). Freezing in response to social threat: A replication. *Psychological Research, 84*(7), 1890–1896. https://doi.org/10.1007/s00426-019-01203-4

O'Keefe, T. (2013). Transformation. In *Survive and prosper: Personal transformation out of crisis* (pp. 127–156). Australian Health & Education Centre.

Ouhalla, J. (1994). *Introducing transformational grammar: From rules to principles and parameters.* Hodder Arnold.

Pease, A., & Pease, B. (2017). *The definitive book of body language.* HQ Non Fiction AU.

Poscheschnik, G., & Crepaldi, G. (2022). Only chance and circumstances? Or, how Freudian are Freudian slips? A review of research literature concerning parapraxes. *Psychoanalytic Psychology, 39*(3), 189–197. https://doi.org/10.1037/pap0000384

Shamim, H., Jean, M., Umair, M., Muddaloor, P., Farinango, M., Ansary, A., Dakka, A., Nazir, Z., White, C., Habbal, A., & Mohammed, L. (2022). Role of metformin in the management of polycystic ovarian syndrome-associated acne: A systematic review. *Cureus, 14*(8), Article e28462. https://doi.org/10.7759/cureus.28462

Taormino, T. (2009). *The big book of sex toys: From vibrators and dildos to swings and slings – playful and kinky bedside accessories that make your sex life amazing.* Quiver.

Chapter 7 References

Aydin, S., Ercan, M., Çaşkurlu, T., Taşçi, A. I., Karaman, İ., Odabaş, Ö., Yilmaz, Y., Ağargün, M. Y., Kara, H., & Sevin, G. (1997). Acupuncture and hypnotic suggestions in the treatment of non-organic male sexual dysfunction. *Scandinavian Journal of Urology and Nephrology, 31*(3), 271–274. https://doi.org/10.3109/00365599709070347

Bryant, R., Hung, L., Dobson-Stone, C., & Schofield, P. (2013). The association between the oxytocin receptor gene (OXTR) and hypnotizability. *Psychoneuroendocrinology, 38*(10), 1979–1984. https://doi.org/10.1016/j.psyneuen.2013.03.002

Carto, C., Pagalavan, M., Nackeeran, S., Blachman-Braun, R., Kresch, E., Kuchakulla, M., & Ramasamy, R. (2022). Consumption of a healthy plant-based diet is associated with a decreased risk of erectile dysfunction: A cross-sectional study of the National Health and Nutrition Examination Survey. *Urology, 161*, 76–82. https://doi.org/10.1016/j.urology.2021.12.021

Cooper, K., Russell, A., Calley, S., Chen, H., Kramer, J., & Verplanken, B. (2022). Cognitive processes in autism: Repetitive thinking in autistic versus non-autistic adults. *Autism, 26*(4), 849–858. https://doi.org/10.1177/13623613211034380

Davis, N. O., & Kollins, S. H. (2012). Treatment for co-occurring attention deficit/hyperactivity disorder and autism spectrum disorder. *Neurotherapeutics, 9*(3), 518–530. https://doi.org/10.1007/s13311-012-0126-9

Dewitte, M., Bettocchi, C., Carvalho, J., Corona, G., Flink, I., Limoncin, E., Pascoal, P., Reisman, Y., & Van Lankveld, J. (2021). A psychosocial approach to erectile dysfunction: Position statements from the European Society of Sexual Medicine (ESSM). *Sexual Medicine, 9*(6), Article 100434. https://doi.org/10.1016/j.esxm.2021.100434

Gerbild, H., Larsen, C. M., Graugaard, C., & Areskoug Josefsson, K. (2018). Physical activity to improve erectile function: A systematic review of intervention studies. *Sexual Medicine, 6*(2), 75–89. https://doi.org/10.1016/j.esxm.2018.02.001

Harrison, A., Gamsiz, E., Berkowitz, I., Nagpal, S., & Jerskey, B. (2015). Genetic variation in the oxytocin receptor gene is associated with a social phenotype in autism spectrum disorders. *American Journal of Medical Genetics Part B: Neuropsychiatric Genetics, 168*(8), 720-729. https://doi.org/10.1002/ajmg.b.32377

Leslie, S., & Sooriyamoorthy, T. (2023). Erectile dysfunction. In *StatPearls*. StatPearls Publishing. https://www.ncbi.nlm.nih.gov/books/NBK562253/

Melis, M. R., & Argiolas, A. (2021). Oxytocin, erectile function and sexual behavior: Last discoveries and possible advances. *International Journal of Molecular Sciences, 22*(19), Article 10376. https://doi.org/10.3390/ijms221910376

Neijenhuijs, K., Holtmaat, K., Aaronson, N., Holzner, B., Terwee, C., Cuijpers, P., & Verdonck-de Leeuw, I. (2019). The International Index of Erectile Function (IIEF)—A systematic review of measurement properties. *The*

Journal of Sexual Medicine, 16(7), 1078–1091. https:// doi.org/10.1016/j.jsxm.2019.04.010

O'Keefe, T. (2000). *Self-hypnosis for life: Mind, body and spiritual excellence.* Extraordinary People Press.

Osterberg, C., Bernie, A., & Ramasamy, R. (2014). Risks of testosterone replacement therapy in men. *Indian Journal of Urology, 30*(1), 2–7. https://doi.org/10.4103/0970-1591.124197

Patel, D. V., Halls, J., & Patel, U. (2012). Investigation of erectile dysfunction. *British Journal of Radiology, 85*(1), S69–S78. https://doi.org/10.1259/bjr/20361140

Rajfer, J. (2000). Relationship between testosterone and erectile dysfunction. *Reviews in Urology, 2*(2), 122–128. https://www.ncbi.nlm.nih.gov/pmc/articles/PMC1476110/

Sadovsky, R. (2002). The role of the primary care clinician in the management of erectile dysfunction. *Reviews in Urology, 4*(Suppl. 3), S54–S63. https://www.ncbi.nlm.nih.gov/pmc/articles/PMC1557658/

Schardein, J., & Hotaling, J. (2022). The impact of testosterone on erectile function. *Androgens: Clinical Research and Therapeutics, 3*(1), 113–124. https://doi.org/10.1089/andro.2021.0033

Schulz, S. E., & Stevenson, R. A. (2019). Sensory hypersensitivity predicts repetitive behaviours in autistic and typically-developing children. *Autism, 23*(4), 1028–1041. https://doi.org/10.1177/1362361318774559

Sheng, Z. (2021). Psychological consequences of erectile dysfunction. *Trends in Urology & Men's Health, 12*(6), 19–22. https://doi.org/10.1002/tre.827

Shoshany, O., Katz, D., & Love, C. (2017). Much more than prescribing a pill – Assessment and treatment of erectile dysfunction by the general practitioner. *Australian Family Physician, 46*(9), 634–639. https://pubmed.ncbi.nlm.nih.gov/28892593/

Stanaland, A., Gaither, S., & Gassman-Pines, A. (2023). When is masculinity "fragile"? An expectancy-discrepancy-threat model of masculine identity. *Personality and Social Psychology Review, 27*(4), 359–377. https://doi.org/10.1177/10888683221141176

Ückert, S., Becker, A., Bannowsky, A., Tsikas, D., & Kuczyk, M. (2020). 312 Endogenous vasoactive peptides in the control of penile erectile tissue: Is there a role of arginine-vasopressin (AVP)? *The Journal of Sexual Medicine, 17*(Suppl. 1), S76. https://doi.org/10.1016/j.jsxm.2019.11.134

Zhang, Z., Gao, X., Zhou, Y., Yu, C., Pimolsettapun, J., Yang, L., & Zhao, Y. (2020). Study on the combination of brief psychodynamic psychotherapy with Viagra in the treatment of non-organic ED. *General Psychiatry, 33*(5), Article e100184. https://doi.org/10.1136/gpsych-2019-100184

Zheng, Z. (2021). Psychological consequences of erectile dysfunction. *Trends in Urology & Men's Health, 12*(6), 19–22. https://doi.org/10.1002/tre.827

Chapter 8 References

Cai, T., Pisano, F., Magri, V., Verze, P., Mondaini, N., D'Elia, C., Malossini, G., Mazzoli, S., Perletti, G., Gontero, P., Mirone, V., & Bartoletti, R. (2014). Chlamydia trachomatis infection is related to premature ejaculation in chronic prostatitis patients: Results from a cross-sectional study. *The Journal of Sexual Medicine, 11*(12), 3085–3092. https://doi.org/10.1111/jsm.12699

Crowdis, M., Leslie, S., & Nazir, S. (2023). Premature ejaculation. In *StatPearls*. StatPearls Publishing. https://www.ncbi.nlm.nih.gov/books/NBK546701/

Dane, L. (Ed.). (2003). *The complete illustrated Kama Sutra.* Inner Traditions.

Facco, E. (2016). Hypnosis and anesthesia: Back to the future. *Minerva Anestesiologica, 82*(12), 1343–1356. https://pubmed.ncbi.nlm.nih.gov/27575449/

Hammond, D. C. (Ed). (2010). *Handbook of hypnotic suggestions and metaphors.* W. W. Norton & Company.

Leung, H., Shek, D., Leung, E., & Shek, E. (2019). Development of contextually-relevant sexuality education: Lessons from a comprehensive review of adolescent sexuality education across cultures. *International Journal of Environmental Research and Public Health, 16*(4), Article 621. https://doi.org/10.3390/ijerph16040621

Mohamed, I., Ahmad, H., Hassaan, S., & Hassan, S. (2020). Assessment of anxiety and depression among substance use disorder patients: A case-control study. *Middle East Current Psychiatry, 27*, Article 22. https://doi.org/10.1186/s43045-020-00029-w

Otunctemur, A., Ozbek, E., Kirecci, S. L., Ozcan, L., Dursun, M., Cekmen, M., & Ozdogan, H. K. (2014). Relevance of serum nitric oxide levels and the efficacy of selective serotonin reuptake inhibitors treatment on premature ejaculation: Decreased nitric oxide is associated with premature ejaculation. *Andrologia, 46*(9), 951–955. https://doi.org/10.1111/and.12179

Rosen, S. (Ed.). (2010). *My voice will go with you: The teaching tales of Milton H. Erickson.* W. W. Norton & Company.

Strassberg, D. S., Mahoney, J. M., Schaugaard, M., & Hale, V. E. (1990). The role of anxiety in premature ejaculation: A psychophysiological model. *Archives of Sexual Behavior, 19*(3), 251–257. https://doi.org/10.1007/BF01541550

Symonds, T., Perelman, M., Althof, S., Giuliano, F., Martin, M., May, K., Abraham, L., Crossland, A., & Morris, M. (2007). Development and validation of a premature ejaculation diagnostic tool. *European Urology, 52*(2), 565–573. https://doi.org/10.1016/j.eururo.2007.01.028

Chapter 9 References

Anğın, A. D., Gün, İ., Sakin, Ö., Çıkman, M. S., Eserdağ, S., & Anğın, P. (2020). Effects of predisposing factors on the success and treatment period in vaginismus. *JBRA Assisted Reproduction, 24*(2), 180–188. https://doi.org/10.5935/1518-0557.20200018

Alwarith, J., Kahleova, H., Rembert, E., Yonas, W., Dort, S., Calcagno, M., Burgess, N., Crosby, L., & Barnard, N. (2019). Nutrition interventions in rheumatoid arthritis: The potential use of plant-based diets. A review. *Frontiers in Nutrition, 6,* Article 141. https://doi. org/10.3389/fnut.2019.00141

Bhardwaj, P., Au, C., Benito-Martin, A., Ladumor, H., Oshchepkova, S., Moges, R., & Brown, K. (2019). Estrogens and breast cancer: Mechanisms involved in obesity-related development, growth, and progression. *The Journal of Steroid Biochemistry and Molecular Biology, 189,* 161–170. https://doi.org/10.1016/j. jsbmb.2019.03.002

Bonazza, F., Politi, G., Leone, D., Vegni, E., & Borghi, L. (2023). Psychological factors in functional hypothalamic amenorrhea: A systematic review and meta-analysis. *Frontiers in Endocrinology, 14,* Article 981491. https:// doi.org/10.3389/fendo.2023.981491

Carlson, K., & Nguyen, H. (2024). Genitourinary Syndrome of Menopause. In *StatPearls.* StatPearls Publishing. https:// www.ncbi.nlm.nih.gov/books/NBK559297/

Chermansky, C. J., & Moalli, P. A. (2016). Role of pelvic floor in lower urinary tract function. *Autonomic Neuroscience, 200,* 43-48. https://doi.org/10.1016/j.autneu.2015.06.003

Cruz, O., Hernández, D. E., & Pérez, M. (2018). Dos casos de liquen plano con tratamiento de hipnosis [Lichen planus submitted to hypnosis treatment: Report of two cases]. *Revista Argentina de Dermatología, 99*(2). https://rad-online.org.ar/2018/06/01/dos-casos-de-liquen-plano-con-tratamiento-de-hipnosis/

Desai, S., & Corley, S. (2023). Treating co-existent genitourinary syndrome of menopause in patients with lichen sclerosus improves symptoms. *International*

Journal of Women's Dermatology, 9(1), e071. https://doi.
org/10.1097/JW9.0000000000000071

Dimoulas, E., Steffian, L., Steffian, G., Doran, A. P.,
Rasmusson, A. M., & Morgan, C. A., III. (2007).
Dissociation during intense military stress is related to
subsequent somatic symptoms in women. *Psychiatry
(Edgmont), 4*(2), 66–73. https://www.ncbi.nlm.nih.gov/
pmc/articles/PMC2922349/

Erickson, M. (1966). The interspersal hypnotic technique for
symptom correction and pain control. *American Journal
of Clinical Hypnosis, 8*(3), 198–209. https://doi.org/10.10
80/00029157.1966.10402492

Farhi, D., & Dupin, N. (2010). Pathophysiology, etiologic
factors, and clinical management of oral lichen
planus, part I: Facts and controversies. *Clinics in
Dermatology, 28*(1), 100–108. https://doi.org/10.1016/j.
clindermatol.2009.03.004

Hacker Hughes, J. G. H., Earnshaw, N. M., Greenberg,
N., Eldridge, R., Fear, N. T., French, C., Deahl, M.
P., & Wessely, S. (2008). The use of psychological
decompression in military operational environments.
Military Medicine, 173(6), 534–538. https://doi.
org/10.7205/MILMED.173.6.534

Kalkur, C., Sattur, A., & Guttal, K. (2015). Role of depression,
anxiety and stress in patients with oral lichen planus: A
pilot study. *Indian Journal of Dermatology, 60*(5), 445–
449. https://doi.org/10.4103/0019-5154.159625

Machin, S., McConnell, D., & Adams, J. (2010). Vaginal
lichen planus: Preservation of sexual function in severe

disease. *BMJ Case Reports*, *2010*. https://doi.org/10.1136/bcr.08.2009.2208

Margolin, L., Cope, D., Bakst-Sisser, R., & Greenspan, J. (2007). The steroid withdrawal syndrome: A review of the implications, etiology, and treatments. *Journal of Pain and Symptom Management, 33*(2), 224–228. https://doi.org/10.1016/j.jpainsymman.2006.08.013

Maseroli, E., Scavello, I., Rastrelli, G., Limoncin, E., Cipriani, S., Corona, G., Fambrini, M., Magini, A., Jannini, E. A., Maggi, M., & Vignozzi, L. (2018). Outcome of medical and psychosexual interventions for vaginismus: A systematic review and meta-analysis. *The Journal of Sexual Medicine, 15*(12), 1752–1764. https://doi.org/10.1016/j.jsxm.2018.10.003

Melnik, T., Hawton, K., & McGuire, H. (2012). Interventions for vaginismus. *Cochrane Database of Systematic Reviews, 2012*(12), Article CD001760. https://doi.org/10.1002/14651858.CD001760.pub2

Mohan, R. P. S., Gupta, A., Kamarthi, N., Malik, S., Goel, S., & Gupta, S. (2017). Incidence of oral lichen planus in perimenopausal women: A cross-sectional study in Western Uttar Pradesh population. *Journal of Mid-life Health, 8*(2), 70–74. https://doi.org/10.4103/jmh.JMH_34_17

Moloney, R., Desbonnet, L., Clarke, G., Timothy, D., & Cryan, J. (2014). The microbiome: Stress, health and disease. *Mammalian Genome, 25*, 49–74. https://doi.org/10.1007/s00335-013-9488-5

Musheyev, Y., Levada, M., Ftiha, F., Garrick, I., Ahasan, H., & Jiang, M. (2022). Panhypopituitarism presents as amenorrhea secondary to post traumatic stress disorder in a 33-year-old patient: A case report. *Cureus, 14*(3), Article e22812. https://doi.org/10.7759/cureus.22812

Myint, K., Jayakumar, R., Hoe, S.-Z., Kanthimathi, M. S., & Lam, S.-K. (2017). Cortisol, β-endorphin, and oxidative stress markers in healthy medical students in response to examination stress. *Biomedical Research, 28*(8), 3774–3779.

Patterson, D. R., & Mendoza, M. E. (2024). *Clinical hypnosis for pain control: A comprehensive approach to management and treatment* (2nd ed.). American Psychological Association.

Pisetsky, D. S. (2023). Pathogenesis of autoimmune disease. *Nature Reviews Nephrology, 19*, 509–524. https://doi.org/10.1038/s41581-023-00720-1

Pithavadian, R., Chalmers, J., & Dune, T. (2023). The experiences of women seeking help for vaginismus and its impact on their sense of self: An integrative review. *Women's Health (London), 19*. https://doi.org/10.1177/17455057231199383

Raday, F., Facio, A., Zelinska, E, Chandrakirana, K., & Aouij, E. (2017, October). *Women's autonomy, equality and reproductive health in international human rights: Between recognition, backlash and regressive trends.* U.N. Working group on the issue of discrimination against women in law and in practice. https://www.ohchr.org/sites/default/files/Documents/Issues/Women/WG/WomensAutonomyEqualityReproductiveHealth.pdf

Raveendran, A. V., & Rajini, P. (2024). Vaginismus: Diagnostic challenges and proposed diagnostic criteria. *Balkan Medical Journal, 41*(1), 80–82. https://doi.org/10.4274/balkanmedj.galenos.2023.2022-9-62

Reissing, E. D., Borg, C., Spoelstra, S. K., ter Kuile, M. M., Both, S., de Jong, P. J., van Lankveld, J. J. D. M., Melles, R. J., Weijenborg, P. Th. M., & Weijmar Schultz, W. C. M. (2014). "Throwing the baby out with the bathwater": The demise of vaginismus in favor of genito-pelvic pain/penetration disorder. *Archives of Sexual Behavior, 43*(7), 1209–1213. https://doi.org/10.1007/s10508-014-0322-2

Shufelt, C. L., Torbati, T., & Dutra, E. (2017). Hypothalamic amenorrhea and the long-term health consequences. *Seminars in Reproductive Medicine, 35*(3), 256–262. https://doi.org/10.1055/s-0037-1603581

Slaoui, A., Benzina, I., Talib, S., Etber, A., Zeraidi, N., Lakhdar, A., Kharbach, A., & Baydada, A. (2020). Congenital vaginal atresia: About an uncommon case. *Pan African Medical Journal, 37*, Article 69. https://doi.org/10.11604/pamj.2020.37.69.21682

Song, H., Fang, F., Tomasson, G., Arnberg, F. K., Mataix-Cols, D., de la Cruz, L. F., Almqvist, C., Fall, K., & Valdimarsdóttir, U. A. (2018). Association of stress-related disorders with subsequent autoimmune disease. *JAMA, 319*(23), 2388–2400. https://doi.org/10.1001/jama.2018.7028

Sprouse-Blum, A., Smith, G., Sugai, D., & Parsa, F. D. (2010). Understanding endorphins and their importance in

pain management. *Hawaii Medical Journal, 69*(3),
70–71. https://www.ncbi.nlm.nih.gov/pmc/articles/
PMC3104618/

Tomova, A., Bukovsky, I., Rembert, E., Yonas, W., Alwarith,
J., Barnard, N. D., & Kahleova, H. (2019). The effects of
vegetarian and vegan diets on gut microbiota. *Frontiers
in Nutrition, 6*, Article 47. https://doi.org/10.3389/
fnut.2019.00047

Vatsyayana, M., Burton, R., & Arbuthnot, F. F. (2012). *The
original Kama Sutra completely illustrated* (V. Jain, Ed.,
13th ed.). Mittal Publishing.

Chapter 10 References

Alinsod, R. M. (2017). Re: Transcutaneous temperature
controlled radiofrequency for orgasmic dysfunction.
Lasers in Surgery and Medicine 2016;48(7): 641–645.
Lasers in Surgery and Medicine, 49(7), 727. https://doi.
org/10.1002/lsm.22643

Bridges, C. F., Critelli, J. W., & Loos, V. E. (1985). Hypnotic
susceptibility, inhibitory control, and orgasmic
consistency. *Archives of Sexual Behavior, 14*(4), 373–376.
https://doi.org/10.1007/BF01550852

Carrellas, B. (2007). *Urban Tantra: Sacred sex for the twenty-
first century*. Celestial Arts.

Casula, C. C. (2022). Stimulating unconscious processes with
metaphors and narrative. *American Journal of Clinical
Hypnosis, 64*(4), 339–354. https://doi.org/10.1080/00029
157.2021.2019670

Dąbrowski, K. (1964). *Positive disintegration*. Little, Brown.

Gérard, M., Berry, M., Shtarkshall, R. A., Amsel, R., & Binik, Y. M. (2021). Female multiple orgasm: An exploratory internet-based survey. *Journal of Sex Research, 58*(2), 206–221. https://doi.org/10.1080/00224499.2020.17432 24

Golmakani, N., Zare, Z., Khadem, N., Shareh, H., & Shakeri, M. T. (2015). The effect of pelvic floor muscle exercises program on sexual self-efficacy in primiparous women after delivery. *Iranian Journal of Nursing and Midwifery Research, 20*(3), 347–353. https://pubmed.ncbi.nlm.nih. gov/26120335/

Heffer, T., & Willoughby, T. (2017). A count of coping strategies: A longitudinal study investigating an alternative method to understanding coping and adjustment. *PLOS ONE, 12*(10), Article e0186057. https://doi.org/10.1371/journal.pone.0186057

Hilgard, E. R., & Hilgard, J. R. (1983). *Hypnosis in the relief of pain*. Brunner/Mazel.

Holstege, G., Georgiadis, J. R., Paans, A. M. J., Meiners, L. C., van der Graaf, F. H. C. E., & Reinders, A. A. T. S. (2003). Brain activation during human male ejaculation. *Journal of Neuroscience, 23*(27), 9185–9193. https://doi. org/10.1523/JNEUROSCI.23-27-09185.2003

Jenkins, L. C., & Mulhall, J. P. (2015). Delayed orgasm and anorgasmia. *Fertility and Sterility, 104*(5), 1082–1088. https://doi.org/10.1016/j.fertnstert.2015.09.029

Johnsson, E., Zolkowska, K., & McNeil, T. F. (2015). Prediction of adaptation difficulties by country of origin, cumulate psychosocial stressors and attitude toward integrating: A Swedish study of first-generation immigrants from Somalia, Vietnam and China. *International Journal of Social Psychiatry, 61*(2), 174–182. https://doi. org/10.1177/0020764014537639ma

Pastore, A. L., Palleschi, G., Fuschi, A., Maggioni, C., Rago, R., Zucchi, A., Costantini, E., & Carbone, A. (2014). Pelvic floor muscle rehabilitation for patients with lifelong premature ejaculation: A novel therapeutic approach. *Therapeutic Advances in Urology, 6*(3), 83–88. https://doi. org/10.1177/1756287214523329

Rodriguez, F. D., Camacho, A., Bordes, S. J., Gardner, B., Levin, R. J., & Tubbs, R. S. (2021). Female ejaculation: An update on anatomy, history, and controversies. *Clinical Anatomy, 34*(1), 103–107. https://doi. org/10.1002/ca.23654

Safron, A. (2016). What is orgasm? A model of sexual trance and climax via rhythmic entrainment. *Socioaffective Neuroscience & Psychology, 6*(1), Article 31763. https:// doi.org/10.3402/snp.v6.31763

Starc, A. (2019). Clinical hypnosis and female sexual dysfunction: A case report. *Journal of Applied Health Sciences, 5*(1), 105–111. https://doi. org/10.24141/1/5/1/10

Wise, N. J., Frangos, E., & Komisaruk, B. R. (2017). Brain activity unique to orgasm in women: An fMRI analysis. *The Journal of Sexual Medicine, 14*(11), 1380–1391. https://doi.org/10.1016/j.jsxm.2017.08.014

Chapter 11 References

Algahtani, F. (2017). Teaching students with intellectual disabilities: Constructivism or behaviorism? *Educational Research and Reviews, 12*(21), 1031–1035. https://doi.org/10.5897/ERR2017.3366

American Psychiatric Association. (2022). *Diagnostic and statistical manual of mental disorders* (5th ed., text rev.). https://doi.org/10.1176/appi.books.9780890425787

Boyer, S. M., Caplan, E. J., & Edwards, L. K. (2022). Trauma-related dissociation and the dissociative disorders: Neglected symptoms with severe public health consequences. *Delaware Journal of Public Health, 8*(2), 78–84. https://doi.org/10.32481/djph.2022.05.010

Bruni, F., & Burkett, E. (2002). *A gospel of shame: Sexual abuse and the Catholic Church.* https://archive.org/details/gospelofshamechi00brun

Carroll, J. (2010, June 9). *Mandatory celibacy at the heart of what's wrong.* National Catholic Reporter. https://www.ncronline.org/news/accountability/mandatory-celibacy-heart-whats-wrong

Committee to Evaluate the Supplemental Security Income Disability Program for Children with Mental Disorders, Board on the Health of Select Populations, Board on Children, Youth, and Families, Institute of Medicine, & Division of Behavioral and Social Sciences and Education. (2015). Clinical characteristics of intellectual disabilities. In T. F. Boat & J. T. Wu (Eds.), *Mental disorders and disabilities among low-income children*

(169–178). The National Academies Press. https://nap.
nationalacademies.org/read/21780/chapter/13

de Sade, M. (1969). *Juliette*. Atlantic Monthly Press.

Ellis, H., Symonds, A., & Kruella, H. (1896). *Das konträre
Geschlechtsgefühl* [The contrary gender feeling]. Wigand.

Erickson, J. C., III. (1994). The use of hypnosis in anesthesia:
A master class commentary. *International Journal of
Clinical and Experimental Hypnosis, 42*(1), 8–12. https://
doi.org/10.1080/00207149408409337

Esdaile, J. (2023). *Mesmerism in India and its practical
application in surgery and medicine*. Legare Street Press.

Foucault, M. (1991). *Discipline and punish: The birth of a
prison*. Penguin.

Gebhard, P. H., Gagnon, J., Pomeroy, W. B., & Christenson, C. V.
(1965). *Sex offenders: An analysis of types*. Harper & Row.

Gold, S. D., Feinstein, B. A., Skidmore, W. C., & Marx, B.
P. (2011). Childhood physical abuse, internalized
homophobia, and experiential avoidance among lesbians
and gay men. *Psychological Trauma: Theory, Research,
Practice, and Policy, 3*(1), 50–60. https://doi.org/10.1037/
a0020487

Hunter, R. (2005). *Hypnosis for inner conflict resolution:
Introducing parts therapy*. Crown House Publishing.

James, E. L. (2012). *Fifty shades of grey*. Vintage books.

Justice for Magdalenes Research. (n.d.). *About the Magdalene
laundries*. http://jfmresearch.com/home/preserving-
magdalene-history/about-the-magdalene-laundries/

Low, G., Jones, D., MacLeod, A., Power, M., & Duggan, C. (2011). Childhood trauma, dissociation and self-harming behaviour: A pilot study. *British Journal of Medical Psychology, 73*(2), 269–278. https://doi.org/10.1348/000711200160363

Marks, I. (1979). Exposure therapy for phobias and obsessive-compulsive disorders. *Hospital Practice, 14*(2), 101–108. https://doi.org/10.1080/21548331.1979.11707486

Rose, T. (2022, November 16). NSW passes law to make coercive control a stand-alone offence in an Australian first. *The Guardian.* https://www.theguardian.com/australia-news/2022/nov/16/nsw-passes-law-to-make-coercive-control-a-stand-alone-offence-in-an-australian-first

Sobanski, T., & Wagner, G. (2017). Functional neuroanatomy in panic disorder: Status quo of the research. *World Journal of Psychiatry, 7*(1), 12–33. https://doi.org/10.5498/wjp.v7.i1.12

Taormino, T. (Ed.). (2012). *The ultimate guide to kink: BDSM, role play and the erotic edge.* Cleis Press.

Unwin, J. D. (1934). *Sex and culture.* Oxford University Press.

Chapter 12 References

AlAwlaqi, A., Amor, H., & Hammadeh, M. E. (2017). Role of hormones in hypoactive sexual desire disorder and current treatment. *Journal of the Turkish German Gynecological Association, 18*(4), 210–218. https://doi.org/10.4274/jtgga.2017.0071

Alesi, S., Forslund, M., Melin, J., Romualdi, D., Peña, A., Tay, C. T., Witchel, S. F., Teede, H., & Mousa, A. (2023). Efficacy and safety of anti-androgens in the management of polycystic ovary syndrome: A systematic review and meta-analysis of randomized controlled trials. *eClinicalMedicine, 63*, Article 102162. https://doi.org/10.1016/j.eclinm.2023.102162

American Psychiatric Association. (2022). *Diagnostic and statistical manual of mental disorders* (5th ed., text rev.). https://doi.org/10.1176/appi.books.9780890425787

Armstrong, J. M., Avant, R. A., Charchenko, C. M., Westerman, M. E., Ziegelmann, M. J., Miest, T. S., & Trost, L. W. (2018). Impact of anabolic androgenic steroids on sexual function. *Translational Andrology and Urology, 7*(3), 483–489. https://doi.org/10.21037/tau.2018.04.23

Blum, K., Badgaiyan, R. D., & Gold, M. S. (2015). Hypersexuality addiction and withdrawal: Phenomenology, neurogenetics and epigenetics. *Cureus, 7*(7), Article e290. https://doi.org/10.7759/cureus.290

Cappelletti, M., & Wallen, K. (2015). Increasing women's sexual desire: The comparative effectiveness of estrogens and androgens. *Hormones and Behavior, 78*, 178–193. https://doi.org/10.1016/j.yhbeh.2015.11.003

Conde, D. M., Verdade, R. C., Valadares, A. L. R., Mella, L. F. B., Pedro, A. O., & Costa-Paiva, L. (2021). Menopause and cognitive impairment: A narrative review of current knowledge. *World Journal of Psychiatry, 11*(8), 412–428. https://doi.org/10.5498/wjp.v11.i8.412

Evers, Y. J., Hoebe, C. J. P. A., Dukers-Muijrers, N. H. T. M., Kampman, C. J. G., Kuizenga-Wessel, S., Shilue, D., Bakker, N. C. M., Schamp, S. M. A. A., Van Buel, H., Van Der Meijden, W. C. J. P. M., & Van Liere, G. A. F. S. (2020). Sexual, addiction and mental health care needs among men who have sex with men practicing chemsex – A cross-sectional study in the Netherlands. *Preventive Medicine Reports, 18*, Article 101074. https://doi.org/10.1016/j.pmedr.2020.101074

Fong, T. W. (2006). Understanding and managing compulsive sexual behaviors. *Psychiatry (Edgmont), 3*(11), 51–58. https://www.ncbi.nlm.nih.gov/pmc/articles/PMC2945841/

Gieselmann, A., Aoudia, M. A., Carr, M., Germain, A., Gorzka, R., Holzinger, B., Kleim, B., Krakow, B., Kunze, A. E., Lancee, J., Nadorff, M. R., Nielsen, T., Riemann, D., Sandahl, H., Schlarb, A. A., Schmid, C., Schredl, M., Spoormaker, V. I., Steil, R., van Schagen, ... Pietrowsky, R. (2019). Aetiology and treatment of nightmare disorder: State of the art and future perspectives. *Journal of Sleep Research, 28*(4), Article e12820. https://doi.org/10.1111/jsr.12820

Hanson, S., Hunter, L. P., Bormann, J. R., & Sobo, E. J. (2009). Paternal fears of childbirth: A literature review. *The Journal of Perinatal Education, 18*(4), 12–20. https://doi.org/10.1624/105812409X474672

Mușină, A. M., Huțanu, I., Scripcariu, D. V., Aniței, M. G., Filip, B., Hogea, M., Radu, I., Gavrilescu, M. M., Panuță, A., Buna-Arvinte, M., Moraru, V. G., & Scripcariu, V. (2020). Surgical management of adrenal gland tumors: Single center experience. *Acta Endocrinologica (Bucharest), 16*(2), 208–215. https://doi.org/10.4183/aeb.2020.208

Park, J., Mcllvain, V., Rosenberg, J., Donovan, L., Desai, P., & Kim, J. Y. (2022). The mechanisms of anabolic steroids, selective androgen receptor modulators and myostatin inhibitors. *The Korean Journal of Sports Medicine, 40*(2), 67–85. https://doi.org/10.5763/kjsm.2022.40.2.67

Torem, M. S. (2007). Mind-body hypnotic imagery in the treatment of autoimmune disorders. *The American Journal of Clinical Hypnosis, 50*(2), 157–170. https://doi.org/10.1080/00029157.2007.10401612

Untersmayr, E., Jensen, A. N., & Walch, K. (2017). Sex hormone allergy: Clinical aspects, causes and therapeutic strategies – Update and secondary publication. *World Allergy Organization Journal, 10*(1), Article 45. https://doi.org/10.1186/s40413-017-0176-x

Vowels, L. M., & Mark, K. P. (2020). Strategies for mitigating sexual desire discrepancy in relationships. *Archives of Sexual Behavior, 49*(3), 1017–1028. https://doi.org/10.1007/s10508-020-01640-y

Vykhodtcev, S., Tregubenko, I., & Fedorova, A. (2022). Women who practice commercial sex and chemsex in St. Petersburg (Russia). *The Journal of Sexual Medicine, 19*(5, Suppl. 2), S202. https://doi.org/10.1016/j.jsxm.2022.03.459

World Health Organization. (2024, May). *International statistical classification of diseases and related health problems (ICD)*. Retrieved July 1, 2024, from https://www.who.int/standards/classifications/classification-of-diseases

Chapter 13 References

Cowan, A., Ashai, A., & Gentile, J. (2020). Psychotherapy with survivors of sexual abuse and assault. *Innovations in Clinical Neuroscience, 17*(1–3), 22–26. https://www.ncbi. nlm.nih.gov/pmc/articles/PMC7239557/

Goleman, D. (2021). *Emotional intelligence: Why it can matter more than IQ* (25th anniversary ed.). Bloomsbury.

Heacox, A. (2015). *Wolves in folklore, religion and mythology.* CreateSpace Independent Publishing Platform.

Jülich, S. (2005). Stockholm syndrome and child sexual abuse. *Journal of Child Sexual Abuse, 14*(3), 107–129. https:// doi.org/10.1300/J070v14n03_06

Kellie, D., Blake, K., & Brooks, R. (2019). What drives female objectification? An investigation of appearance-based interpersonal perceptions and the objectification of women. *PLOS ONE, 14*(8), Article e0221388. https://doi. org/10.1371/journal.pone.0221388

Lawson, D. (2018, March). Understanding and treating survivors of incest. *Counseling Today.* https://www. counseling.org/publications/counseling-today-magazine/article-archive/article/legacy/understanding-treating-survivors-incest

O'Keefe, T. (2013). *Inspiration for survive and prosper: Personal transformation out of crisis.* Australian Health & Education Centre.

Pease, A., & Pease, B. (2017). *The definitive book of body language.* HQ Non Fiction AU.

Rothbaum, B. O., Foa, E. B., Riggs, D. S., Murdock, T. B., & Walsh, W. (1992). A prospective examination of post-traumatic stress disorder in rape victims. *Journal of Traumatic Stress, 5*(3), 455–475. https://doi.org/10.1002/jts.2490050309

Sagone, E., Commodari, E., Indiana, M. L., & La Rosa, V. L. (2023). Exploring the association between attachment style, psychological well-being, and relationship status in young adults and adults—A cross-sectional study. *European Journal of Investigative Health Psychology and Education, 13*(3), 525–539. https://doi.org/10.3390/ejihpe13030040

Saradjian, J., & Hanks, H. (1996). *Women who sexually abuse children: From research to clinical practice.* John Wiley & Sons.

Thomas, J. C., & Kopel, J. (2023). Male victims of sexual assault: A review of the literature. *Behavioral Sciences, 13*(4), Article 304. https://doi.org/10.3390/bs13040304

Timms, R., & Connors, P. (2008). Adult promiscuity following childhood sexual abuse: An introduction. *The Psychotherapy Patient, 8*(1–2), 19–27. https://doi.org/10.1300/J358v08n01_03

Ullman, S. E., & Filipas, H. H. (2001). Predictors of PTSD symptom severity and social reactions in sexual assault victims. *Journal of Traumatic Stress, 14*(2), 369–389. https://doi.org/10.1023/A:1011125220522

Walker, J., Archer, J., & Davies, M. (2005). Effects of male rape on psychological functioning. *British Journal of Clinical Psychology, 44*(3), 445–451. https://doi.org/10.1348/014466505X52750

Wenninger, K., & Heiman, J. (1998). Relating body image to psychological and sexual functioning in child sexual abuse survivors. *Journal of Traumatic Stress, 11*(3), 543–562. https://doi.org/10.1023/A:1024408830159

Chapter 14 References

Allen, N. E., Appleby, P. N., Davey, G. K., & Key, T. J. (2000). Hormones and diet: Low insulin-like growth factor-I but normal bioavailable androgens in vegan men. *British Journal of Cancer, 83*, 95–97. https://doi.org/10.1054/bjoc.2000.1152

Bahner, J., Johansson, R., & Svanelöv, E. (2024). Who counts as a sexual subject? The impact of ableist rhetoric for people with intellectual disability in Sweden. *Sexuality Research and Social Policy*, 21, 161–176. https://doi.org/10.1007/s13178-023-00873-5

Barrett, O. E. C., Mattacola, E., & Finlay, K. A. (2023). "You feel a bit unsexy sometimes": The psychosocial impact of a spinal cord injury on sexual function and sexual satisfaction. *Spinal Cord, 6*, 51–56. https://doi.org/10.1038/s41393-022-00858-y

Baumann, F., Reike, A., Hallek, M., Wiskemann, J., & Reimer, V. (2018). Does exercise have a preventive effect on secondary lymphedema in breast cancer patients following local treatment? A systematic review. *Breast Care (Basel), 13*(5), 380–385. https://doi.org/10.1159/000487428

Bogart, K., & Dunn, D. (2019). Ableism special issue introduction. *Journal of Social Issues, 75*(3), 650–664. https://doi.org/10.1111/josi.12354

Callen, K. (2020). Disabled sexualities: A theoretical review of sociological approaches and a call to problematize the normative/non-normative dialectic. *Sexualities, 25*(5–6), 502–522. https://doi.org/10.1177/1363460720973892

Gillespie, T., Sayegh, H., Brunelle, C., Daniell, K., & Taghian, A. (2018). Breast cancer-related lymphedema: Risk factors, precautionary measures, and treatments. *Gland Surgery, 7*(4), 379–403. https://doi.org/10.21037/gs.2018.05.04

Heyne, S., Esser, P., Geue, K., Friedrich, M., & Mehnert-Theuerkauf, A. (2021). Frequency of sexual problems and related psychosocial characteristics in cancer patients—Findings from an epidemiological multicenter study in Germany. *Frontiers in Psychology, 12*, Article 679870. https://doi.org/10.3389/fpsyg.2021.679870

Liu, X., Li, C., Fan, X., Kuang, Y., Zhang, X., Chen, L., Song, J., Zhou, Y., Takahashi, E., He, G., & Li, W. (2020). Nicotinamide, a vitamin B3, ameliorates depressive behaviors independent of SIRT1 activity in mice. *Molecular Brain, 13*, Article 162. https://doi.org/10.1186/s13041-020-00703-4

O'Keefe, T. (2000). *Self-hypnosis for life: Mind, body & spiritual excellence.* Extraordinary People Press.

O'Keefe, T. (2018). *Stop drug and alcohol addiction: A guide for clinical hypnotherapists.* Australian Health & Education Centre.

Paul, P., & Whitelaw, G. (2010). *Hearing and deafness: An introduction for health and education professionals.* Jones & Bartlett Publishers.

Shakespeare, T., & Richardson, S. (2018). The sexual politics of disability, twenty years on. *Scandinavian Journal of Disability Research, 20*(1), 82–91. https://doi.org/10.16993/sjdr.25

Shindel, A., Xin, Z., Lin, G., Fandel, T., Huang, Y., Banie, L., Breyer, B., Garcia, M., Lin, C.-S., & Lue, T. (2010). Erectogenic and neurotrophic effects of icariin, a purified extract of horny goat weed (Epimedium spp.) in vitro and in vivo. *Journal of Sexual Medicine, 7*(4), 1518–1528. https://doi.org/10.1111/j.1743-6109.2009.01699.x

Smith, B. (2012). Inappropriate prescribing. *Monitor on Psychology, 43*(6), 36. https://www.apa.org/monitor/2012/06/prescribing

Streur, C. S., Corona, L., Smith, J. E., Lin, M., Wiener, J. S., & Wittmann, D. A. (2022). Sexual function of men and women with spina bifida: A scoping literature review. *Sexual Medicine Reviews, 9*(2), 244–266. https://doi.org/10.1016/j.sxmr.2020.09.001

Turabian, J. (2021). Psychotropic drugs originate permanent biological changes that go against resolution of mental health problems: A view from general medicine. *Journal of Addictive Disorders and Mental Health, 1*(3). https://unisciencepub.com/wp-content/uploads/2021/12/Psychotropic-Drugs-Originate-Permanent-Biological-Changes-that-go-Against-of-Resolution-of-Men.pdf

Wolinsky, S., & Ryan, M. (2007). *Trances people live: Healing approaches in quantum psychology*. Bramble Books US.

World Health Organization. (2024, march 13). *Breast cancer*. Retrieved September 16, 2024, from https://www.who.int/news-room/fact-sheets/detail/breast-cancer

Zelicha, H., Yang, J., Henning, S. M., Huang, J., Lee, R.-P., Thames, G., Livingston, E. H., Heber, D., & Li, Z. (2024). Effect of cinnamon spice on continuously monitored glycemic response in adults with prediabetes: A 4-week randomized controlled crossover trial. *The American Journal of Medicine, 119*(3), 649–657. https://doi.org/10.1016/j.ajcnut.2024.01.008

Chapter 15 References

Bird, E., Piccirillo, M., Garcia, N., Blais, R., & Campbell, S. (2021). Relationship between post-traumatic stress disorder and sexual difficulties: A systematic review of veterans and military personnel. *The Journal of Sexual Medicine, 18*(8), 1398–1426. https://doi.org/10.1016/j.jsxm.2021.05.011

Carrellas, B. (2017). *Urban Tantra: Sacred sex for the twenty-first century* (2nd ed.). Clarkson Potter/Ten Speed.

Comfort, A. (2017). *The joy of sex: A gourmet guide to love making* (B. Hindley & J. Keeble, Narr. ; 50th anniversary facsimile ed.) [Audiobook]. Octopus Publishing Group.

Dewitte, M., Carvalho, J., Corona, G., Limoncin, E., Pascoal, P., Reisman, Y., & Štulhofer, A. (2020). Sexual desire discrepancy: A position statement of the European

Society for Sexual Medicine. *Sexual Medicine*, 8(2), 121–131. https://doi.org/10.1016/j.esxm.2020.02.008

Flynn, K., Lin, L., Bruner, D. W., Cyranowski, J., Hahn, E., Jeffery, D., Reese, J. B., Reeve, B., Shelby, R., & Weinfurt, K. (2016). Sexual satisfaction and the importance of sexual health to quality of life throughout the life course of U.S. adults. *The Journal of Sexual Medicine*, *13*(11), 1642–1650. https://doi.org/10.1016/j.jsxm.2016.08.011

Friday, N. (1998). *Men in love: Men's sexual fantasies: The triumph of love over rage*. Random House Publishing Group.

Friday, N. (2008). *My secret garden: Women's sexual fantasies*. Gallery Books.

Gentry, C., & Fredsti, D. (2010). *What women really want in bed: The surprising secrets women wish men knew about sex*. Quiver Books.

Grace, A. (2023, September 8). *Your partner is probably fantasizing about someone else during sex: New study*. New York Post. https://nypost.com/2023/09/08/almost-half-of-americans-think-about-someone-else-during-sex-study/

Hariton, E. B., & Singer, J. L. (1974). Women's fantasies during sexual intercourse: Normative and theoretical implications. *Journal of Consulting and Clinical Psychology*, *42*(3), 313–322. https://doi.org/10.1037/h0036669

James, E. L. (2015). *Fifty shades of grey* (Film Tie-in ed.). Cornerstone Digital.

Mersy, L. F., & Vencill, J. A. (2023, August 22). *Desire: An inclusive guide to navigating libido differences in relationships*. Beacon Press.

San Martín, C., Simonelli, C., Sønksen, J., Schnetzler, G., & Patel, S. (2012). Perceptions and opinions of men and women on a man's sexual confidence and its relationship to ED: Results of the European Sexual Confidence Survey. *International Journal of Impotence Research, 24*(6), 234–241. https://doi.org/10.1038/ijir.2012.23

Sprinkle, A., & Stephens, B. (2017). *The explorer's guide to planet orgasm: For every body* (YuDori, Illus.). Greenery Press.

Toledano, R., & Pfaus, J. (2006). The Sexual Arousal and Desire Inventory (SADI): A multidimensional scale to assess subjective sexual arousal and desire. *The Journal of Sexual Medicine, 3*(5), 853–877. https://doi.org/10.1111/j.1743-6109.2006.00293.x

Vatsyayana, M., Burton, R., & Arbuthnot, F. F. (2012). *The original Kama Sutra completely illustrated* (V. Jain, Ed., 13th ed.). Mittal Publishing.

Wareham, R. J. (2022). The problem with faith-based carve-outs: RSE policy, religion and educational goods. *Journal of Philosophy of Education, 56*(5), 707–726. https://doi.org/10.1111/1467-9752.12700

Resources

I have made the following documents that I use in my clinic available for you to use as a guide to create your own. You can access them at the website URL provided below:

- Terms of therapy contract for hypnosis and sex therapy
- Sex therapy contract
- Client history-taking form
- Sexual history questionnaire
- Mental health questionnaire

Download these documents as PDFs and amend them for your own use from:

www.doctorok.com/sextherapybookresources

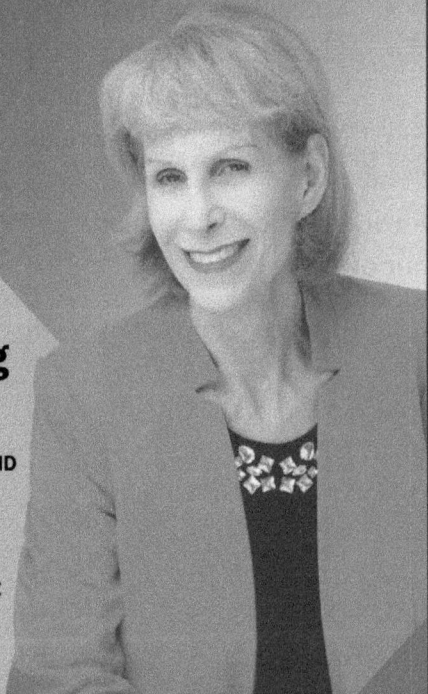
498

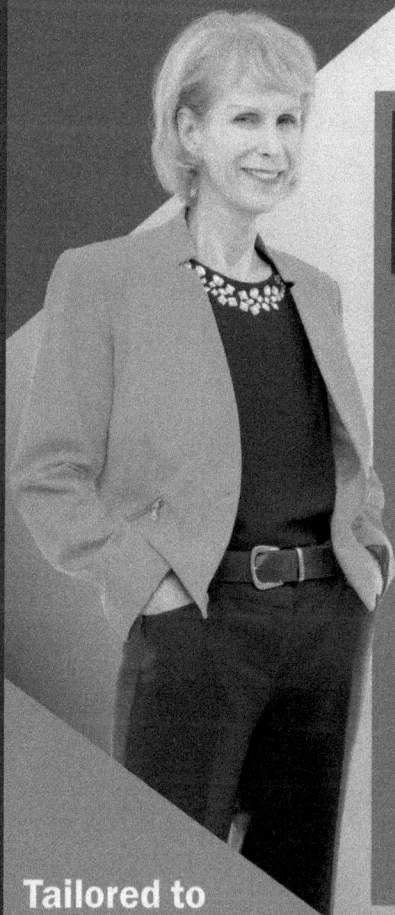
499

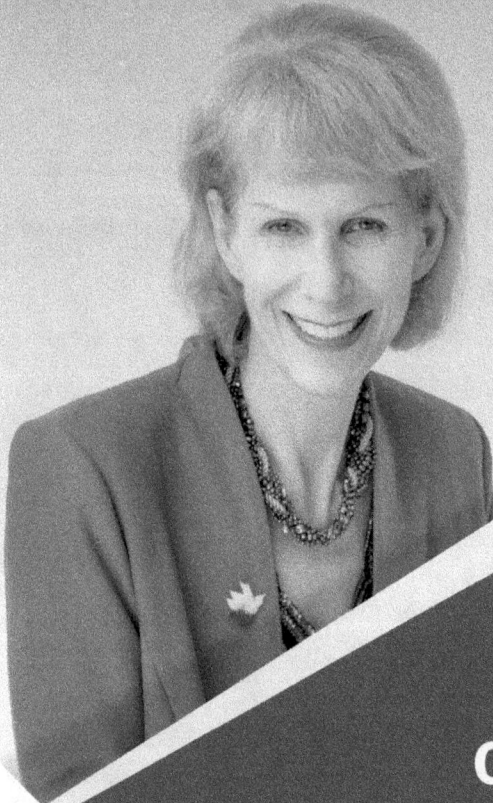

Clinical
Mental Health
Supervision in
Sex Therapy

for Healthcare Professionals

Conducted online

Available globally

With Dr Tracie O'Keefe DCH, BHSC, ND

www.doctorok.com/1-hour-clinical-supervision/

500